R00069 59833

Medical and Biologic Effects of Environmental Pollutants

ARSENIC

NATIONAL RESEARCH COUNCIL

Committee on
Medical and Biologic Effects of
Environmental Pollutants

DIVISION OF MEDICAL SCIENCES
ASSEMBLY OF LIFE SCIENCES
NATIONAL RESEARCH COUNCIL

NATIONAL ACADEMY
OF SCIENCES
WASHINGTON, D.C.   1977

Other volumes in the Medical and Biologic Effects of Environmental Pollutants series (formerly named Biologic Effects of Atmospheric Pollutants):

ASBESTOS (ISBN 0-309-01927-3)
CHLORINE AND HYDROGEN CHLORIDE (ISBN 0-309-02519-2)
CHROMIUM (ISBN 0-309-02217-7)
COPPER (ISBN 0-309-02536-2)
FLUORIDES (ISBN 0-309-01922-2)
LEAD (ISBN 0-309-01941-9)
MANGANESE (ISBN 0-309-02143-X)
NICKEL (ISBN 0-309-02314-9)
OZONE AND OTHER PHOTOCHEMICAL OXIDANTS (ISBN 0-309-02531-1)
PARTICULATE POLYCYCLIC ORGANIC MATTER (ISBN 0-309-62027-1)
SELENIUM (ISBN 0-309-02503-6)
VANADIUM (ISBN 0-309-02218-5)
VAPOR-PHASE ORGANIC POLLUTANTS (ISBN 0-309-02441-2)

NOTICE: The project that is the subject of this report was approved by the Governing Board of the National Research Council, whose members are drawn from the Councils of the National Academy of Sciences, the National Academy of Engineering, and the Institute of Medicine. The members of the Committee responsible for the report were chosen for their special competences and with regard for appropriate balance.

This report has been reviewed by a group other than the authors according to procedures approved by a Report Review Committee consisting of members of the National Academy of Sciences, the National Academy of Engineering, and the Institute of Medicine.

The work on which this publication is based was performed pursuant to Contract No. 68-02-1226 with the Environmental Protection Agency.

International Standard Book Number 0-309-02604-0

Library of Congress Catalog Card No. 77-81690

Available from
Printing and Publishing Office, National Academy of Sciences
2101 Constitution Avenue, N.W., Washington, D.C. 20418

Printed in the United States of America

SUBCOMMITTEE ON ARSENIC

ORVILLE A. LEVANDER, Agricultural Research Center, Beltsville, Maryland, *Chairman*
ROY E. ALBERT, New York University Medical Center, New York
R. K. BOUTWELL, University of Wisconsin, Madison, Wisconsin
WILLIAM B. BUCK, Iowa State University, Ames, Iowa
ANTHONY CALABRESE, National Marine Fisheries Service, Milford, Connecticut
CORLETTE C. CALVERT, Agricultural Research Center, Beltsville, Maryland
ALDEN S. CRAFTS, University of California, Davis, California
CYRUS FELDMAN, Oak Ridge National Laboratory, Oak Ridge, Tennessee
MICHAEL FLEISCHER, U.S. Geological Survey, Washington, D.C.
KURT J. IRGOLIC, Texas A&M University, College Station, Texas
PHILIP C. KEARNEY, Agricultural Research Center, Beltsville, Maryland
LYMAN MOORE, Bureau of Land Management, Salt Lake City, Utah
S. A. PEOPLES, University of California, Davis, California
JOSEPH H. SOARES, JR., University of Maryland, College Park, Maryland
WARREN E. C. WACKER, Harvard University, Cambridge, Massachusetts
DOROTHY B. WINDHORST, Hoffmann–La Roche, Inc., Nutley, New Jersey
EDWIN A. WOOLSON, Agricultural Research Center, Beltsville, Maryland
RALPH A. ZINGARO, Texas A&M University, College Station, Texas

T. D. BOAZ, JR., Division of Medical Sciences, National Research Council, Washington, D.C., *Staff Officer*

COMMITTEE ON MEDICAL AND BIOLOGIC EFFECTS OF ENVIRONMENTAL POLLUTANTS

HERSCHEL E. GRIFFIN, Graduate School of Public Health, University of Pittsburgh, Pittsburgh, Pennsylvania, *Chairman*
RONALD F. COBURN, University of Pennsylvania School of Medicine, Philadelphia, Pennsylvania
T. TIMOTHY CROCKER, University of California College of Medicine, Irvine, California
CLEMENT A. FINCH, University of Washington School of Medicine, Seattle, Washington
SHELDON K. FRIEDLANDER, California Institute of Technology, Pasadena, California
ROBERT I. HENKIN, Georgetown University Hospital, Washington, D.C.
IAN T. T. HIGGINS, School of Public Health, University of Michigan, Ann Arbor, Michigan
JOE W. HIGHTOWER, Rice University, Houston, Texas
HENRY KAMIN, Duke University Medical Center, Durham, North Carolina
ORVILLE A. LEVANDER, Agricultural Research Center, Beltsville, Maryland
DWIGHT F. METZLER, Kansas State Department of Health and Environment, Topeka, Kansas
I. HERBERT SCHEINBERG, Albert Einstein College of Medicine, New York, New York
RALPH G. SMITH, School of Public Health, University of Michigan, Ann Arbor, Michigan
ROGER P. SMITH, Dartmouth Medical School, Hanover, New Hampshire

T. D. BOAZ, JR., Division of Medical Sciences, National Research Council, Washington, D.C., *Executive Director*

Acknowledgments

This document represents a coordinated effort on the part of the members of the Subcommittee on Arsenic, who reviewed and revised each other's work. Hence, it is more than a compilation of separate items written by separate authors. The contributions of individual authors are shown below. The summary, conclusions, and recommendations represent a consensus of the members of the Subcommittee.

Chapter 1, the introduction, was written by Dr. Orville A. Levander, chairman of the Subcommittee. Chapter 2, on the chemistry of arsenic, was the work of Drs. Kurt J. Irgolic, Warren E. C. Wacker, and Ralph A. Zingaro. Chapter 3, on the distribution of arsenic in the environment, contains the contributions of several authors, Dr. Edwin A. Woolson being responsible for its development. Mr. Lyman Moore and Drs. Michael Fleischer and Woolson prepared the section on natural sources. Drs. Philip C. Kearney and Woolson were responsible for the section on man-made sources, except the material on feed additives, which was prepared by Dr. William B. Buck; that on drugs and on war gases and riot-control agents, by Dr. S. A. Peoples; and that on disposal, by Dr. Corlette C. Calvert.

The section on plants in Chapter 4, on the metabolism of arsenic, was the responsibility of Dr. Alden S. Crafts, but the remainder of the chapter was prepared by Dr. Peoples. For Chapter 5, on the biologic effects of arsenic on plants and animals, Dr. Levander contributed the sections on microorganisms and laboratory animals, Dr. Crafts the section on plants, Dr. Buck that on domestic animals, Dr. Anthony Calabrese that on aquatic organisms, and Dr. Joseph H. Soares, Jr., that on wildlife. In Chapter 6, on the biologic effects of arsenic on man, the section on toxicity was written by Dr. Dorothy B. Windhorst, except for the part dealing with occupational episodes of toxicity, which was the work of Dr. Roy E. Albert; Dr. R. K. Boutwell contributed the sections on teratogenesis and on mutagenesis; and Drs. Albert and Boutwell were jointly responsible for the sections on carcinogenesis and evaluation.

Dr. Woolson compiled the material appearing in Appendix A, on the arsenic content of plants and plant products, and in Appendix B, on the arsenic content of animals. Mr. Cyrus Feldman was the author of Appendix C, on the determination of arsenic in natural materials.

Ms. Joan Stokes checked all the bibliographic references for accuracy and compiled the consolidated reference list. The manuscript was edited by Mr. Norman Grossblatt, who also compiled the glossary in coordination with Dr. Irgolic.

Free use was made of the resources available at the National Library of Medicine, the National Agricultural Library, the Library of Congress, and the Air Pollution Technical Information Center of the Environmental Protection Agency. Also acknowledged is the assistance given to the Subcommittee by the National Research Council's Advisory Center on Toxicology, the National Academy of Sciences Library, the Environmental Studies Board, and various units of the National Research Council.

ERRATUM

On page 55, the paragraph that begins "The World Health Organization reported . . ." contains an incorrect statement and requires a qualification. The paragraph should read as follows:

The World Health Organization reported that average arsenic intakes for Canada, the United Kingdom, the United States, and France varied from 25 to 33 µg/kg of body weight per day; specific values ranged from 7 to 60 µg/kg of body weight per day.[881] These intakes are much higher than those currently being reported in the United States (Jelinek, C. F., and P. E. Corneliussen. Levels of arsenic in the United States food supply. Environ. Health Perspect. 19:83-87, 1977).

Arsenic
ISBN 0-309-02604-0

Contents

1 Introduction
2 Chemistry of Arsenic
3 Distribution of Arsenic in the Environment
4 Metabolism of Arsenic
5 Biologic Effects of Arsenic on Plants and Animals
6 Biologic Effects of Arsenic on Man
7 Summary and Conclusions
8 Recommendations

Appendix A: Arsenic Content of Plants and Plants
Appendix B: Arsenic Content of Animals
Appendix C: Determining Traces of Arsenic in Materials

Glossary

References

Index

1

Introduction

PROLOGUE

I am an evil, poisonous smoke . . .
But when from poison I am freed,
   Through art and sleight of hand,
Then can I cure both man and beast,
   From dire disease ofttimes direct them;
But prepare me correctly, and take great care
   That you faithfully keep watchful guard over me;
For else I am poison, and poison remain,
   That pierces the heart of many a one.

(Valentini, 1694[845])

The alchemists' symbol for arsenic, a menacing coiled serpent, probably symbolizes very well the element's prevailing evil reputation. Anxiety about arsenic is not difficult to comprehend, inasmuch as arsenic compounds were the preferred homicidal and suicidal agents during the Middle Ages and arsenicals have been regarded largely in terms of their poisonous characteristics in the nonscientific literature. For example, an almost clinical description of acute arsenic poisoning appears in the novel *Madame Bovary*.[255] Flaubert's extensive account of Emma Bovary's prolonged death throes must have made a vivid impression on many a reader. Arşenic has also been referred to in more recent literature, such as Kesselring's drama, *Arsenic and Old Lace*.[423] Although arsenic was only one of three poisons used by the Brewster sisters to dispatch their guests, "Strychnine and Old Lace" or "Cyanide and Old Lace" would not have had as great an impact on the public.

A famous case of hypothetical arsenic poisoning was the alleged attempt to do away with Napoleon Bonaparte on several occasions during his exile on St. Helena. After analyzing compilations of Napoleon's signs and symptoms during his later years, Forshufvud et al.[259] concluded that the Emperor had suffered intermittently from chronic and acute arsenic poisoning. Neutron-activation analysis of hair reputedly taken from Napoleon's head showed considerably more arsenic than samples from unexposed people. An editorial concerning this controversial hypothesis[577] set off a large measure of debate.[105,132,337,370,666,667,865] The original hypothesizers later analyzed additional hair samples attributed to Napoleon and found a distribution of arsenic along the length of the hair shaft that indicated a periodicity of exposure that coincided relatively well with the course of his disease.[260,744] However, the evidence of chronic arsenic poisoning of the Emperor was described as "unsatisfactory, irritating, and tortuous."[104] Another viewpoint was that Napoleon may indeed have received arsenic, but "only in an honest endeavour to help him."[836]

The possibility that arsenic compounds were prescribed for Napoleon reveals another side of arsenic—its widespread use in eighteenth- and nineteenth-century medicine as a tonic, or "alterative." At about the same time that Flaubert was writing *Madame Bovary*, there were a half-dozen "official" arsenicals listed in the U.S. Dispensatory.[870] The prevailing professional opinion at that time concerning the medicinal use of arsenic was summarized as follows:[29] "Arsenic is *a safe medicine*; none of the respondants having found it permanently detrimental. When given in a judicious manner, it did not even induce serious temporary effects. In the few cases apparently leading to a contrary inference, there was sufficient evidence of ignorant administration, or injudicious perseverance on the part of the patient." The heyday of arsenical chemotherapeutics occurred in the early part of the twentieth century, when Ehrlich discovered Salvarsan (arsphenamine), which was effective in treating human venereal diseases; but the use of these compounds declined after World War II, with the advent of the more specific antibiotics.

The complex folklore surrounding arsenic might provide us with an

Introduction

example of man's supposed ability to tolerate the element, inasmuch as peasants in the Styrian Alps of Austria during the nineteenth century were said to consume arsenic habitually as a means of promoting physical stamina.[30] The origins of this custom are difficult to trace. One of the best early accounts was that of Roscoe,[673] who concluded: "I. That arsenious acid is well known to and widely distributed amongst the peasants of Styria. II. That arsenious acid is taken regularly into the system, by certain persons in Styria, in quantities usually supposed sufficient to produce immediate death." Maclagan[507] had reached similar conclusions. The nineteenth-century medical establishment, however, especially in the English-speaking world, remained highly skeptical of the phenomenon: "Upon the whole, it is not improbable that the accounts received of the habitual use of arsenic by the peasants of Styria are either untrue or greatly exaggerated."[870] Maclagan[508] later claimed that two habitual arsenic-eaters took their dose in the presence of a scientific meeting on the Continent, thereby providing "public testimony to the accuracy of the observations previously made." Unfortunately, this is one aspect of the biochemistry of arsenic that will probably never be totally resolved.

Although the earlier medicinal uses and criminal abuses of arsenicals provide a helpful background of information about these compounds, the primary purpose of this report is not to determine the human hazards of such large direct exposures. Rather, this report is concerned primarily with assessing a more indirect hazard—the possibility of man's harming himself by contaminating his environment with arsenicals. There are potential ecologic dangers, in that large quantities of arsenicals are injected into the environment as a result of industrial and especially agricultural activities. Paris green (copper acetoarsenite) was the first pesticide widely used in modern agriculture (see Whorton[856] for an account of early agricultural experience with this and other arsenicals), and several arsenic compounds continue to be used today (see Chapter 3). Moreover, recent studies have again raised the question of the carcinogenicity of inorganic arsenic compounds (see Chapter 6). For some applications, there appear to be no suitable substitutes for the arsenicals. Therefore, we must learn to manage carefully the toxic yet useful compounds of arsenic.

2

Chemistry of Arsenic

The chemistry of arsenic is a very extensive subject.[735] This chapter is limited to a description of the chemistry of arsenic compounds that have potential environmental importance. A list of these compounds is given in Table 2-1.

In the natural environment, arsenic is rarely encountered as the free element. More frequently it is a component of sulfidic ores, in which it occurs as metal arsenides, e.g., nickel diarsenide, cobalt diarsenide, nickel arsenide, cobalt arsenide sulfide, copper arsenide sulfide, and iron diarsenide. Arsenates of aluminum, barium, bismuth, calcium, cobalt, copper, iron, lead, magnesium, manganese, uranium, and zinc also occur naturally, along with arsenic trioxide, which is formed as the weathering product of arsenides. Realgar (tetraarsenic tetrasulfide) and orpiment (arsenic trisulfide) are naturally occurring sulfides of arsenic.[765] In one form or another, arsenic is present in rocks,[603] in soils,[307] in water,[435] and in living organisms[92] in concentrations of parts per billion to parts per million. The commercial use and production of inorganic and organic arsenic compounds have raised local concentrations of this element in the environment much above the natural background concentrations.

TABLE 2-1 Arsenic Compounds of Environmental Importance

Arsenic trioxide	Arsenic pentasulfide	4-Nitrophenylarsonic
Arsenic pentoxide	Methanearsonic acid	acid
o-Arsenous acid	Cacodylic acid	Carbarsone
o-Arsenic acid	Trimethylarsine oxide	Melarsoprol
m-Arsenous acid	Methyldihydroxyarsine	Bis(carboxymethylmer-
Salts of arsenous acid:	Dimethylhydroxyarsine	capto) (p-carbamoyl-
arsenites	Trimethylarsine	phenyl) arsine, disodium
Salts of arsenic acid:	Arsanilic acid	salt
arsenates	3-Nitro-4-hydroxyphenyl-	10,10-Bis-(phenoxarsine)
Tetraarsenic tetrasulfide	arsonic acid	oxide
Arsenic trisulfide		

ARSENIC TRIOXIDE

Arsenic trioxide is the primary product of arsenic smelters. This oxide has direct applications in industry—e.g., as a glass decolorizing agent. Other commercially useful organic and inorganic arsenic derivatives are prepared from it.

Arsenic trioxide has been reported to exist in three allotropic modifications. The cubic form, arsenolite, is stable below −13° C. At higher temperatures, there is the monoclinic form, claudetite. An amorphous, glassy modification can also be prepared. Because the rate of conversion of the low-temperature cubic form to the monoclinic form is so low, it is possible to heat arsenolite to its melting point of 272° C. Claudetite melts at 313° C. A boiling-point range of 457–465° C has been reported for arsenic trioxide.[32] Arsenolite is made up of As_4O_6 molecules in which four arsenic atoms occupy the corners of a tetrahedron, with each pair of arsenic atoms joined by a bridging oxygen atom. The As_4O_6 molecules in arsenolite are arranged in such a manner that their centers occupy the lattice points of a diamond structure. According to Becker and co-workers,[59] there are apparently two monoclinic forms of arsenic trioxide (claudetite I and II), in which alternate arsenic and oxygen atoms are linked into sheets, resulting in the formation of open macromolecular structures. In the amorphous, glassy form, the macromolecular structure is similar to that of claudetite, but irregular.

The cubic form is slightly soluble in water. The solubility of arsenic trioxide in 100 g of water is 1.2 g at 0° C, 2.1 g at 25° C, and 5.6 g at 75° C. It is claimed that the aqueous solutions have a sweet, metallic taste.[664] The rate of dissolution is very low, and several weeks are required to achieve equilibrium. The rate of dissolution of the amorphous, glassy form is higher than that of claudetite. Arsenic trioxide is slightly soluble in glycerol.[32] The compound is not hygroscopic.

Arsenic trioxide begins to sublime at 135° C. Vapor-pressure data[32] for cubic arsenic trioxide are summarized in Table 2-2.

When metallic arsenides or arsenic-containing sulfides are roasted in air, and when arsenic-containing coal is burned, arsenic trioxide is formed. The vapors condense in the flues and on the walls of the stacks as a powder commonly called "white arsenic." Some arsenic trioxide finds its way into the air. Condensation of the vapors on a surface at temperatures above 250° C forms the glassy modification, which slowly changes to the crystalline, monoclinic form.[32]

ARSENIC PENTOXIDE

Oxidation of elemental arsenic or arsenic trioxide by nitric acid, followed by evaporation of the resulting mixture and dehydration of the residue, yields white hygroscopic crystals of arsenic pentoxide. Thermal decomposition of the pentoxide converts it to the trioxide with concurrent loss of oxygen. The pentoxide, in contrast with the trioxide, is very soluble in water; 630 g of arsenic pentoxide dissolve in 100 g of water.[32]

ARSENOUS AND ARSENIC ACIDS

Presumably, when arsenic trioxide is dissolved in water, the solution contains o-arsenous acid, H_3AsO_3. When As_4O_6 was dissolved in an acidic aqueous solution, only the undissociated species, $As(OH)_3$, was detected.[745] Raman spectral and nuclear-magnetic-resonance studies[481] indicate that, unlike the phosphorous acid molecule, which has both hydrogen–phosphorus and hydrogen–oxygen bonds, all the hydrogen atoms in arsenous acid are linked to oxygen atoms. Arsenous acid cannot be isolated. On evaporation of its solutions, arsenic trioxide is obtained. The successive pK_a values for $As(OH)_3$ have been reported as 9.23,[103] 12.13, and 13.40.[434] In alkaline solution, the anions $AsO(OH)_2^-$, $AsO_2(OH)^{-2}$, and AsO_3^{-3} might be present. However, it has been claimed that the m-arsenite ion, AsO_2^-, is also present in such solutions.[32]

o-Arsenous acid and m-arsenous acid could form as products of the hydrolysis of As_4O_6. By analogy with the phosphorus compound, the *meta* acid would be expected to be polymeric. However, the arsenic–

TABLE 2-2 Vapor Pressure of Cubic Arsenic Trioxide^a

Temperature, °C	Vapor Pressure, torr
100	0.000266
120	0.00180
140	0.01035
160	0.0473
180	0.186
200	0.653
220	2.065
240	5.96
260	15.7

^{a}Data from Gmelins Handbuch.[32]

oxygen–arsenic bond is known to possess extreme hydrolytic instability. Hence, the monomeric *ortho* form would be expected to be the predominant species.[481,745] This question merits additional investigation.

The existence of the As^{+3} cation in aqueous solution does not appear to have any experimental support. Reactions of the type shown below conceivably occur, but experimental evidence is lacking, even in strongly acidic solution.[170]

$$H_2O + HO^- + AsO^+ \leftarrow As(OH)_3 \rightarrow As^{+3} + 3OH^-.$$

The extraction of arsenous acid from water by amyl alcohol has been reported.[32]

The hydroxides of iron(II) or iron(III), chromium, and aluminum readily absorb arsenous acid.[32]

o-Arsenic acid, H_3AsO_4, can be prepared in the form of a white crystalline solid, $H_3AsO_4 \cdot \frac{1}{2}H_2O$. This is the product formed when arsenic trioxide is dissolved in nitric acid and the solution is evaporated. It is a fairly strong acid, with pK_a values reported as 2.20, 6.97, and 11.53.[256] Arsenic acid is an oxidizing agent in acid solution, with an E° value of 0.56 V for the reaction:[169]

$$H_3AsO_4 + 2H^+ + 2e^- \rightleftarrows HAsO_2 + 2H_2O. \quad (1f\ HCl^*)$$

*1 formal hydrogen chloride.

It is generally agreed that trivalent arsenic is considerably more toxic than pentavalent arsenic, so the question of whether arsenic exists in aqueous media in the form of arsenite or arsenate—i.e., AsO_3^{-3} or AsO_4^{-3}—is very important. Thermodynamic calculations[732] indicate that, in oxygenated ocean water, the ratio of the activity of arsenate to that of arsenite should be $10^{26} : 1$. An Eh-pH stability diagram has been published (Figure 2-1). However, the ratios found in ocean water[393] were in the range $0.1 : 1$ to $10 : 1$. Several reports have claimed that bacteria are capable of reducing arsenate to arsenite in fresh and ocean water.[393]

ARSENITES AND ARSENATES

Arsenites of the formulas MH_2AsO_3, M_2HAsO_3, and M_3AsO_3 are known. In these formulas, M represents a univalent metal cation or one

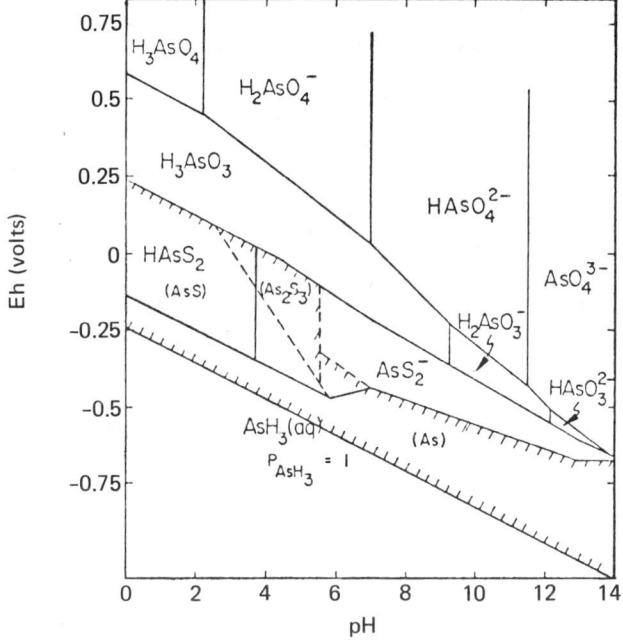

FIGURE 2-1 The Eh-pH diagram for arsenic at 25° C and 1 atm, with total arsenic 10^{-5} mol/liter and total sulfur 10^{-3} mol/liter. Symbols for solid species are enclosed in parentheses in crosshatched area, which indicates solubility less than 10^{-5} mol/liter. Eh = standard oxidation–reduction potential. Reprinted with permission from Ferguson and Gavis.[249]

equivalent of a multivalent cation. The alkali-metal arsenites are freely soluble in water, the alkaline-earth arsenites are slightly soluble, and the heavy-metal arsenites are insoluble. Scheele's green (cupric arsenite), whose formula has been reported to be $Cu(AsO_2)_2$ and $CuHAsO_3$, is an example of an insoluble arsenite.

Arsenic acid forms a corresponding series of salts that have similar solubility properties. Commercial lead arsenate, used as an insecticide, consists of $PbHAsO_4$ and some $Pb_3(AsO_4)_2$. The pH of a saturated solution of $PbHAsO_4$ containing 0.22 mg/liter at 25° C is 4–5. The solubility product constant[83] for $Pb_3(AsO_4)_2$ has been reported to be 10^{-35}. Commercial calcium arsenate, also used as an insecticide, consists of 61% calcium arsenate and 9% calcium arsenite (of variable composition).[34]

Condensed arsenates or arsenites, which are salts of polyarsenic or polyarsenous acids or a corresponding *meta* acid, are known in the solid state, such as dipotassium hydrogen arsenate, tetrapotassium diarsenate, and potassium *m*-arsenate. The arsenic–oxygen–arsenic bond in these compounds has extreme hydrolytic instability. It is therefore very unlikely that any species containing an arsenic–oxygen–arsenic group can be present in aqueous media in appreciable concentration.[745] The above-mentioned hydrolytic instabilities are important and must be taken into account whenever the replacement of the biologically ubiquitous phosphate groups by arsenate is considered.

ESTERS OF ARSENOUS AND ARSENIC ACIDS

Neutral esters of arsenous acid or arsenic acid, such as triorganyl arsenite and triorganyl arsenate, can be prepared, provided that the reaction products are protected from the action of moisture and acidic compounds.[745] The arsenic–oxygen–carbon bond also has considerable hydrolytic instability. Esters of these acids are therefore not stable in aqueous media. Because these acids have three hydroxyl groups that can react with alcohols, three series of esters could be formed—$ROAs(OH)_2$, $(RO)_2AsOH$, and $(RO)_3As$. It seems, however, that monoesters and diesters of arsenous acid and of arsenic acid have never been isolated.[745] 1,2-Dihydroxyalkanes and 1,3-dihydroxyalkanes react with arsenic trioxide to form cyclic esters.[234]

Because there are similarities between arsenic acid and phosphoric acid, the possibility that arsenate can replace the important phosphate group in biologically essential molecules (such as the monosaccharide phosphates and adenosine triphosphate) must be considered. However, arsenic acid esters are much more easily hydrolyzed than phosphoric acid esters. It has been postulated[211,869] that the glucose–enzyme complex, which generally reacts with phosphate to produce glucose-1-phosphate, can also interact with arsenate. The glucose arsenate thus formed is immediately hydrolyzed, regenerating glucose that cannot take part in further reactions unless it is rephosphorylated. The competition between arsenate and phosphate has been proposed in many other enzymatic reactions.[484,815]

ARSENIC SULFIDES

Because of the low solubility of arsenic sulfides under conditions prevalent in anaerobic aqueous and sedimentary media containing hydrogen sulfide, these compounds may accumulate as precipitates and thus remove arsenic from the aqueous environment. The most important sulfides of arsenic are realgar, orpiment, and arsenic pentasulfide. Realgar occurs in nature as an arsenic ore. The arsenic trisulfide and pentasulfide are formed when hydrogen sulfide reacts with trivalent or pentavalent inorganic arsenic compounds in the presence of hydrochloric acid. Saturated solutions in distilled water contain sulfide at approximately 4×10^{-6} mol/liter. The solubility in water containing hydrogen sulfide is somewhat lower, but of the same order of magnitude. In alkaline solution, the sulfides dissolve, with formation of thioarsenites or thioarsenates. These sulfides are decomposed by cold water in the absence of hydrogen sulfide within several days, mainly with formation of arsenic oxides, hydrogen sulfide, and sulfur.

The sulfides are generally stable in air at room temperature, but realgar is highly susceptible to attack by oxygen under illumination. At higher temperatures, the sulfides of arsenic react with oxygen.[33]

ORGANIC ARSENIC COMPOUNDS

A very large number of arsenic compounds that contain one or more arsenic–carbon bonds have been synthesized. The large variety of compounds is made possible by the property of the arsenic atom to bond from one to five organic groups, aromatic or aliphatic. The valences not used in bonding organic groups can be linked to other atoms and groups. Such compounds may contain trivalent or pentavalent arsenic atoms or be onium derivatives of arsenic. Table 2-3 lists the most important general types of organic arsenic compounds.

Chemistry of Arsenic

TABLE 2-3 Important Classes of Organic Arsenic Compounds

$RAsX_2$ } R_2AsX	X = H, halogen, NR_2, OR, SR, SeR, alkali metal, pseudohalogen
R_3As	Triorganylarsine
$[R_4As]^+X^-$	Tetraorganylarsonium salt (X = uninegative anion)
R_5As	Pentaorganyl arsenic
$(RAsY)_n$	Y = O, S, NH, NR
R_2As-X-AsR_2	X = O, S, Se, NR
R_3AsY	Y = O, S, Se, Te, NR
R_3AsX_2	X = halogen
$RAsO(OH)_2$	Arsonic acid
$R_2AsO(OH)$	Diorganylarsinic acid

The organic arsenic compounds that have environmental importance are those that contain methyl groups, the aromatic arsenic derivatives used as feed additives and in veterinary medicine, and a few others that may be important in biologic cycles.

METHYLATION OF ARSENIC COMPOUNDS

It has been known for almost 100 years that inorganic arsenic compounds, such as cupric arsenite and copper acetoarsenite, can emit a poisonous gas.[136] This gas, trimethylarsine, is formed by the action of molds. Challenger demonstrated that *Penicillium brevicaule* can convert arsenic trioxide and arsenites to trimethylarsine.[138,139] With alkylarsonic and dialkylarsinic acids, mixed alkylmethylarsines were obtained.[137,140]

The reduction and methylation of arsenate by *Methanobacterium* under anaerobic conditions were reported by McBride and Wolfe.[527] The arsenate is presumably reduced to arsenite, which is then methylated to methylarsines. Wood[872] studied the synthesis of dimethylarsine from arsenate in a reaction that requires methylcobalamin and methane synthetase. Schrauzer et al.[707] showed that methylarsine, dimethylarsine, arsine, and methane were produced from methyl-(aquo)cobaloxime-As_2O_3-DTE in water. Methylarsine was also obtained from H_3AsO_4-DTE-methyl(aquo)cobaloxime in the presence of Zn/NH_4Cl. These authors suggested a reaction between As^{+3} and CH_3^- (from the cobaloxime) to produce CH_3As^{+2}. However, because the existence of As^{+3} cations in aqueous solution is very unlikely, a displacement reaction of the following type appears to be more likely:

$$CH_3^- + As(OH)_3 \rightarrow CH_3As(OH)_2 + OH^-.$$
methyldihydroxyarsine

METHANEARSONIC ACID

Methanearsonic acid is an herbicide for some grass species. Very little is known about the molecular interaction of this acid or its salts with biologically important compounds. The known chemistry of methanearsonic acid is outlined in Figure 2-2 to point out which compounds could be formed from it.

Methanearsonic acid is a dibasic acid[465] with pK_a values of 4.1 and 8.7 and can form neutral and acidic salts. The alkali-metal salts are soluble, whereas the heavy-metal salts are insoluble in neutral and mildly acidic media. Methanearsonic acid undergoes dehydration above 130° C to a polymeric anhydride.[56] Differential thermal analysis of disodium methanearsonate showed that complete combustion was achieved at 660° C.[421] Arsonic acids can be esterified with alkanols and diols under anhydrous conditions. The esters are very easily hydrolyzed. It should be noted that aliphatic arsonic acids react with hydrogen sulfide to give

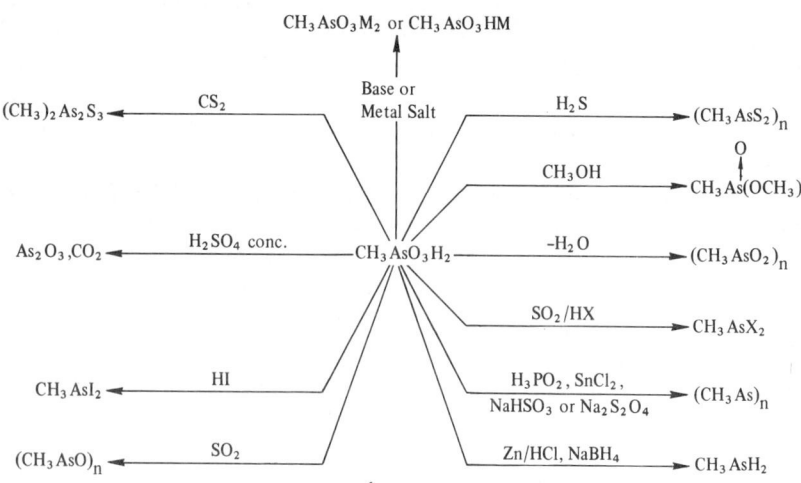

FIGURE 2-2 Reactions of methanearsonic acid.

sulfur-containing arsenic compounds. Thiols have been shown to convert arsonic acids to organylbis(alkylthio)arsines (K. J. Irgolic, personal communication). This reaction merits serious consideration. It is known that trivalent arsenic compounds interact with protein thiol groups (as discussed later), inactivating, for instance, enzymes. Pentavalent arsenic compounds, such as methanearsonic acid, have thus far not been shown to react with thiol groups in biologic systems, but might be able to. If the conversion of methanearsonic acid to methylbis(alkylthio)arsine, which has been carried out in the test tube (K. J. Irgolic, unpublished results), also occurs in a cell, disturbance of enzyme activities is very likely. For methanearsonic acid to be transformed to dimethylarsine or trimethylarsine, a reduction of the pentavalent compound within the biologic system must occur. Very little is known about the mechanism of this reduction.

DIMETHYLARSINIC ACID

Dimethylarsinic acid (cacodylic acid) and its salts find widespread use as postemergence contact herbicides. It is very similar in its reactions to methylarsonic acid. The arsenic–carbon bonds are very stable, but are cleaved by heating with solid sodium hydroxide[39] or chromium trioxide.[117] The acid has a pK_a value of 6.2.[41] In strongly acidic solution, cacodylic acid exhibits basic properties and forms adducts with mineral acids.[396] The reactions of cacodylic acid are summarized in Figure 2-3. It has been pointed out that cacodylic acid reacts with

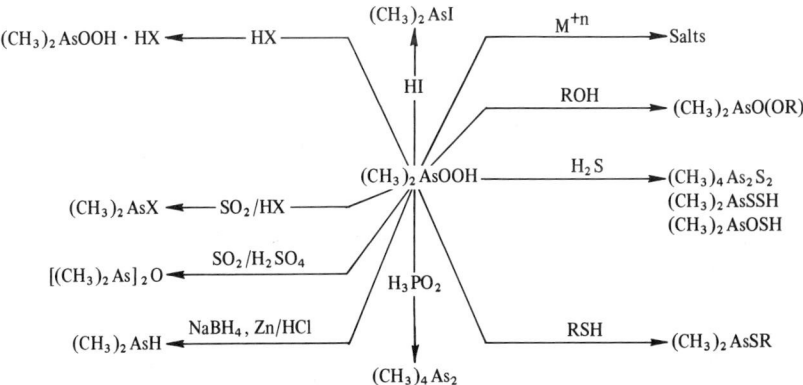

FIGURE 2-3 Reactions of cacodylic acid.

$HSCH_2CONH_2$[48] and $HSCH_2CH(NH_2)COOH$[424] to produce the trivalent arsenic derivatives R_2As-SR'.

ALKYLARSINES AND DIALKYLARSINES

Alkylarsines and dialkylarsines have been detected as products formed by the reduction and methylation of inorganic and methylarsenic acids. They have also been used in experiments to elucidate their effects on biologic systems.[383] Methylarsine is a gas at room temperature. The alkylarsines are sensitive to oxygen but are not spontaneously flammable in air.[200,619] They are unreactive to water.[199] A saturated solution of methylarsine in water contains arsine at 80 ppm.[198] Alkali-metal hydroxides have no effect on alkylarsines.[199,332] In the absence of oxygen, alkylarsines are thermally stable. Methylarsine was kept at 240° C for 3 h without decomposition.[199] The products of oxidation of alkylarsines are $(RAs)_n$, $(RAsO)_n$, and $RAsO_3H_2$, depending on the reaction conditions.

Dimethylarsine is an air-sensitive liquid that boils at 36° C. It bursts into flame on contact with air.[618] The oxidation products are arsenic acid and arsenic trioxide.

ALKYLDIHALOARSINES AND DIALKYLHALOARSINES

Alkyldihaloarsines are distillable liquids. They are strongly desiccant and irritating to the nose, throat, and bronchi.[467] Because of these properties, 2-chlorovinyldichloroarsine (lewisite), which has been reported to have the odor of geraniums,[177] has received considerable attention as a compound suitable as a war gas. Lewisite and similar compounds cause painful, slow-healing blisters on the skin, violent sneezing, and severe pain in the throat and chest.[309] Castro[131] found that ethyldichloroarsine inhibits cholinesterase in human plasma.

Alkyldihaloarsines hydrolyze on contact with water or moist air,[752] probably forming alkyldihydroxyarsines. However, only arsenosoalkanes have been isolated from the reaction mixtures.

It is important to note that the arsenic–halogen bond hydrolyzes very slowly. This is to be contrasted with the extremely rapid hydrolysis of the phosphorus–chlorine and antimony–chlorine bonds. Hence, the chlorides of arsenic, both organic and inorganic, are unique among the group VA elements. The painful, slow-healing burns caused when arsenic chlorides come into contact with the skin or the mucous membranes might be explained as follows: The arsenic halide contacts the tissues and penetrates rapidly and deeply. The arsenic–chlorine bond then undergoes very slow hydrolysis, with the release of hydrogen chloride. The hydrogen chloride released causes the tissue damage. Hence, the arsenic itself may not be the toxic agent in lewisite and related compounds, but it may exacerbate the effect of hydrogen chloride produced.

Of great biologic importance are the facile reactions that alkyldihaloarsines, alkyldihydroxyarsines, and arsenosoalkanes undergo with thiols. All these compounds easily condense with the sulfhydryl groups to form alkylbis(organylthio)arsines:[841,884]

$$RAsX_2 + 2HSR' \rightarrow RAs(SR')_2 + 2HX.$$

With 1,2-dithiols and 1,3-dithiols, the very stable 2-arsa-1,3-dithiacyclopentane and hexanes are produced.[761,858] Such reactions may very well take place with the thiol groups of proteins. If thiol groups are present in enzymes, trivalent arsenic compounds can form stable bonds with them, thus preventing the enzymes from functioning properly. The likely reaction between lipoic acid, a building block of the enzyme pyruvate oxidase, and a trivalent alkyldihaloarsine is the following:

British antilewisite (dimercaprol, BAL) reacts similarly with trivalent arsenic compounds.[761] Dialkylhaloarsines and dialkylhydroxyarsines react similarly with thiols, but cannot form the stable neutral ring compounds with dithiols.

3

Distribution of Arsenic in the Environment

NATURAL SOURCES

Earth's Crust

Arsenic ranks twentieth among the elements in abundance in the earth's crust. The abundance of arsenic in the continental crust of the earth is generally given as 1.5–2 ppm. Thus, it is relatively scarce. Nevertheless, it is a major constituent of no fewer than 245 mineral species. Arsenic is found in high concentration in sulfide deposits, where it is present as the native element or alloys (four minerals), arsenides (27 minerals), sulfides (13 minerals), sulfosalts (sulfides of arsenic with metals, such as lead, copper, silver, and thallium, 65 minerals), and the oxidation products of the foregoing (two oxides, 11 arsenites, 116 arsenates, and seven silicates). Of these minerals, arsenopyrite is by far the most common. In addition, many sulfides contain appreciable amounts of arsenic in solid solution; the most important of these is pyrite, which has a maximal arsenic content of about 5% (common range, 0.02–0.5%). The arsenic-bearing sulfides and sulfosalts oxidize readily; under surface conditions, oxidation proceeds to arsenic trioxide and to the arsenate stage.

Distribution of Arsenic in the Environment

TABLE 3-1 Arsenic in Igneous Rocks[a]

Rocks	No. Analyses	Arsenic Concentration, ppm	
		Range Usually Reported	Average
Ultrabasic	37	0.3–16	3.0
Basalts, gabbros	146	0.06–113	2.0
Andesites, dacites	41	0.5–5.8	2.0
Granitic	73	0.2–13.8	1.5
Silicic volcanic	52	0.2–12.2	3.0

[a]Estimated on the basis of data of Onishi[602] and Boyle and Jonasson.[94]

Igneous and Sedimentary Rock

Concentrations of arsenic in igneous rocks are listed in Table 3-1. No trend of concentration is apparent with respect to content of silica or other major elements. The limited data available indicate rather uniform distribution of arsenic among the major constituent minerals, except for slight enrichment in the sulfide minerals of igneous rocks.

Data on the concentration of arsenic in sedimentary rocks are summarized in Table 3-2. Shales, clays, phosphate rocks, and sedimen-

TABLE 3-2 Arsenic in Sedimentary Rocks[a]

Rocks	No. Analyses	Arsenic Concentration, ppm	
		Range Usually Reported	Average
Limestones	37	0.1–20	1.7
Sandstones	11	0.6–120	2.0
Shales and clays	324	0.3–490	14.5[b]
Phosphorites	282	0.4–188	22.6
Sedimentary iron ores	110	1–2,900	400?
Sedimentary manganese ores	—	(up to 1.5%)	—
Coal	1,150	0–2,000	13[c]

[a]Estimated on the basis of data of Onishi[602] and Boyle and Jonasson.[94]
[b]Excluding one sample with arsenic at 490 ppm.
[c]Boyle and Jonasson[94] gave 4 ppm.

tary iron and manganese oxides are notably enriched in arsenic. The data of Tourtelot[794] indicate that most of the arsenic in nonmarine clays and shales is associated with the clay minerals, whereas a considerable proportion of the arsenic in offshore marine samples is present as pyrite. Tourtelot, Schultz, and Gill[795] found a correlation between the arsenic and organic carbon concentrations. A similar correlation was observed by Ruch, Kennedy, and Shimp[689] for unconsolidated sediments of Lake Michigan; they attributed this arsenic to man's activities—the arsenic content in surface sediments (0–6 cm) averaged more than twice that at depths greater than 20 cm (12.4 vs. 5.3 ppm).

It should be noted that a higher than average content of arsenic is commonly found in sandstones, shales, and coals associated with uranium mineralization in Utah, Colorado, Wyoming, and South Dakota; this suggests considerable mobility of arsenic.

High concentrations of arsenic (maximum, 2,100 ppm; average, 115 ppm; median, 60 ppm) have also been noted in sediments from the area of hot brines in the Red Sea.[345,408]

Most of the analyses for phosphorites[316,797] are related to samples from the United States (Table 3-3). There is considerable variation in arsenic content, even from a single area, and no correlations with concentrations of phosphorus pentoxide, organic matter, or other major constituents are proved. Gulbrandsen[316] suggested a correlation of arsenic with organic matter for the phosphorites of the Phosphoria Formation (Montana, Wyoming, and Idaho); Stow[764] found no such correlation for Florida land-pebble phosphate, but found a positive correlation with iron content. The available analyses have been made on whole rock; consequently, correlations of arsenic with other constituents can be made with confidence only if the purified phosphate mineral and associated clay material are determined. It would be especially desirable to conduct such studies on samples of high arsenic content.

Soil

Arsenic is present in all soils, and the geologic history of a particular soil determines its arsenic content.[308] The natural arsenic content in virgin soils varies from 0.1 to 40 ppm. The average is about 5–6 ppm, but it varies considerably among geographic regions.[159] Soils overlying sulfide ore desposits commonly contain arsenic at several hundred parts per million; the reported maximum is 8,000 ppm. This arsenic may be present in unweathered sulfide minerals or in an inorganic anion state. The most common sulfide is arsenopyrite, although arse-

TABLE 3-3 Arsenic in Phosphorites[a]

Locality and Type of Rock	No. Analyses	Arsenic Concentration, ppm		
		Range	Average	Median
South Carolina, river rock	4	56.8–88.1	68.4	64.3
South Carolina, land rock	4	9.2–27.5	17.4	15.9
Florida, hard rock	8	1.4–9.6	5.4	5.7
Florida, land pebble	31	3.6–21.2	11.9	11.6
Florida, soft rock	6	0.4–18.6	7.5	5.7
Tennessee, blue rock	7	8.4–37.7	20.4	19.8
Tennessee, brown rock	25	5.1–56.1	14.6	12.5
Tennessee, white rock	3	4.8–21.7	10.6	5.2
Kentucky	3	6.7–12.7	9.9	10.3
Arkansas	8	14.6–188.2	61.0	43.8
Oklahoma	3	15.6–19.3	17.6	17.9
Montana	25	<10–106	40.0	30
Idaho	27	8.4–60	18.5	15
Wyoming	17	<10–150	26.4	17
Utah	14	8.4–43.2	16.0	14
British Columbia	1	—	28.3	28.3
Europe	10	7.6–54.8	25.1	20.8
North Africa	13	7.0–36.7	17.4	16.3
Israel	?	20–40	?	?
Insular (West Indies, Pacific)	21	5.1–76.2	16.3	12.0
Southern Australia	2	20.3–24.3	22.3	22.3

[a] Summarized mainly from Tremearne and Jacob[797] and Gulbrandsen.[316]

nosulfides of almost any metal cation can be found. Inorganic arsenate may be bound to iron and aluminum cations or oxides or to any other cation present (such as calcium, magnesium, lead, and zinc).

Arsenic may also be bound to the organic matter in soils, in which case it is released into the soil solution as the organic matter is oxidized and is then available for plant uptake or fixation by soil cations.[675] Some arsenic from other inorganic forms is also available for plant uptake, inasmuch as the slightly soluble iron and aluminum arsenates and the soil solution are in equilibrium. The amount released for plant uptake is a function of the particular chemical and physical forms of individual arsenic compounds. The amount of available arsenic (extracted with 0.05 N hydrochloric acid and 0.025 N sulfuric acid) is small in virgin soils and averages about one-tenth of the total arsenic present in most cultivated soils.[159,308,311]

Water

The cycle of arsenic in natural waters has recently been reviewed by Ferguson and Gavis.[249] Data on the arsenic content of waters and sediments are summarized in Tables 3-4 and 3-5. Sugawara and Kanamori[768] showed that the ratio of As(V) to total arsenic was close to 0.8 : 1 in ocean water. Braman[97] reported ratios of 0.56 : 1 and 0.81 : 1 for a tidal flat and saline bay water, respectively. He also found that As(III), methanearsonic acid, and cacodylic acid were present. The ratio of As(V) to As(III), based on thermodynamic calculations, should be 10^{26} : 1 for oxygenated seawater at a pH of 8.1. In reality, it is 0.1 : 1 to 10 : 1. This unexpectedly high As(III) content is caused, at least in part, by biologic reduction in seawater.[393] The content of arsenic in seawater is a small fraction (perhaps 0.1%) of the amount calculated to have been carried into the sea. Nearly all the arsenic has been precipitated or adsorbed on marine clays (probably most important), phosphorite, and hydrous oxides of iron and manganese. The scavenging of arsenic from solution by coprecipitation with hydrous oxides of iron and manganese in laboratory experiments is well known, but its occurrence in natural waters has not been studied in detail. Moenke[551] noted that spring waters (pH, 5.1) of high arsenic content precipitated about 80% of their arsenic in iron-rich sediments within 160 m of the source of entry.

The high content of arsenic in hot springs is notable; fumarolic gases have been reported to contain arsenic at up to 0.7 ppm. Extremely high arsenic concentrations have been reported in some groundwaters from areas of thermal activity,[312,448] from areas of rocks with high arsenic content,[86,294,883] and in some waters of high dissolved-salt content.[478,851] Most of the other high values reported in rivers and lakes and in sediments (Tables 3-4 and 3-5) are probably due to industrial contamination. Angino and others[18] have shown that household detergents (mostly of the high-phosphate type) widely used in the United States contained arsenic at 1–73 ppm; their use probably contributes significant amounts of arsenic to surface waters. Sollins,[751] however, felt that, after dilution during use, the concentration would be well below the recommended maximum and constitute no particular hazard. It has been generally assumed that surface waters, like the ocean, are "self-purifying" with respect to arsenic—i.e., that the arsenic is removed from solution by deposition with sediments; but quantitative studies are lacking. Sediments are always higher in arsenic than the waters with which they are associated.

The data on ground waters are inadequate. About 3% of the analyses show arsenic at more than 50 ppb, the 1962 maximal permissible

Distribution of Arsenic in the Environment

TABLE 3-4 Arsenic in Fresh Waters

Water	Arsenic Concentration, µg/liter (ppb)	Reference
United States, lakes:		
New York, Chautauqua	3.5–35.6	474
Michigan	0.5–2.4	720
Superior	0.1–1.6	720
Wisconsin	4.0–117	141
California, Searles	198,000–243,000	851
California	0.0–100^a	478
	0.0–2,000^b	478
Florida, Echols	3.58	99
Florida, Magdelene	1.75	99
United States, rivers:		
Hillsborough	0.25	99
Withlacoochee	0.42	99
Fox (polluted watershed)	100–6,000	107
Yellowstone	4.5	231
Narrow	0.90	659
Providence	0.75–0.90	659
Seekonk	2.48–3.45	659
Sugar Creek (contaminated)	<10–1,100	224, 859
Columbia	1.6	602
Schuylkill	30–180	436
United States, canals:		
Florida	<10–20	305
United States, well water:		
California	≤10–<2,000	296
Florida	0.68	99
Minnesota (contaminated)	11,800–21,000	244
Washington	5.0–6.0	241
Oregon	0.00–1,700	294
United States, Puget Sound	1.5–1,200	186, 187
United States, rainwater:		
Rhode Island	0.82	659
Washington, Seattle	17	186
Argentina, Cordoba, drinking water	480–1,490	315
	traces–300	42
Bosnia, Shebrenica, spring	4,607	385
Canada, well water	0.5–15	302
	<2.3–7.500	883
Chile	800	86

TABLE 3-4 (*Continued*)

Water	Arsenic Concentration, µg/liter (ppb)	Reference
Italy, Modena Province:		
Groundwater	3.0–5.0	824
Subsurface	<0.4–2.1	155
Japan:		
Rain	0.01–13.9	405
Rivers (40)	0.25–7.7	405
Aomori Prefecture	30–3,950	588
Lakes	0.16–1.9	602
Germany:		
Elbe River	20–25	602
Rhine River	3.1	432
Greece, lakes	1.1–54.5	602
Formosa, well water	800	242
New Zealand, rivers:		
Waikato River[c]	5–100	448
Waiotapu Valley	trace–276,000	312
Yagnob, Daiyee River, suspended	100–300	445
Sweden:		
Rivers	0.2–0.4	602
Glacial ice	2.0–3.8	847
Antarctica	0.60–0.75	405
Spring waters,[d] California, Kamchatka, U.S.S.R., New Zealand	130–1,000	851
Oil- and gas-field waters, California, Louisiana, Hungary	0.0–5,800	851
Thermal waters, Wyoming, Nevada, California, Alaska, Iceland	20–3,800	851
Spring waters,[e] U.S.S.R., Wyoming, Algeria, Iceland	30–500	851

[a]Dissolved solids, <2,000 ppm.
[b]Dissolved solids, >2,000 ppm.
[c]High in bicarbonate; of geothermal origin.
[d]High in bicarbonate and boron.
[e]Deposit travertine.

Distribution of Arsenic in the Environment

TABLE 3-5 Arsenic in Sediments

Locality	Arsenic Concentration, ppm	Reference
United States:		
New York, Chautauqua	0.5–306.0	694
Texas	3.6	3
	0.8–8.0	654
Winyah Bay	8.0–12.0	394
Lake Michigan	5.0–30.0	689
	7.2–28.8	720
Lake Superior	2.8–5.4	720
Lakes, Wisconsin	0.1–45.0	727
Sugar Creek (contaminated)	4,470–66,700	859
Puget Sound	2.9–10,000	186
Washington, rivers		
Skagit	15–34	186,187
Stillaguamish	17–48	186,187
Snohomish	22–74	186,187
Duwamish	15–40	186,187
Puyallup	2.6–7.5	186,187
Nisqually	4.5–12	186,187
Dosewallips	7.4	186,187
Duckabush	6.8	186,187
Japan	0.0–93.4	405
Minamata area	4.7–60	319
Netherlands, Rhine Delta	ND–310	197
New Zealand:		
Waiotapu Valley muds	51–14,250	312
Marine	6.6	652
Pelagic	40	819
England	<2–5,000	38,456,789

ND = Not detected.

concentration in drinking water.[808,813] In view of recent reports of chronic arsenic poisoning attributed to the use of such waters in Chile[86] and in Oregon,[294] further study is imperative. The volcanic rocks from which the arsenic-rich waters come in Oregon are of a type that is common in the western United States.[262]

Plants

Arsenic is ubiquitous in the plant kingdom. Its concentration varies from less than 0.01 to about 5 ppm (dry-weight basis). Appendix A lists the arsenic concentrations of some plants and plant products. Differences in arsenic content probably reflect species differences in plants and, in a larger sense, environmental and edaphic factors in a particular geographic region. Plants growing in arsenic-contaminated soils generally have higher residues than plants grown in normal soils. Arsenic concentrations are less than 5.0 ppm (dry wt) or 0.5 ppm (fresh wt) for untreated vegetation, whereas treated plants may have much higher concentrations. However, values for some nontreated plants are as high as or higher than those for plants that were treated with arsenic or grown in arsenic-contaminated soil. Natural variations among plants, plant species, available soil arsenic, and growing conditions are all responsible in part for these discrepancies. There appears to be little chance that animals would be poisoned by consuming plants that contain arsenic residues from contaminated soils, because plant injury occurs before toxic concentrations could appear.

Marine plants, particularly algae and seaweed, may have extremely high arsenic contents. In 11 varieties of British seaweed examined, a range of 5.2 ppm (in *Chondrus crispus*) to 94 ppm (in *Laminaria digitata*) was recorded.[398] In green algae, the amount of arsenic varied inversely with the apparent chlorophyll content, from 0.05 to 5.0 ppm on a dry-weight basis.[519] For brown algae, values of around 30 ppm have been reported.

Animals and Humans

Arsenic is present in all living organisms (Appendix B). Marine fish may contain up to 10 ppm; coelenterates, some mollusks, and crustaceans may contain higher arsenic concentrations. Freshwater fish contain up to about 3 ppm, although most values are less than 1 ppm. Domestic animals and man generally contain less than 0.3 ppm on a wet-weight basis. The total human body content varies between 3 and 4 mg and tends to increase with age. With the exception of hair, nails, and teeth, analyses have revealed that most body tissues contain less than 0.3 ppm.

The median arsenic content in 1,000 samples of human hair was 0.51 ppm, as determined by neutron-activation analysis.[743] The median concentrations for males and females were 0.62 and 0.37 ppm, respectively. Arsenic content of hair has served as an indicator in incidents of suspected poisoning. Values greater than about 2–3 ppm indicate possible poisoning, although higher concentrations have been recorded in occupational surveys. For example, a survey of workers in a copper processing plant in Czechoslovakia showed mean arsenic contents of 178 ppm in 21 persons exposed to air containing arsenic trioxide at 1.01–5.07 mg/m^3 and 56.6 ppm in 18 persons exposed to air containing 0.08–0.18 mg/m^3; a control (nonexposed) group had 0.149 ppm.[651] In such occupational surveys, it is important to distinguish between exogenous arsenic from atmospheric pollution and cosmetics and that from ingestion. Nail clippings from a patient with acute polyneuritis from arsenic poisoning contained arsenic at 20–130 ppm.[818] The normal arsenic content of nails is 0.43–1.08 ppm.[380]

The arsenic content of urine can vary normally from 0.1 to 1.0 ppm. Great daily variations exist and depend on the amount of arsenic in various foodstuffs. It is generally high after consumption of seafood. When arsenic is ingested, the amount excreted increases over several days to a maximum and then declines to normal.

Some of the highest concentrations of arsenic in biota are encountered in marine organisms. The average arsenic content of freshwater fish—including shad, gar, carp, bullhead, pickerel, bluegill, black bass, white bass, buffalo, and horned dace—varied up to 2.1 ppm.[233] The average oil content of these fish was only 2.49%, but the oil carried 22.8% of the total arsenic present. The arsenic in the liver oil of the large-mouthed black bass averaged 30 ppm. These values are generally lower than those reported for marine fish, which range up to 32.4 ppm for cod. Shrimp contain arsenic at 3.8–128 ppm on a dry-weight basis.[172] A survey of canned seafood showed the following arsenic concentrations: clams, 15.9 ppm; oysters, 16.0 ppm; smoked oysters, 45.8 ppm; lobsters, 22.1 ppm; and shrimp, 19.9 ppm.[203]

Air

Trace amounts of arsenic may be present in air. Although no 24-h maximal atmospheric concentration has been set in the United States, 3 μg/m^3 has been recommended in the U.S.S.R. and Czechoslovakia.[676] The threshold limit recommended for industrial workers is 500 μg/m^3 for arsenic and its compounds and 200 μg/m^3 for arsine.[425] Exposure standards for inorganic arsenic have recently been proposed by the Occupational Safety and Health Administration.[809] They limit air concentration to "4 μg As/m³ of air averaged over an eight hour period." A ceiling limit of 10 μg/m³ is proposed for any 15-min period during a work shift.

Data on emission of arsenic to the atmosphere have been summarized by Sullivan[770] and by Davis and Associates[196] and are discussed at the end of this chapter. Arsenic content in air and dust is summarized in Table 3-6. In areas remote from industrial contamination, air concentrations of arsenic generally are less than 0.02 μg/m³, whereas in urban areas they vary from less than 0.01 to 0.16 μg/m³. Two of the air values reported as "United States, Miscellaneous" were 2.50 μg/m³ in Anaconda, Montana, in 1961–1962 (the maximum) and 1.40 μg/m³ in El Paso, Texas, in 1964.[770]

MAN-MADE SOURCES

Production

Data on domestic and world production, imports, and domestic consumption of arsenic from 1964 to 1973, as shown in Table 3-7, were obtained from the Bureau of Mines, *Minerals in the U.S. Economy*.[811] Much of the arsenic processed in the United States is imported in copper ore and concentrates. An equal amount is imported as arsenic compounds. Agriculture is the largest user of arsenic, accounting for about 80% of the demand. Figure 3-1 indicates sources of arsenicals by country and type of material in 1973. Tables 3-8, 3-9, and 3-10 show U.S. imports for consumption of white arsenic (arsenic trioxide), U.S. imports of arsenicals by class, and world production of white arsenic.[812]

In the United States, arsenic is produced entirely as a by-product of the smelting of nonferrous-metal ores. Domestic production of arsenic has been adversely affected since the 1920's, when very large quantities of imported by-product arsenic became available from a copper mine in Sweden whose ore contained a high proportion of arsenic. The demand for arsenic was reduced after World War II by the advent of organic substances developed during and after the war that were used as pesticides and for other purposes for which arsenic had previously been used. The resulting surplus of by-product arsenic kept the price of white arsenic (77% arsenic metal) at 6.25–6.75 cents/lb (13.8–14.9 cents/kg) from July 1968 through 1973. However, in early 1974, the price increased to 13 cents/lb (28.7 cents/kg).

Arsenic is a troublesome contaminant in ores. Some arsenic com-

Distribution of Arsenic in the Environment

TABLE 3-6 Arsenic in Air and Dust

Locality	Arsenic Concentration Air, μg/m³	Dust, ppm	Reference
United States:			
Maryland	0.005–0.012	—	23
Washington, D.C.	0.02	—	23
Miscellaneous	0.01–2.50	—	770
Tacoma, Wash.	—	1,300[a]	543
Tacoma, Wash.	—	70[b]	543
Fly ash	—	680–1,700	580
Australia	—	10–12[c]	161
Czechoslovakia	—	14.0[d]	64
	—	750–3,800[a]	651
England	0.041–0.078	—	301
Japan	0.012–0.066	—	513
	—	0.012–0.19[e]	514
Mexico	0.005	—	582
Russia:			
Rostov	0.8–6.0	—	74
3,000–5,000 m from copper smelter	58–160	—	687
300–4,000 m from power plant	3.8–24.8	—	687
Germany	—	1.0–297	706

[a]Dust from copper smelter.
[b]Dust remote from copper smelter.
[c]Dust from cattle dipping.
[d]Near power plant.
[e]Airborne.

pounds volatilize during smelting and must be removed from smelter exhaust gases. Its presence in metals reduces electric conductivity and malleability to below commercial specifications for most uses. The cost of removing arsenic during smelting and refining exceeds its value. Arsenic was last produced for its own value during World War II, when

TABLE 3-7[a] Arsenic Supply–Demand Relationships, 1964-1973 (Short Tons)

	1964	1965	1966	1967	1968	1969	1970	1971	1972	1973
World production:										
United States	2,600	5,000	2,900	1,800	1,400	2,500	2,300	2,100	1,900	2,100
Rest of the world	49,900	50,600	50,800	53,200	56,700	50,900	52,200	49,700	47,000	48,000
Total	52,500	55,600	53,700	55,000	58,100	53,400	54,500	51,800	48,900	50,100
Components of U.S. supply:										
Domestic mines	2,600	5,000	2,900	1,800	1,400	2,500	2,300	2,100	1,900	2,100
Contained in imported copper ore and concentrates	5,100	7,300	6,500	3,200	4,700	7,800	8,600	5,400	8,400	8,100
Imports, compounds	14,000	12,000	14,400	20,800	19,300	14,000	14,400	13,300	10,500	8,850
Imports, metal	155	180	180	300	400	400	500	540	670	640
Industry stocks, Jan.	4,600	1,500	1,300	1,000	400	2,300	6,400	11,900	13,600	16,100
Total U.S. supply	26,455	25,980	25,280	27,100	26,200	27,000	32,200	33,240	35,070	35,790
Distribution of U.S. supply:										
Industry stocks, Dec. 31	1,500	1,300	1,000	400	2,300	6,400	11,900	13,600	16,100	11,600
Demand	24,955	24,680	24,280	26,700	23,900	20,600	20,300	19,640	18,970	24,190
U.S. demand pattern:										
Agriculture	20,800	20,500	20,500	21,800	19,900	16,300	16,100	15,600	15,100	19,700
Ceramics and glass	1,500	1,900	1,800	2,000	2,100	2,100	2,100	2,000	1,900	2,000
Chemicals	1,100	1,000	800	1,000	900	1,000	1,000	970	940	1,200
Pharmaceuticals	755	580	480	900	300	500	500	500	480	490
Other	800	700	700	1,000	700	700	600	570	550	800
U.S. primary demand	24,955	24,680	24,280	26,700	23,900	20,600	20,300	19,640	18,970	24,190

[a]Reprinted from *Minerals in the U.S. Economy*, Bureau of Mines, 1975.[811]

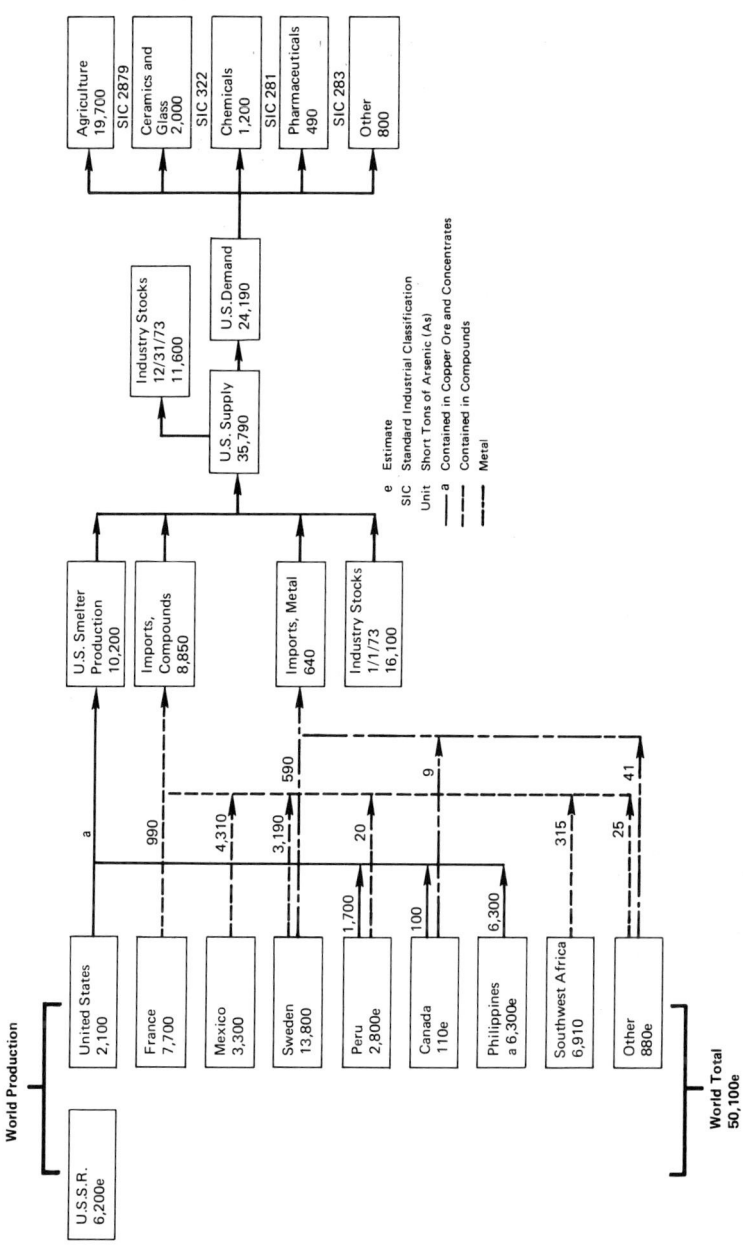

FIGURE 3-1 Arsenic supply–demand relationship. Reprinted from *Minerals in the U.S. Economy*, Bureau of Mines, 1975.[811]

TABLE 3-8 U.S. Imports of Arsenic Trioxide, by Country[a]

	Arsenic							
	1970		1971		1972		1973	
Exporting Country	Tons[b]	Value, $1,000	Tons[b]	Value, $1,000	Tons[b]	Value, $1,000	Tons[b]	Value, $1,000
Mexico	7,750	867	8,316	980	3,552	462	5,605	760
Sweden	8,142	870	7,276	968	8,184	1,228	4,144	706
France	2,650	274	1,425	180	1,556	184	1,281	190
Republic of South Africa	111	13	196	23	285	44	409	50
Peru	110	65	68	27	24	27	25	1
Other countries	—	—	25	9	12	11	32	7
Total	18,763	2,089	17,306	2,187	13,613	1,956	11,496	1,714

[a]Derived from 1973 Bureau of Mines *Minerals Yearbook*, "Minor Metals," 812tp.2 Includes small amounts of arsenous acid.
[b]2,000-lb tons; to convert to metric (1,000-kg) tons, or tonnes, multiply by 0.907.

TABLE 3-9 U.S. Imports of Arsenicals, by Class[a]

Class	Arsenic							
	1970		1971		1972		1973	
	Tons[b]	Value, $1,000	Tons[b]	Value, $1,000	Tons[b]	Value, $1,000	Tons[b]	Value, $1,000
Arsenic trioxide	18,762.5	2,089	17,306	2,187	13,613	1,956	11,496	1,714
Metallic arsenic	456	1,876	536	1,260	665.5	1,790	643	2,630
Sulfide	8.5	5	—	—	1	<0.5	2	414
Sodium arsenate	93	23	124	35	239.5	69	263	74
Lead arsenate	—	—	2	1	—	—	—	—
Other arsenic compounds	21	50	0.5	26	<0.5	19	<0.5	21

[a]Derived from 1973 Bureau of Mines *Minerals Yearbook*, "Minor Metals."[812(p.2)]
[b]2,000-lb tons; to convert to metric (1,000-kg) tons, or tonnes, multiply by 0.907.

TABLE 3-10 World Production of Arsenic Trioxide[a]

Country	Arsenic Production, tons[b]			
	1970	1971	1972	1973(p)
Brazil	328	163	181	76
Canada	71	50	30	—
France	11,236	8,844	10,000(e)	10,000
Germany, West	408	40	491	520(e)
Japan	974	1,054	471	500(e)
Mexico	10,075	12,658	5,618	4,828
Peru	851	723	1,123	1,200(e)
Portugal	209	205	15	22
South-West Africa, Territory of[c]	4,478	4,080	2,612	8,981
Sweden	18,078	19,290	17,857	18,200(e)
U.S.S.R.(e)	7,880	7,880	7,940	7,990
United States	w	w	w	w
Total, excluding United States	54,588	54,987	46,338	52,317

[a] Derived from *Minerals Yearbook 1973*, "white arsenic (arsenic trioxide)."[812(p.1360)] Including calculated trioxide equivalent for output reported as elemental arsenic and arsenic compounds other than trioxide. In addition to countries listed, Argentina, Austria, Belgium, People's Republic of China, Czechoslovakia, East Germany, Finland, Hungary, Southern Rhodesia, Spain, the United Kingdom, and Yugoslavia have produced arsenic or arsenic compounds in previous years, but information is inadequate to ascertain whether such production has continued and, if so, to what extent.
[b] 2,000-lb tons; to convert to metric (1,000-kg) tons, or tonnes, multiply by 0.907.
[c] Output of Tsumeb Corp., Ltd., for year ending June 30; values given are for white arsenic equivalent of reported black arsenic production.

p = preliminary
e = estimated
w = withheld to avoid disclosing individual company confidential data

military uses increased demand and supplies from Sweden were interrupted. Substantial resources of high-grade arsenic ore are available in the United States, in case arsenic production again becomes necessary.

Arsenic is present in appreciable amounts in many lead–zinc and copper ores; therefore, emission of arsenic may be a problem at any smelter treating such ores. However, the only U.S. plant recovering arsenic from those ores is a copper smelter in Tacoma, Washington. This facility is equipped to smelt copper ores and concentrates containing a considerable proportion of arsenic and to complete smelting of intermediate products—such as flue dust, speiss, and various residues of high arsenic content—received from other smelters.

At the Tacoma plant, the high-arsenic ores and concentrates treated

Distribution of Arsenic in the Environment

usually contain 3–15% arsenic, and the speiss and flue dust 5–30% or even more. The charge is first roasted with reducing fluxes to drive off as much arsenic as possible. Fluxing is necessary to ensure vaporization of arsenic, because arsenic pentoxide forms stable arsenates with common metallic oxides. Pyrite, galena, or carbonaceous material added to the charge reduces the pentoxide to trioxide, which sublimes at 193° C. The arsenic compounds are collected in cooling flues or chambers, where the temperatures of the gas and vapor are controlled. They enter the first chamber at approximately 220° C; by the time the gas and vapor reach the last chamber, they have been cooled to 100° C or less. The condensed crude product is 90–95% arsenic trioxide. Exhaust from the cooling flues passes through baghouses and Cottrell precipitators to remove any remaining arsenic trioxide or other dust. The calcine, now low in arsenic, is smelted for copper and other metals. The impure trioxide is resublimed and recondensed to remove impurities, until a product with the required purity is obtained.[746,812]

The arsenic-containing ore from U.S. mines received at Tacoma originates mainly in the Butte, Montana, and Coeur d'Alene, Idaho, districts. However, most of the arsenic feed material comes as concentrates from foreign mines for treatment at the Tacoma copper smelter or is an intermediate product from the treatment of ores at other U.S. smelters.

Since 1971, federal and state regulations have been adopted that will greatly limit atmospheric discharges of particulate matter and sulfur from metal smelters, power generating stations, and other industrial plants. Large construction programs were in progress during 1974 at nearly all nonferrous smelters and at most coal-fired electric generating plants to install equipment that will remove about 99% of the particulate matter from smelter exhausts and will treat all stack gases in acid plants or other sulfur-removing facilities to lower the sulfur content of the final discharge to a harmless concentration. As larger percentages of particulate matter and sulfur dioxide are removed from effluent gases, so also should the amount of arsenic emitted be lowered.

Uses

Approximately 97% of the arsenic produced enters end-product manufacture in the form of white arsenic, and the remaining 3% as metal for metallurgic additives in special lead and copper alloys.[812]

In an expanding agricultural market, agricultural uses accounted for about 81% of total consumption of arsenic in 1973 (Table 3-7). Arsenic trioxide is the raw material for arsenical pesticides, including lead arsenate, calcium arsenate, sodium arsenite, and organic arsenicals. These compounds are used in insecticides, herbicides, fungicides, algicides, sheepdips, wood preservatives, and dyestuffs and for the eradication of tapeworm in sheep and cattle.

Insecticides

The names, uses, and toxic dosages of several important arsenical pesticides are listed in Table 3-11. Compounds like Paris green (copper acetoarsenite) used to be popular insecticides in orchards, but are of minor importance today.[787] Likewise, lead arsenate and calcium arsenate have been used extensively in the United States for insect control on fruits, tobacco, cotton, and some vegetables, but current use is slight. The U.S. Department of Agriculture (USDA) used to be responsible for registering arsenical pesticides; today, all uses of arsenical pesticides for crop protection are registered by the Environmental Protection Agency.

Lead arsenate was first used about 1892.[787] It has been used chiefly for controlling codling moths, weevils, grasshoppers, Japanese beetles, cankerworms, leaf rollers, tomato fruitworms, bud worms, scale, plum curculio, cabbageworms, potato bugs, and tobacco hornworms. Lead arsenate is a stomach poison, with very little contact activity when used on chewing insects. Calcium arsenate is more effective than lead arsenate in combating the cotton bollworm.[451]

Pesticides related to lead arsenate include lead arsenite, used to a limited extent as an insecticide and fungicide; lead *m*-arsenate; and monolead *o*-arsenate and trilead arsenate, used as insecticides.

Magnesium arsenate was first used as an insect stomach poison on the Mexican bean beetle around 1920–1930, but its use is now very limited. Zinc arsenate has been used as an insecticide since about 1920 and controls many of the same pests as lead arsenate. It has been used in place of lead arsenate, because it leaves no lead residue. Compounds related to zinc arsenate used as pesticides include zinc fluoroarsenate, to control codling moths, and zinc *m*-arsenite, used to a limited extent as a wood preservative. Zinc arsenite has been used as an insecticide against chewing insects since about 1900, mainly on potatoes; it is too phytotoxic to use on orchards, bush crops, or other forage crops.

Sodium arsenite came into use as an insecticide between 1920 and 1930, mainly as a bait and as a livestock dip. As an insecticide, it must be used very carefully because of its extreme phytotoxicity; consequently, it is applied around the base of plants to prevent contact with the foliage. As a cattle dip, it is used to control ticks, fleas, and

Distribution of Arsenic in the Environment

TABLE 3-11 Names and Properties of Some Important Arsenical Pesticides[a]

Pesticide	Application Rates and Methods	Commercial Uses	Toxicity, LD_{50}, mg/kg
Arsenic acid	1½ qt/acre (0.0035 m³/ha) of the 75% concentrate	Cotton desiccant to facilitate mechanical harvesting	48 (young rats) 100 (older rats)
Cacodylic acid	3–10 lb/acre (3.4–11.2 kg/ha)	Lawn renovation and general weed control in noncrop areas	830 (rats)
DSMA	Directed after emergence on cotton at 2.25 lb/acre (2.52 kg/ha); 2–3.8 lb/acre (2.24–4.26 kg/ha) for lawn and ornamental uses	Cotton and noncrop areas; crabgrass	1,800 (rats)
MSMA	Directed after emergence on cotton at 2.25 lb/acre (2.52 kg/ha); 2–3.8 lb/acre (2.24–4.26 kg/ha) for lawn and ornamental uses	Cotton and noncrop areas; crabgrass	1,800 (rats)
Calcium arsenate	1½–3 lb/acre (1.68–3.36 kg/ha) in 100 gal (0.38 m³) of water or dust at 2–25 lb/acre (2.24–28 kg/ha)	Cotton insecticide; fruits, vegetables, and potatoes	150
Lead arsenate	3–60 lb/acre (3.36–67.3 kg/ha) or 1–60 lb/100 gal (1.2–72 kg/m³) of water	Fruits, vegetables, nuts, turf, and ornamentals	100
Paris green	1–16 lb/acre (1.12–17.9 kg/ha)	Baits and mosquito larvicide	22
Sodium arsenite	1–20 lb/acre (1.12–22.4 kg/ha) in dry baits	Baits and a livestock dip; a nonselective herbicide, rodenticide, desiccant, and aquatic weed killer	10

[a] Data from *Herbicide Handbook*[347,844] and Thompson.[787]

lice. Unfortunately, many children and domestic animals have been harmed accidentally by sodium arsenite.

The USDA took action to reduce the hazards from some arsenical pesticides intended for use in and around homes. In a press release dated November 24, 1967, the USDA proposed to decrease the percentage of sodium arsenite and arsenic trioxide in products for home use. Specifically, the following actions were recommended: products containing more than 2.0% sodium arsenite or 1.5% arsenic trioxide would not be registered for use around the home, and labels for arsenical products registered for agricultural, commercial, or industrial use would be required to display prominently the statements "Do not use or store in or around the home" and "Do not allow domestic animals to graze treated area." A press release dated July 17, 1969, gave notice that these restrictions were put on arsenical products for home use.

Herbicides

The inorganic arsenicals, primarily sodium arsenite, have been widely used since about 1890 as weedkillers, particularly as nonselective soil sterilants.[178] Consequently, sodium arsenite found use around military and commercial installations—along roadsides and on railroad rights-of-way. Its use for the control of crabgrass (*Digitaria sanguinalis*) expanded rapidly from only a few hundred tons a year in the early 1950's to 5,000 tons (4,536 tonnes) in 1959.

The use of organic arsenical herbicides—MSMA (monosodium methanearsonate), DSMA (disodium methanearsonate), and cacodylic acid—has grown rapidly in the last decade. MSMA and DSMA have been used as selective herbicides for the postemergence control of crabgrass, Dallisgrass (*Paspalum dilatatum*), and other weedy grasses in turf.[4] They are currently used extensively as selective postemergence herbicides in cotton and noncrop areas for the control of Johnsongrass (*Sorghum halepense*), nutsedge (*Cyperus* spp.), watergrass, sandbur (*Cenchrus* spp.), foxtail (*Echinochloa* spp.), cocklebur (*Xanthium* spp.), pigweed (*Amaranthus* spp.), and grasses in noncrop areas.[844] DSMA was first used for cotton weed control in 1961 to enhance the activity of another herbicide, 3',4'-dichloro-2-methylacrylanilide.[786] In 1963, 71,000 acres (about 29,000 ha) in Mississippi were treated with DSMA as a directed spray, and more than 329,000 acres (about 133,000 ha) were treated in 1964.[534]

The need for the selective herbicides for cotton production in the United States is particularly critical.[265] Johnsongrass, a hardy perennial species, is extremely difficult to control[427,545] and is estimated to infest approximately 4.3 million acres (about 1.74 million hectares) of cotton-producing soils. The methanearsonates are selective economic herbicides for Johnsongrass control.[321-324] Unfortunately, no complete estimates are available on the amounts of MSMA and DSMA being used in the United States. In 1969, Baker *et al.*[46] estimated that the annual use in the United States ranged from 6,000 to 8,000 tons (5,400 to 7,300 tonnes). An informal survey conducted by the National Cotton Council from reports submitted by different state specialists resulted in an estimate of 4.5 million acres (1.82 million hectares) that received MSMA and DSMA salts.[579] Assuming two applications of 2 lb/acre (2.2 kg/ha), an estimate of 9,000 tons (8,200 tonnes) of MSMA and DSMA would appear to be reasonable. It must be emphasized that these are only estimates. Nevertheless, they do indicate that substantial amounts of these organic arsenicals are finding widespread use in major cotton-growing regions. The National Cotton Council's survey also indicated that severe economic repercussions would be felt in the American cotton industry if these substances were lost to the farmer, because of losses in yield due to weed competition.[579] In 1972, it is estimated that 9,500 tons (8,600 tonnes) of MSMA was consumed in the United States.[829]

Cacodylic acid is a contact herbicide that will defoliate or desiccate a wide variety of plant species. It has been used as a crop destruction agent (Agent Blue) in South Vietnam. Cacodylic acid is not registered for use on agricultural commodities. It is registered as a silvicide (forest pesticide) and for lawn renovation.

Desiccants

Arsenic acid is used extensively as a cotton desiccant in the Black Prairie of Texas, the rolling plains of Oklahoma and Texas, and the high plains of Texas. The use of arsenic acid as a cotton desiccant began about 1955. The use of desiccants has increased rapidly in these cotton-growing regions, owing to the widespread use of mechanical pickers. About 85% of the treated acreage is in Texas. In 1971, over 98% of the U.S. cotton crop was harvested by machines. There are two types of mechanical harvesters—the cotton picker and the cotton stripper. Desiccants are used to prepare cotton plants for stripper harvesting by depleting the leaves and other plant parts of moisture. The reduction in moisture improves harvesting efficiency and prevents degradation of fiber quality that results from leaf staining. In addition, the earlier harvest results in less insect damage and lower insecticide use. Because of the lower harvesting costs, cotton harvest by stripping is rapidly expanding. In Texas, about 75% of the cotton was machine-stripped and about 25% machine-picked in 1970.

It was reported that 2,500 tons (2,300 tonnes) of arsenic was used as desiccants on 1,222,000 acres (about 495,000 ha) of U.S. cotton in 1964. In 1971, it is estimated that Texas alone treated over 2,000,000 acres (about 810,000 ha) with arsenic acid as a desiccant. Arsenic acid is applied once at a rate equivalent to 1.5 quarts (0.0014 m^3) of 75% o-arsenic acid per acre. This rate of application represents a maximum of about 4.5 lb (2.0 kg) of the actual technical chemical per acre during any one season. On the basis of figures for Texas in 1971, this would amount to over 4,500 tons (4,100 tonnes) of arsenic acid used as a desiccant.

Wood Preservatives

Compared quantitatively with the organic liquid wood preservatives (pentachlorophenol and creosote), arsenic is of less importance. The use of the principal wood preservatives in the United States in 1968–1973 is shown in Table 3-12. Use of chromated copper arsenate has

TABLE 3-12 Use of Principal Wood Preservatives, United States[a]

Preservative	1968	1969	1970	1971	1972	1973
Liquids, 1,000 gal[b]						
Creosote	136,799	128,226	125,624	116,553	110,499	97,582
Petroleum	73,588	68,071	75,624	81,122	85,664	79,986
Coal tar	20,469	19,618	21,903	21,449	21,670	17,063
Total	230,856	215,915	223,151	219,124	217,833	194,631
Solids, 1,000 lb[c]						
Pentachlorophenol	26,389	25,542	28,461	32,039	36,546	38,837
Fluor chrome arsenate phenol	3,971	4,539	2,687	2,169	1,914	1,683
Chromated zinc chloride[d,e]	1,526	1,384	1,462	1,336	1,774	1,949
Acid copper chromate	1,139	872	755	1,178	1,238	1,635
Chromated copper arsenate[d,f]	3,215	4,668	6,033	8,572	9,748	11,667
All others	1,554	1,050	820	749	999	1,270
Total	37,794	38,055	40,218	46,043	52,219	57,041

[a]Data from U.S. Department of Agriculture.[803]
[b]To convert to cubic meters, multiply values in table by 3.8.
[c]To convert to kilograms, multiply values in table by 453.6
[d]Includes copperized.
[e]Includes fire-retardant use.
[f]Includes Bolidensalts.

Distribution of Arsenic in the Environment

increased threefold in that period. Pentavalent arsenic compounds are used alone or mixed with other substances. Lansche has summarized the uses of some of the compounds, including Wolman salts (25% sodium arsenate) and Osmosalts (25% sodium arsenate).[451] There are three "Bolidensalts" (which probably derived their name from the Boliden mining operation in Sweden), including the following tradename products: Bolidensalt BIS, Bolidensalt BIS Copperized, and Bolidensalt K33. The zinc and chromium arsenates are used in a water solution in wood preservative plants and are applied to wood under vacuum and pressure. They are precipitated in the wood fibers, making the treated wood resistant to leaching.

Feed Additives

Four organic arsenicals (arsanilic acid, 3-nitro-4-hydroxyphenylarsonic acid, 4-nitrophenylarsonic acid, and 4-ureidophenylarsonic acid, or carbarsone), all substituted phenylarsonic acids, have qualified for feed-additive use under the Food Additive Law of 1958 (see Chapter 5). A food-additive petition demonstrating safety and efficacy of each is on record with the Food and Drug Administration (FDA). Drug combinations that include one of the arsenicals require separate petitions. These are to be found in the Federal Register and in the *Feed Additive Compendium*, a Miller Publishing Co. adjunct to *Feedstuffs*, a news journal for the feed industry.[587] Three of the pentavalent organic arsenicals were marketed in the early 1950's and described in an FDA-sponsored symposium.[274] The discussion also included the coccidiostat, arsenosobenzene, a trivalent organic arsenical (later abandoned with the advent of the Food Additive Law). The arsenical feed additives were further discussed in a second symposium on drugs in feeds sponsored by the National Academy of Sciences.[628] The recommended uses and safety considerations are discussed in Chapter 5 of the present report.

Less arsenic is used in feed additives than in pesticides, defoliants, or herbicides. In a typical year, the following are manufactured or sold: arsanilic acid, 1,360 tonnes; carbarsone, 450 tonnes; 3-nitro-4-hydroxyphenylarsonic acid, 900 tonnes; and combinations, 450 tonnes.

Concern was expressed about the fate of the various arsonic acids excreted by animals. Although these have been shown to undergo no degradation or only minor structural alteration before excretion, it is not known to what extent they accumulate in poultry litter or manure. Morrison reported that commercial use of 3-nitro-4-hydroxyphenylarsonic acid yielded arsenic at 15–30 ppm in the litter, but the concentrations of arsenic in the poultry tissues and feathers were not high.[562] Indeed, the tissue concentrations in birds raised on the litter did not appear to differ from those in birds raised on wire. At the recommended fertilization rate for poultry litter, 4–6 tons/acre (0.002–0.003 kg/ha), the addition of arsenic to soil was calculated as 1–2 ppm per year. The arsenic concentrations of soil, cover crops, and alfalfa crops fertilized for up to 20 years with arsenical poultry litter were not increased. Drainage water after 20 years of such fertilization was reported to contain arsenic at 0.29 ppm.

Drugs

Inorganic arsenic compounds have been used in medicine since the dawn of history and have been claimed to be effective in many diseases or where a tonic was indicated. The introduction of Salvarsan (arsphenamine) by Ehrlich at the turn of the century gave rise to intense activity on the part of the organic chemists, and it is estimated that more than 32,000 arsenic compounds were synthesized.

These drugs were active primarily against the parasites causing syphilis, yaws, relapsing fever, trichomonal vaginitis, trypanosomiasis, and amebic dysentery. With the advent of penicillin, the use of these drugs has been largely discontinued, although some are still in common use. (Some of these compounds have been reintroduced for other purposes—e.g., as feed additives and herbicides—and their dosages when used as drugs should be recalled when their toxicity for man and animals is considered.) Sodium cacodylate was used as a tonic and given by injection (because of its poor absorption when given orally) at 0.03–0.10 g every 2–3 days. It often produced the odor of garlic in the urine, breath, and sweat. DSMA (then called Arrhenal) was used for the same purpose and in the same dosage. The phenylarsonate Atoxyl (sodium arsanilate) was once used hypodermically in trypanosomiasis at 0.03–0.06 g/day.

The following drugs are in current use in human and veterinary medicine:

- Glycobiarsol[278]—used in intestinal amebiasis, trichomoniasis, and moniliasis; toxicity rare, because only 4% is absorbed.
- Carbarsone—used in intestinal amebiasis in man[278] and blackhead in turkeys[849] and chickens;[623] toxicity rarely reported; lacks effect on optic nerve reported for other p-NH_2 arsenobenzenes.
- Melarsoprol—used in trypanosomiasis[278,512] and filariasis;[22,518] occasional reactive encephalitis, usually fatal.

- Tryparsamide—used in syphilis and trypanosomiasis with cerebral involvement;[278,512] can cause retinitis with optic atrophy.
- Neoarsphenamine—used in eperythrozoonosis of swine and *Spirillum minus* infections (rat-bite fever) in man.[512]
- Dichlorophenarsine—used in dirofilariasis (heartworm infection) in dogs.[402,442]
- Caparsolate—used in filariasis in dogs[214,386,611,612] and lungworm infection in dogs.[206,611,612]
- Lead arsenate—used in monieziasis in sheep and goats.[512]
- Melarsonyl—used in filariasis in dogs[221] and trypanosomiasis.[278]

War Gases and Riot-Control Agents

The war gas lewisite was used in World War I and was highly effective in producing casualties, because it caused skin lesions that were difficult to heal.

Arsenic compounds are still in use that are less toxic than lewisite but that are highly irritating to the skin, eyes, and respiratory tract, thereby causing dermal pain, lacrimation, sneezing, and vomiting. (The commonly used tear gas and mace apparently are not arsenicals, but alkylating agents related to chloroacetophenone.) Information on these compounds, both chemical and pharmacologic, is difficult to obtain, because research data on them are classified or for other reasons.[283] Some such compounds are listed in Table 3-13. Ruchhoft *et al.*[690] were interested in the possibility that the use of these compounds would contaminate city water supplies, and they studied some of them with that possibility in mind. Rothberg[680] was interested in the possibility that these compounds could cause sensitization and tested the alkylating agents CS (O-chlorobenzilide malononitrile), CN (α-chloroacetophenone), and BBC (α-bromotolunitrile) and the arsenical compound DM (phenylarsazine chloride) in guinea pigs. He found that CS and CN caused sensitization, but that DM and BBC did not.

In summary, several arsenical compounds are available for use as riot-control agents that act as severe irritants to the skin and mucus membranes. Information about their other pharmacologic and toxicologic effects is not available in the literature.

Other Minor Uses

Because of its semimetallic properties, arsenic has metallurgic applications as an additive metal. Addition of 0.5–2% to lead improves the

TABLE 3-13 Arsenic Compounds Used or Developed for Use as Chemical-Warfare or Riot-Control Agents[a]

Chemical	Solubility, mg/liter H_2O at 20° C	Chemical-Warfare Symbol
Methyldichloroarsine	1,000	MD
Ethyldichloroarsine	1,000	ED
Lewisite	500	M1
Phenyldichloroarsine	Insoluble	PD
Diphenylchloroarsine	14.4	DA
Phenylarsazine chloride	15.7	DM
Diphenylcyanoarsine	Sparingly soluble	DC
Diphenylaminocyanoarsine	?	—

[a] Data from Gates et al.[283] and Ruchhoft et al.[690]

sphericity of lead shot. The addition of up to 3% arsenic to lead-base bearing alloys improves their mechanical properties, particularly at high temperatures. A small amount of arsenic is added to lead-base battery grid metal and cable sheathing to increase their hardness.

Addition of smaller amounts of arsenic improves the corrosion resistance and raises the recrystallization temperature of copper. At 0.15–0.50%, it improves the high-temperature properties of copper parts used for locomotive staybolts, firebox straps, and plates. At 0.02–0.05%, it minimizes or prevents dezincification of brass. It has been claimed that small additions of arsenic to brass minimize "season cracking" (failure of stressed material in a corrosive environment).

High-purity arsenic (exceeding 99.999%) is used in semiconductor technology. This material may be produced from the reduction of purified arsenic compounds, such as arsenic trioxide and arsenic trichloride, with hydrogen or the thermal dissociation of arsine. Specifically, it is used to make gallium arsenide, which is used in such semiconductor devices as diodes, transistors, and lasers. Indium arsenide is used for infrared detectors and in Hall effect applications. Small quantities are also used as a dopant in germanium and silicon devices. High-purity arsenic trichloride and arsine are used in the production of epitaxial gallium arsenide. A series of low-melting-point glasses containing high-purity arsenic have been developed for semiconductor and infrared applications.

Nearly all glass contains arsenic as an additive. It aids in the formation of glass and is a fining agent for removing gases, an oxidizing–reducing agent, and a decolorizing agent. The arsenic content of glass is normally 0.2–1%.

Arsenic is also used as a catalyst in the hydrogenation–cracking of hydrocarbons in the presence of olefins, in the manufacture of paper pulp and chloromethylsilane, in the oxidation of propene to acrolein, and in the ozonization of cyanides. Arsenic finds use in the Giammarco–Vetrocoke hydrogen sulfide removal process for treating coke-oven gas, synthesis gas, and high-pressure gas streams.[510] Alkaline arsenites and arsenates are used to react with hydrogen sulfide and absorb it from gas.

Residues

Arsenic, which occurs ubiquitously in nature, may also enter the biosphere through unintended contamination from industrial activity or through desired use, e.g., as a pesticide, medicine, or feed additive. Some of the arsenic is easily recycled in nature (that from pesticides, medicines, etc.), but other arsenic (such as that used as additives in metal and glass) is not easily recycled. The following sections discuss the residues that occur in the biosphere as a result of man's activity.

Soils

Soils are usually contaminated with arsenic through the use of pesticides, although some contamination occurs from smelting operations, burning of cotton wastes, and fallout from the burning of fuel. An excellent review of arsenic behavior in soil has recently been published.[837] Arsenic in the environment can undergo oxidation, reduction, methylation, and demethylation in soil.

Large residues have been found on orchard soils that received 30–60 lb of lead arsenate per acre (34–67 kg/ha) per year from pesticide applications, which began in the early 1900's. The soils have therefore received 1,800–3,600 lb of lead arsenate per acre (2,020–4,035 kg/ha). This is equivalent to an arsenic concentration of 194–389 ppm, if the arsenate remains in the top 6 in. (15.24 cm) of soil. Arsenic was accumulated at up to 2,500 ppm in a fine soil.[877] It contained high concentrations of hydrous iron and aluminum oxides or their cations. Little arsenic accumulates in sandy soils that are low in available iron and aluminum compounds. Soils removed from orchard production after these concentrations of arsenic are reached are generally phytotoxic, although the toxicity may decrease with time.[822] If a tree is to be replanted in areas with such concentrations, the soil may be excavated and replaced by new soil to promote growth.

High-arsenic soil may be toxic to plant life.[181] However, different soils with the same total arsenic content do not have the same toxicity to plants,[7] unless they have similar contents of iron, aluminum, organic matter, and phosphate and similar pH and unless the plants grown on them are under the same environmental stresses. Woolson et al.[876] have shown that various chemical forms of arsenic have different phytotoxicities. Thus, soils with high concentrations of easily soluble arsenic (soils low in reactive iron and aluminum) will be more toxic to plants than soils with low concentrations of easily soluble arsenic, although the total arsenic contents may be similar. Because plants growing in high-arsenic soils have very little growth, human consumption of high arsenic residues through the plant food chain is unlikely. Plant growth is reduced as arsenic content increases.[28,71] For instance, a total arsenic content of about 300 ppm equivalent to extracted available arsenic at about 30 ppm in an average soil will reduce growth of many crops by about 50%. Seedlings shown to contain arsenic at 15 ppm on a dry-weight basis have suffered a 50% reduction in growth; this is equivalent to about 1.5 ppm on a fresh-weight basis, which is below the tolerances set by the FDA for arsenic in fruits. Sensitive crops, such as green beans, are adversely affected by extracted available arsenic at as low as 5 ppm.[873]

The use of different fertilizer materials and fertilization practices also influences the soluble arsenic content of soils and the arsenic content of the harvested crop.[757] A high phosphate application to soils receiving arsenicals increases the arsenic content of corn foliage, but apparently not of corn seed. Schweizer[715] showed the effects of phosphate fertilization on DSMA residues with cotton bioassay. The toxicity depended on the amount of phosphate applied and on the soil type. Phosphate fertilizers may contain arsenic at up to 1,200 ppm, but at normal application rates, "it seems highly improbable that the arsenic in domestic phosphate fertilizer exerts any toxic effects, even with very large annual applications of the fertilizer over extended periods of time."[797]

Arsenic may be leached downward in sandy soils. In heavier soils, little leaching is likely.[530] High phosphate contents and excess phosphate fertilization increase the rate of arsenic leaching. Arsenate in solution at saturation follows the order: sodium arsenate > calcium arsenate ($10^{-5} M$) > aluminum arsenate ($10^{-7} M$) > iron arsenate ($10^{-9} M$).[151,152] Thus, the more soluble arsenates (sodium and calcium) will leach from a soil more readily than the less soluble (aluminum and

Distribution of Arsenic in the Environment

iron) forms. When a soil was subjected to leaching conditions with potassium biphosphate, the percentage of aluminum arsenate (extractable with 0.5 N ammonium fluoride) decreased and percentage of the more insoluble iron arsenate (extractable with 0.1 N sodium hydroxide) increased.[878] Thus, the arsenic that remains after phosphate treatment and subsequent leaching is itself less phytotoxic.

Total soil arsenic does not accurately reflect the form that is available to plants. Arsenic phytotoxicity decreases in this order: water-soluble > calcium arsenate ≃ aluminum arsenate > iron arsenate. Toxicity is probably related to the solubility constant of the individual compound. Extractants used to test for available nutrients (Bray P-1, 0.5 N sodium bicarbonate, and a mixed acid—0.05 N hydrochloric acid + 0.025 N sulfuric acid) more accurately reflect amounts of arsenic that are available for uptake at the root surface. Extractable arsenic at 5 ppm is toxic to sensitive species.

The behavior of the organoarsenic herbicides in soil has been reviewed by Hiltbold.[354] The organoarsenic herbicides are used in foliar treatment at lower rates than the inorganic arsenic insecticides. Methanearsonic acid (MAA) and its salts (MSMA and DSMA) are selective herbicides used to control specific weeds. Cacodylic acid is a general contact desiccant used to defoliate or destroy unwanted vegetation.

Organic aliphatic arsenic compounds behave very much like the inorganic arsenic salts in soil.[395] The methanearsonic acids are fixed in soil and are only gradually leached through the soil profile.[204,355] Both the amount and rate of leaching are increased when soil is coarse and its reactive iron and aluminum content is low. Cacodylic acid is likewise fixed by iron and aluminum in the soil, although not as strongly as inorganic arsenate or MAA. Metabolism of organic arsenicals occurs in soil with inorganic arsenate as the major metabolite under aerobic conditions. A volatile organoarsenic compound, possibly dimethylarsine (cacodyl hydride), is generated in soil under both aerobic and anaerobic soil conditions from cacodylic acid.[412,879] Trimethylarsine has also been isolated above grass.[97] Residue accumulation in cotton soils should be slower than that in orchard soils, because less arsenic is applied with the organic arsenicals (1–2 ppm) than was applied with lead arsenate (3.3–6.6 ppm). In addition, the aliphatic arsenicals are reduced to arsines more readily than is arsenate and will be lost from the site of application as a gas.

Large accumulations occur around smelters.[541] A survey of the Helena Valley indicated that soil samples collected from the upper 10.2 cm within 1.6 km of the smelter stack contained arsenic at up to 150 ppm. The arsenic content decreased with distance from the stack for a distance of 8–16 km. A calculated total of 780 tonnes of arsenic has been added to the soil at a distance of 1.07–16 km from the stack during 80 years of operation. Accumulations up to 380 ppm occurred around the Tacoma smelter.[188]

It should be noted that continued additions of arsenicals, regardless of the source, may result in soils that are too toxic to support some forms of plant life. The constant turnover of organic matter and the resulting microbial reduction and volatilization (see Figure 3-2) will tend to reduce high concentrations of arsenicals. This will result in a reduction in toxicity. Arsenicals will accumulate in soil when greater amounts are added than are removed in harvested plants, through volatilization, and through leaching.

Water

As noted earlier, arsenic is found in all waters. The U.S. Geological Survey reported that 79% of 727 samples examined from across the

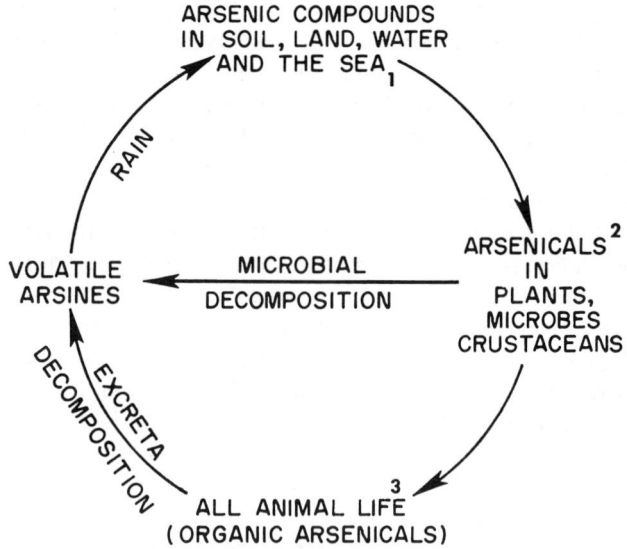

FIGURE 3-2 A proposed arsenic cycle. 1, the cycle in nature involves organic arsenicals; few identified. 2, marine algae may contain arsenic at up to 9 ppm, land plants generally at less than 0.5 ppm. 3, edible tissues of food animals contain, on average, below 0.5 ppm; fish, 0.5–3 ppm; and crustaceans, 3–100 ppm. Reprinted with permission from Frost.[268]

Distribution of Arsenic in the Environment

United States contained arsenic at less than 10 µg/liter (the 1962 recommended drinking-water concentration), 21% at greater than 10 µg/liter, and 2% at greater than 50 µg/liter (the 1962 maximal allowable arsenic content for drinking water).[224] The highest concentration (1,100 µg/liter) was found in South Carolina in a sample downstream from an industrial complex in North Carolina that contained an arsenical-producing company. At the next sampling station downstream, the concentration was 10 µg/liter. The EPA has recently published primary interim standards for drinking water. The maximal allowable arsenic content remains 50 µg/liter.[811]

Arsenic can be removed from industrial waste by several methods before the waste is discharged into the water system. Among the methods reported are precipitation by calcium oxide and ferric chloride, basic anion-exchange resins, passage through lime and ashes, and flocculation with chlorine-saturated water and ferrous sulfate.

Questions have been raised over the arsenic added to the environment through phosphate detergents. Angino found that water treated with cold lime contained arsenic at 0.4 ppb.[18] Water at the intake contained 2.6–3.6 ppb before treatment. The arsenic in water returned to the Kansas River after sewage treatment ranged from 1.5 to 2.1 ppb, which is lower than the concentration at the intake. Angino felt that arsenic in detergents added significant quantities of arsenic to the river system; others have felt that there was little danger.[622,751]

Most arsenic in water is added through industrial discharges. The highest concentrations, other than those occurring naturally in spring waters, are usually in areas of high industrial activity.

Rivers seem to be self-cleansing relative to soluble arsenic. The arsenic concentration in solution decreases with the distance from the source of pollution. Arsenic decreased to background concentrations in river waters 400–1,300 m from the source of pollution. However, the rate of disappearance was a function of stream characteristics. Arsenates and arsenites presumably form insoluble salts with cations in the water and settle out in the sediments of these rivers. Arsenic was detected at 75 ppm in sediments of polluted waterways, compared with 11 ppm in clean waterways.

Endemic contamination of freshwater supplies has been reported in Argentina, Reichenstein, Silesia, and Antofagasta, Chile. In Silesia, the contamination arose through leaching of arsenic wastes from mining operations into spring water. In Chile, arsenic in drinking water decreased from 800 ppb to 30 ppb after the installation of a water-treatment plant.[86] In New Zealand, dairy cattle have been poisoned by arsenic in mineral springs. Wells in Lane County, Oregon, were contaminated with arsenic naturally and had high pH and high sodium and bicarbonate contents.[294]

Concentrations found in water, ice, and oceans are presented in Table 3-4. Waters with known contamination are generally high in arsenic, although many waters not contaminated by man are also high in arsenic. The latter are generally alkaline, with very high sodium and bicarbonate contents. Mud downstream from a source of contamination may also contain high concentrations of arsenic residues.

Plants

Plants are affected by arsenic applied intentionally as pesticides and accidentally from smelter fallout. The effects are usually dose-related, but are strongly modified by a host of variables, including plant species, geographic region, soil type, and climatic conditions. Two important dose-related effects measurable in plants are arsenic residues and phytotoxicity.

The detailed studies have been conducted on paired crop soil residues in tobacco. Arsenicals were removed in 1952 from the list of recommended insecticides for control of hornworms on tobacco (the arsenic insecticide had been added directly to the leaf), and a sharp decrease in the arsenic content of cigarettes was later reported. The concentration of arsenic in the cured leaf of field-grown tobacco was generally less than 2 ppm where no arsenic was applied to soils. In general, there was an increase in arsenic content in tobacco with increasing rates applied to soils, but this response is greatly modified by soil type. The previous use of arsenic pesticides in tobacco had been challenged as a possible health hazard. It was proposed that tobacco can be expected to contain high concentrations of arsenic because of absorption from soil. Results of Small and McCants appeared to refute this hypothesis.[738] In an extensive survey of arsenic residues in soils and in cured leaves collected from major flue-cured tobacco-producing regions of North Carolina, soil arsenic concentrations ranged from 1 to 5 ppm (average, 2.8 ppm), and leaf residues, from 0.5 to 3.5 ppm (average, 1.5 ppm). The arsenic content of these soils appears to be within the natural limits for virgin soils, and that of the resulting leaves, within natural background limits. Apparently, previous arsenic spray applications had not contributed significantly to soil residues. With low concentrations of arsenic in soils, soil type and other variables may be more important in determining plant arsenic content than small increases in soil arsenic concentration.

Vegetables do not have significant arsenic content when grown in soils containing high concentrations of applied arsenic trioxide.[532] Soils in New Jersey were subjected to applications of lead arsenate at 250, 500, and 1,000 lb/acre (280, 560, and 1,121 kg/ha), and vegetables grown in these soils were analyzed for arsenic (Table 3-14). Arsenic uptake varied between plant species and increased with increasing amounts of applied arsenic. No plants exceeded tolerance limits where limits existed. Soils around smelters contain high concentrations of arsenic.[185,541] This results in vegetation with increased arsenic content.[357] In the East Helena area, arsenic was found at 0.05 ppm or less in apples, kohlrabi, onions, radishes, and string beans and at up to 3.3 ppm in fresh sunflower leaves. Residues in field crops varied from 0.05 ppm or less in wheat to 14.3 ppm in fresh barley straw. For this type of contamination, the amount of arsenic present decreases in the order of pasture grasses, alfalfa, garden plants, and small grains.

There is no correlation between the selenium and arsenic contents of soils and those of plants growing in the soils.[600] The arsenic content of seleniferous soils from South Dakota varied from 7.1 to 18.4 ppm, and the selenium content, from 1.15 to 5.00 ppm. With a few exceptions, however, indigenous plants contained more selenium than arsenic. The selenium content of plants varied from 0 to 266.7 ppm, and the arsenic content, from 1 to 4.2 ppm.

TABLE 3-14 Arsenic Content of Vegetables Grown in Soils Treated with Lead Arsenate[a]

Vegetable	Arsenic, ppm, in Vegetables Grown in Soil Treated with Lead Arsenate at:		
	250 lb/acre (280 kg/ha)	500 lb/acre (560 kg/ha)	1,000 lb/acre (1,121 kg/ha)
Lettuce	0.08	0.10	0.12
Eggplant	Trace	Trace	Trace
Tomatoes	Trace	Trace	Trace
Carrots	Trace	Trace	Trace
Broccoli	Trace	Trace	Trace
Baby beet roots	0.08	0.08	0.12
Baby beet tops	0.08	0.08	0.13
Peppers (seeds removed)	Trace	Trace	Trace
Snap beans	None	Trace	Trace
Radish tops	0.17	0.33	0.60
Radish roots	0.02	0.17	0.22

[a]Derived from McLean et al.[532]

It is important to note the large variability in the relationships among soil arsenic content, plant arsenic content, injury symptoms, and phytotoxicity reported by different investigators. Vandecaveye et al.[817] reported that alfalfa and grasses grown on a soil having soluble arsenic at less than 2.5 ppm contained arsenic at 20–30 ppm on a dry-weight basis. MacPhee et al.[509] analyzed pea and bean plants grown in pesticide-persistence plots at Kentville, Nova Scotia. The soil plots contained arsenic at 126–157 ppm. Most of the arsenic in the plants was found in vines (2.1 ppm) and pods (0.88 ppm), with small amounts in seeds (0.18 ppm). Reed and Sturgis analyzed rice plants grown on arsenic-treated soils.[662] They reported arsenic at up to 5.0 ppm in the rice head and 2.5 ppm in the straw. Woolson[873] correlated extractable arsenic with plant growth and plant residues for six vegetable crops. Available arsenic concentrations of 6.2–48.3 ppm were necessary to reduce growth by 50%. At these concentrations, edible dry plant contained arsenic at 0.7–76.0 ppm.

There is evidence in the literature of beneficial effects on plant growth from relatively high arsenic concentrations in soils. Stewart and Smith[759] found that a concentration of 25 ppm in soils enhanced the growth of peas, radishes, wheat, and potatoes, whereas beans showed a steady decrease in growth when the arsenic content increased. MacPhee et al.[509] reported an increase in turnip yields with a total arsenic content of 150 ppm in soils. This effect was attributed to control of the turnip root maggot. However, there was a yield decrease in other crops tested, including peas and beans. A beneficial effect on several crops was noted when fields were treated with high concentrations of calcium arsenate. The concentrations of total arsenic in soil where yield decreases were first noted for vetch, oats, and barley were 94, 188, and 283 ppm, respectively (calcium arsenate applied at 500, 1,000, and 1,500 lb/acre, or 560, 1,121, and 1,681 kg/ha).[163] When arsenic applied was below these toxic concentrations, the soils treated with calcium arsenate yielded more than the untreated soils. For example, the yields of rye from soil treated with calcium arsenate at 188 ppm (1,000 lb/acre, or 1,121 kg/ha) were greater than the yields from the same soil if untreated. Wheat yields were increased at 1,131 ppm (6,000 lb/acre, or 6,725 kg/ha), the highest concentration used. In another soil type, corn, sorghum, soybeans, and cotton showed yield increases from applications of 188 ppm (1,000 lb of calcium arsenate per acre, or 1,121 kg/ha).[164]

The increasing use of the methanearsonate herbicides MSMA and DSMA to control weeds in cotton has led to an extensive survey of cottonseed for arsenic residues. Possible sources of methanearsonates for human consumption, owing to their use in cotton, are cottonseed flour and cottonseed oil and, indirectly, milk, meat, and eggs from cows and chickens fed cottonseed meal. Reports compiled by the National Agricultural Chemicals Association (NACA) Industry Task Force for Agricultural Arsenical Pesticides[270] showed that methanearsonates cause no significant arsenic residues in cottonseed if applied to cotton after it has reached a height of 3 in. (7.6 cm) and before early bloom. They cause significant arsenic residues in cottonseed if applied as a directed spray after early bloom.[336] Apparently, either DSMA or MSMA translocated from leaves and stems to the immature ovule if applied at flowering, reached a maximum if applied when the seed was growing most rapidly, and decreased to a low concentration if applied to open cotton. On the basis of these and other results, the registered label restricts use of the methanearsonates from the time cotton is 3 in. (7.6 cm) high until first bloom. It permits no more than two directed applications of DSMA or MSMA of up to 3 or 2 lb/acre (3.4 or 2.2 kg/ha), respectively, per application. Within the specified limits of growth stage, application rates, and application methods, arsenic residues in raw undelinted cottonseed vary from 0 to 0.2 ppm above controls. The analysis of a large number of cottonseed samples from control fields has shown background arsenic concentrations varying from the limit of detection of the method (about 0.05 ppm) to about 0.3 ppm. Therefore, the total arsenic content of samples from treated fields varies from 0.05 to about 0.5 ppm. The report of the NACA Industry Task Force on Tolerance for Methanearsonates[705] therefore requested an arsenic tolerance of 0.5 ppm in cottonseed. The same report illustrates the human exposure likely to occur from this amount of arsenic in cottonseed flour. The average human would have to consume about 1.5 lb (0.68 kg) of cottonseed flour per day to reach 0.3 mg of arsenic from this source, assuming the cottonseed flour all contained the maximum of 0.5 ppm (0.3 mg is a 2,000-fold safety factor based on no-effect feed concentrations for rats). The average concentration of arsenic in cottonseed flour, assuming both added and background arsenic, is about 0.15 ppm. At this concentration, about 5 lb (2.3 kg) of cottonseed flour could be safely consumed per day. In reality, however, very little cottonseed flour is used in baking.

Residues in plants and plant products grown in soils that had been treated with arsenic or in material that had been sprayed itself are listed in Appendix A. Residues are highest in samples taken soon after spraying or dusting. The highest residues in hops came from treating them with impure sulfur. Cotton leaves contained high concentrations of arsenic, probably from being sprayed with arsenic acid before harvest. The treatment is used to defoliate cotton plants before mechanical harvesting. Grass had high concentrations from a sodium arsenite spray. Most other residue values were not very different from those in plant material grown on untreated soil. Although residues may have been high on food crops (e.g., apples) in the past, current surveys indicate that arsenic contamination is not significant. As mentioned previously, arsenic acid is used as a desiccant in Texas and parts of Oklahoma. The FDA analyzed cottonseed products and various commodities from areas where arsenical defoliation was known to be practiced.[96] The arsenic content of various commodities analyzed is shown in Table 3-15. Of another 159 cottonseed product samples

TABLE 3-15 Arsenic (as As_2O_3) in Various Commodities, Texas, 1963[a]

Product	No. Counties Sampled	No. Samples	No. Samples Positive for As_2O_3[b]	As_2O_3 Concentration, ppm[c]	
				Average	Maximum
Potatoes	1	2	2	0.02	0.02
Mustard greens	3	5	4	0.01	0.08
Turnip greens	2	4	3	0.03	0.04
Cabbage	3	7	2	0.01	0.01
Sweet potatoes	1	1	0	—	—
Radishes and tops	1	1	1	0.01	0.01
Lettuce	3	27	12	0.01	0.08
Carrot tops	1	1	1	0.16	0.16
Carrots	3	10	9	0.03	0.05
Corn	1	1	0	—	—
Bell peppers	2	2	0	—	—
Nonfat dry milk	1	1	1	0.01	0.01
Tomatoes	1	1	1	0.01	0.01
Peaches	2	6	6	0.07	0.08
Rough rice	1	4	4	0.16	0.22
Raw unshelled peanuts	1	2	2	0.01	0.01
Wheat	1	3	2	0.03	0.03
Cucumbers	1	2	2	0.03	0.03
Soybean oil	1	2	2	0.09	0.10
Cottonseed oil	6	13	12	0.13	0.52
Cottonseed meal	5	9	9	0.90	3.72
Spinach	1	1	1	0.04	0.04
Collards	2	2	1	0.01	0.01

[a] Derived from Bradicich et al.[96]
[b] Sensitivity of method, 0.01 ppm.
[c] Not corrected for average recovery of 71%.

Distribution of Arsenic in the Environment

tested, 143 were positive; three samples were above the established arsenic trioxide tolerance of 4 ppm allowed by the FDA, and the overall average was less than 0.9 ppm. The report concluded that "these results indicate that levels of arsenic in cottonseed products for human consumption from areas in which arsenical defoliation is practiced are well below established tolerances."

Animals

Arsenic, because of its ubiquity, is eaten or drunk by all animals. The amounts of arsenic found in some animal tissues as a result of normal exposure are presented in Appendix B. Arsenic in abnormal amounts may be ingested by eating plants or drinking water contaminated with arsenic, breathing arsenic-containing dusts, or ingesting arsenic as a medicine or poison. Little arsenic is currently used in human medicine, although it was used extensively in the eighteenth and nineteenth centuries. Phenylarsonic formulations are used as feed additives to enhance growth in poultry and swine.

Arsenic concentrations in animals that have been subjected to high exposure are presented in Appendix B. The highest residues in man are generally in the hair and nails; high concentrations in other portions of the body are transitory. The highest residues—particularly in the stomach, intestines, liver, and kidneys—were from known cases of arsenic poisoning.

Animals subjected to arsenic pollution in the Helena Valley contained higher than normal arsenic residues, mainly in hair.[466] Horse hair contained up to 5.9 ppm, with the higher values in horses living closest to the smelter exhaust stack and eating locally grown hay. Organ analysis of a horse that died of unknown causes revealed residues of 0.7 ppm in the lung, 0.1 ppm in the liver, 0.11 ppm in flank muscle, 2.0 ppm in hair, and a trace in the kidney. Concentrations of cadmium, lead, and mercury were also high. Other miscellaneous animal products from within 3 km of the stack were analyzed. The results were: chicken muscle, trace; rabbit muscle, 0.6 ppm; whole milk, trace; beef liver, 0.2 ppm; beef muscle, 0.05 ppm; beef kneebone, not detected; swine heart, trace; and sausage, trace.

Arsenic concentrations may be increased in chickens and chicken products if they have received arsenic feed additives up to slaughter. Residues, however, decrease rapidly after additive withdrawal. Eggs apparently do not contain detectable residues.[50]

Starlings, sampled as part of a nationwide monitoring program, contained low arsenic concentrations.[524] Only one sample (0.21 ppm) exceeded 0.05 ppm; most contained arsenic at 0.01–0.02 ppm on a wet-weight basis.

Fish and fish products contain the highest concentrations of the animal kingdom, although they are exposed to arsenic only in the sea or rivers. Crustacea generally have the highest arsenic concentrations of the seafood species, and oil from fish contains more arsenic than the flesh.

Bees have often been subject to injury wherever arsenic compounds are used, because only 4–5 µg of arsenic is necessary to cause death. However, analysis of dead bees and contents within a hive have often revealed high arsenic concentrations.[226,228]

Foods

The FDA has conducted surveillance and monitoring programs on pesticides in food. In one survey, arsenic in foods was monitored in samples collected from 30 markets in 29 cities for the period June 1966–April 1967.[523] The sensitivity of the method for arsenic, as As_2O_3, was 0.1 ppm. In this survey, 33 of 360 composite samples collected were positive for arsenic (range, 0.1–0.40 ppm). In the survey covering the period June 1968–April 1969,[166] 57 of 360 composite samples were positive for arsenic (range, 0.1–1.0 ppm). A breakdown of commodities, indicating the numbers of positive samples and the concentrations (or ranges), is as follows: meat, fish, and poultry, 15, 0.1–1.0 ppm; grain and cereal, 7, 0.1–0.2 ppm; fruit, 5, 0.1 ppm; sugar and adjuncts, 5, 0.1 ppm; dairy products, 2, 0.1 ppm; potatoes, 3, 0.1 ppm; leafy vegetables, 4, 0.1 ppm; legume vegetables, 3, 0.1 ppm; root vegetables, 3, 0.1 ppm; garden vegetables, 4, 0.1 ppm; oils, fats, and shortenings, 2, 0.1 ppm; and beverages, 3, 0.1 ppm. Detailed analysis of these data is not possible; however, it is interesting that the highest concentrations occurred in meat, fish, and poultry. The seaport city of Baltimore reported the highest concentrations in this category (four samples and a range of 0.2–1.0 ppm), whereas the inland cities of Kansas City and Minneapolis reported only three samples at 0.1 ppm. Arsenic from seafoods may account for the high concentrations in samples collected from Baltimore.

Arsenic in a sample institutional diet amounted to about 400 µg/day.[709] The amounts of arsenic found in an institutional diet containing no seafood are shown in Table 3-16. Arsenic in various foods is shown in Appendixes A and B. Very little arsenic is currently found in food products other than fish and fish products. The estimate

TABLE 3-16 Arsenic in Institutional Diet[a]

Meal	Diet Weight, g	Arsenic Concentration, μg/g (wet)	Arsenic Concentration, μg/g (dry)	Total Arsenic, μg
Breakfast	766	0.06	0.23	46.0
Dinner	861	0.34	1.85	292.7
Supper	899	0.08	0.42	71.9
Total	2,526	—	—	410.6
Mean	—	0.16	0.83	—

[a]Derived from Schroeder and Balassa.[709]

of Schroeder and Balassa[709] appears to be high in relation to other estimates that are available on total arsenic consumption per day.

The World Health Organization reported that average arsenic intakes for Canada, the United Kingdom, the United States, and France varied from 25 to 33 μg/day; specific values ranged from 7 to 60 μg/day.[881]

A survey of food made in Great Britain indicated that 100 μg of arsenic would be consumed daily from all sources.[320] Analysis for arsenic resulted in the following values for foodstuffs: cereals, 0.18 ppm; fats, 0.05 ppm; fruits and preserves, 0.07 ppm; root vegetables, 0.08 ppm; milk, 0.05 ppm; meat, 0.10 ppm; and fish, 2.0 ppm. The Japanese consume between 70 and 170 μg of arsenic per day.[576] Food products in Canada are low in arsenic, only roots and garden fruits averaging arsenic residues higher than 0.01 ppm in 1971.[740] In 1970, meats, potatoes, and roots averaged greater than 0.01 ppm—0.18, 0.15, and less than 0.18 ppm, respectively. It is clear that the general population receives little arsenic in its food.[741]

Several instances of accidental arsenic poisoning through contaminated foodstuffs have been reported in Japan. Soy sauce, which contained arsenic at 5.6–71.6 μg/ml, was implicated in a toxicity outbreak. The arsenic was in the amino acids (260–275 μg/ml) used in making the sauce; hydrochloric acid may have been the source of arsenic in the preparation of the amino acids.[589] Contaminated powdered milk was implicated in a similar outbreak in Japan. It contained arsenic at 13.5–21 ppm.[426] Contamination of the milk was from sodium phosphate (7.11% arsenic) used in its manufacture.[431]

Air

There are three major sources of arsenic in air: smelting of metals; burning of coal, vegetation, and agricultural wastes; and use of arsenical pesticides.

Almost all arsenic produced for commercial use is recovered as a by-product in the smelting of lead, copper, and gold ores. It is removed from the smelter exhaust gases. These are treated to remove dangerous or valuable substances, many of which are emitted as dusts, including arsenic trioxide, metal and metal oxide particles, and fly ash. Arsenic trioxide is volatile, and nearly all of it is expelled from the ore as a sublimate during smelting. Crude flue dust is usually recycled to the furnace, with a consequent buildup of arsenic, sometimes to as much as 30%. The arsenic-rich flue dust and other arsenic-containing residues from domestic smelters are shipped to a single copper smelter, where the arsenic is separated by controlled roasting and processed to a commercial form. The arsenic-free calcine is smelted to recover other metals.

Even in the smelters where arsenic is not recovered for commercial use, the quantities involved are very large. A reverberatory furnace, for example, may smelt as much as 1,900 tonnes of charge per day and in doing so burn 218 tonnes of coal. The furnace would produce about 2,550,000 m³ of gas per day, containing up to 163 tonnes of solids. This means that it would be necessary to dispose of 5.4–54 tonnes of arsenic each day, with the lower value being more common.[425,520]

Arsenic is brought into the air by a combustion process and exists as an oxide. However, arsenic is removed from the air by settling or rainfall, and atmospheric concentrations do not build up. Air samples may contain arsenic—for example, rural England, 0.4—6.4 ng/kg,[133] an industrial area of Osaka, Japan, 25–90 ng/m³;[515] urban United States, 20 ng/m³;[804] and rural Canada, 0.27—4.7 ng/m³.[657] Nonurban areas had a maximal average concentration of 20 ng/m³, with most values less than 10 ng/m³.[770] Concentrations of arsenic in fly ash increase by a factor of 10 as particle size decreases from 74 to 1.1–2.1 μg. Particles that escape most existing particle-collecting systems (less than 5 μg) contain high arsenic concentrations.[580] Large cities generally have a higher arsenic concentration in the air than do small cities, because of fuel combustion for electricity and heating. An air arsenic content of 30 ng/m³ was calculated on the basis of the amount of coal burned in New York City. This agrees well with the observed air concentrations for New York City.[770]

Air quality data taken in 1950, 1953, 1961, and 1964 for 133 stations showed that the average arsenic content ranged from below detection to 750 ng/m³; the average for all stations was about 30 ng/m³. The Montana State Board of Health reported ambient air concentrations for some cities in Montana in 1961–1962.[766] The highest concentration in the state was 2,500 ng/m³ in Anaconda, the site of the smelter that treats most of the arsenical ore mined in the United States.

Two serious incidents of air pollution by arsenic from smelters in the United States have been recorded in the literature. The first incident took place in Anaconda, Mont.,[328,338] where the rate of emission of arsenic trioxide was 26,884 kg/day (in 64,563 m³ of air per day) while the smelter was processing 9,070 tonnes of copper ore per day. Although no atmospheric concentrations were recorded, edible plants contained arsenic trioxide at up to 482 µg/g. The second incident occurred in a small western town near a gold-smelter.[79] (The exact location was not mentioned.) The mine had been operated intermittently since 1934. In 1962, the operation was resumed with a process that required converting sulfur and arsenic to sulfur dioxide and arsenic trioxide. The smelter processed sufficient ore to produce about 91 tonnes of sulfur dioxide and 36 tonnes of arsenic trioxide per day. The dust-collecting system designed to collect approximately 90% of the toxic dusts failed to operate as expected, and toxic fumes escaped into the atmosphere. These two episodes indicate that there may be some degree of arsenical air pollution at every smelter that treats arsenical ores, especially when dust-collecting equipment is inadequate or not working properly. An example of the arsenical pollution potential estimated for Colorado is shown in Table 3-17. The quantities of arsenic recovered in the concentrates and deposited in the mill tailings were not reported.

TABLE 3-17 Arsenical Pollution Potential from Mills in Colorado[a]

Metal	Average Arsenic Content, %	Quantity of Ore, tons[b]	Potential Arsenic Pollution, tons[b]
Zinc (eight mines)	0.07	48,109	34
Lead (eight mines)	0.08	19,918	16
Copper (one mine)	0.28	4,169	12
Total	—	72,196	62

[a]Data from Kirk and Othmer.[425]
[b]To convert to tonnes, multiply values by 0.9.

Arsenicals are used for weed control and as desiccants for cotton plants before machine picking. Thus, dust and gases emitted from cotton gins contain arsenic. At a distance of 46–91 m downwind from a west Texas cotton gin, concentrations of 600–141,000 ng/m³ were detected. The amount found was inversely proportional to the distance from the source.[805]

The burning of cotton trash from a cotton gin is also a source of arsenic. Approximately 37% of the gins incinerate their trash, 58% return it to the land, and 5% handle it in some other manner. Arsenic emission from incineration is not known.

Arsenical pesticides constitute one of the primary uses of arsenic. From 1937 to 1940, the U.S. Public Health Service studied the effects of lead arsenate on orchard workers.[583] The amounts of lead and arsenic to which they were exposed in the air varied with the operation being performed. The arsenic concentration was highest when they were burning the containers (16,670 μg/m³), followed by mixing (1,850 μg/m³), picking the fruit (880 μg/m³), spraying (140 μg/m³), and thinning the fruit (80 μg/m³). It is noteworthy that the highest arsenic concentration in air came from burning the containers.

Disposal

The problems and methods of waste disposal associated with each of the major arsenic uses and processes are discussed in this section. Much of the available information on waste from the manufacture and use of arsenic compounds is in a profile report on disposition of hazardous wastes prepared for the EPA in 1973,[610] which was used extensively in the preparation of this section.

Waste from Agricultural Uses of Pesticides and Herbicides

• *Cacodylic acid:* Cacodylic acid is a contact herbicide used to defoliate or desiccate a wide variety of plant species and was used as a defoliant for crop destruction in South Vietnam. It is registered for use in lawn renovation or as a silvicide. Ottinger *et al.* indicated that the major source of waste from the agricultural use of cacodylic acid was pesticide residue left in empty containers after use.[610] Residues from plant leaves or material sprayed or applied directly on the soil become bound to soil particles and are not readily leached from the soil or taken up by plant root systems. The present registered uses of the cacodylates preclude their application to food crops, so plant residues are not expected to enter the food chain. However, burning or other types of disposal of material from sprayed areas, as well as erosion of soil from sprayed sites, could constitute a potential hazard. The cacodylates are normally formulated as liquid solutions containing 2–3 lb of cacodylate per gallon of solution (about 240–360 kg/m³). Stojanovic et al. have estimated that 2.2–2.8% of the original contents is left in "empty pesticide containers."[763] An average of 2.5% of the estimated annual use of 1,200,000 gal (4,540 m³) of cacodylate solutions—30,000 gal (114 m³)—is left in containers.[610] The safe and economical disposal of pesticide-contaminated containers is a serious problem that has not been solved.[610]

- *Arsenic acid:* Arsenic acid is used extensively as a cotton desiccant. The amount produced has been estimated at roughly 9,000,000 lb (4,080,000 kg) in 1971.[579] As expected from the use of arsenic acid as a cotton defoliant, residues are associated with the disposal of cotton wastes from cotton gins. Sullivan reported that dust from the ginning operation can have an adverse effect on vegetation downwind of cotton gins.[770] Also, about 37% of the gins burn trash that releases arsenic into the environment. The amounts released are not known. Bag filters and electrostatic precipitators are reasonably adequate for control of dust and particles from the burning of cotton trash. No specific information is available on the removal of arsenic acid residues remaining in containers after use, but it can be assumed that a small percentage of solution will remain. It is also unlikely that any adequate control program is in operation for the collection and disposal of empty arsenic acid containers.

- *Disodium methanearsonate and monosodium methanearsonate:* DSMA and MSMA are used extensively in cotton-producing areas for selective weed control. There is no specific information on the disposal of used pesticide containers and crop residues contaminated with arsenic, but the potential problems with these compounds are probably the same as those with the cacodylates and arsenic acid. The magnitudes of the problems appear to be similar, because the estimated amounts of material used appear to be similar. The potential for contamination of the cotton plant or gin trash may be somewhat less with DSMA and MSMA, because the use of these compounds is restricted to the period between the time the plant is 3 in. (7.6 cm) high and the first bloom.

- *Arsenates (calcium, copper, lead, sodium, zinc, and manganese):* Only two of these compounds, calcium arsenate and lead arsenate, are used extensively as agricultural pesticides. The remaining arsenates are not prepared for agricultural or any other use in any significant quantity. Approximately 2,000,000 lb (907,185 kg) of calcium arsenate and 7,700,000 lb (3,493,000 kg) of lead arsenate were produced in 1969.[802] In 1972, the EPA stopped the registration of lead arsenate, so its use is expected to decrease to the point of insignificance in the very near future.[610] Strict government controls on the use of calcium arsenate are expected to reduce its use in the near future. The three major sources of arsenate wastes are residues in empty containers; surplus pesticides stored by government agencies (the Department of Defense and the EPA), state and municipal facilities, and manufacturing plants; and soil contaminated from extensive use of arsenate pesticides. The latter constitutes the most important waste problem with respect to the arsenates. There is no wholly satisfactory procedure for the recovery of contaminated soils, except removal and mixing with clean soil to dilute the arsenic. Because calcium arsenate and lead arsenate are almost always formulated as dusts, granules, or wettable powder and shipped in siftproof, multiwall paper bags, there is less residue in empty containers. Nevertheless, disposal of empty paper bags could pose a problem, particularly if large quantities are burned or buried in landfills. There are no recommended procedures for the disposal of these kinds of pesticide containers. There is no information on the possible problems related to the disposal of contaminated crop residues. However, Table 3-14 indicates that, even with high application rates of lead arsenate, the residues in vegetable crops would probably be minimal.

• *Copper acetoarsenite and sodium arsenite:* The production and use of these two compounds is not great. The production of copper acetoarsenite (Paris green) is estimated to be at least 100,000 lb/year (45,000 kg/year).[610] One of the uses of sodium arsenite is in livestock dips for cattle tick control. There are strict government controls on the use of these compounds, and the extent of use is expected to remain about the same or possibly to decrease. One of the major problems with the disposal of arsenite wastes involves the disposition of empty containers. The arsenites are generally shipped and stored as liquid solutions, and the problem is handling and disposing of metal and plastic containers. No satisfactory collection and disposal procedures have been devised, but, in view of the low volume of use (in comparison with other arsenicals) and its expected decrease, the problem is not particularly great. Disposal of sodium arsenite cattle dips has created some localized problems, because of the large volumes of liquid and the high concentration of arsenic involved. No totally satisfactory method for disposal is available, but landfill in very tight clay soil has been suggested.

Waste from Use of Arsenical Feed Additives

Arsanilic acid, 3-nitro-4-hydroxyphenylarsonic acid (Roxarsone), 4-nitrophenylarsonic acid, and 4-ureidophenylarsonic acid (carbarsone) are approved for use in animal feeds as therapeutic or growth-promoting agents. These compounds are packaged and sold by a variety of feed ingredient and pharmaceutical manufacturers under many different trade names. Most are sold either pure or mixed with diluents—such as corn germ meal, corn cobs, and calcium carbonate—and are sold directly to feed manufacturers or individual farmers for mixing in poultry or swine feeds or for addition to the drinking water.[587]

Because these materials are fed to animals, the major concern with respect to disposal has to do with the amounts that may be found in animal wastes. FDA regulations require that these arsenic compounds be withdrawn from animals 5 days before slaughter. There is evidence that almost all residues are depleted during this period, and evidence accumulated by Peoples[628] and Calvert[126] indicated that only about 10-15% of ingested arsenic is absorbed by the animals. Thus, it is very likely that nearly all the arsenic fed will eventually appear in animal excreta. It is unknown whether the amounts fed to animals and eventually excreted constitute a disposal problem.

As shown by Morrison, arsenic in animal wastes did not accumulate in soil or ground water after 20 years of poultry manure application.[562] The manure contained arsenic at 15-30 ppm, and the application rate was 4-6 tons/acre (9.0-13.5 tonnes/ha) per year. Messer et al.[540] reported that some poultry litter samples analyzed contained arsenic at up to 75 ppm (dry-weight basis), and Calvert[126] reported up to 45 ppm in dried broiler manure.

In many instances, swine and poultry wastes are stored in anaerobic lagoons for long periods before disposal. If these animals are fed arsenic for therapeutic or growth-promoting purposes, all the arsenic-containing compounds fed may accumulate in waste lagoons. In a recent study,[108] arsenic concentrations were measured in lagoons under swine fed arsanilic acid at 0, 90, and 180 g/ton (0, 99.2, and 198.4 g/tonne) of feed. The wastes were collected during the growing period (31-198 lb, or 14-90 kg) and retained for 120 days in experimental anaerobic lagoons. The only two significant effects observed in these lagoons were total arsenic contents (on a wet-sample basis) of 0.26, 5.77, and 10.60 ppm for 0-, 90-, and 180-g/ton feeding concentrations, respectively, and dry-matter contents in the lagoons of 6.20, 3.57, and

2.89%, respectively. No studies have been conducted on arsenic contents of lagoons used for long periods; inasmuch as lagoons may well be used for some 10–15 years, there may be significant accumulations of arsenic. The effects of these accumulations on microbial activity in the lagoons and on later disposal are unknown.

On the basis of the amount of these arsenicals used each year, estimated at a total of 3,000 tons (2,722 tonnes), and the fact that the manure will probably contain arsenic at only 75–100 ppm, it is unlikely that manure application will create any problem with regard to arsenic contamination of soil. Morrison indicated that, even to approach amounts of arsenic that might affect plant growth, application rates of manure containing arsenic at 30 ppm would need to be about 2,000 tons/acre (4,480 tonnes/ha).[562]

There might be a more serious problem when animal wastes are approved for use as animal feeds. Arsenic in poultry and swine wastes in some instances may be incorporated into diets of animals for which no FDA clearance has been established. Studies by Calvert,[126] by Fontenot,[258] and by Long et al.[485] indicated that arsenic in manure fed to cattle and sheep can be detected in tissues and that a short withdrawal period was sufficient to reduce tissue arsenic to acceptable concentrations.

Waste from Industrial Uses of Arsenic

• *Arsenic trioxide:* The American Smelting and Refining Company (ASARCO) accepts and refines flue dust from a large part of the U.S. copper, gold, zinc, and lead smelting industry. The principal methods for collection of flue dusts are discussed elsewhere in this report. The flue dust is treated with other high-arsenic material to sublime off arsenic oxide, which is condensed in a series of condensing chambers. This dust and dust that remains in the stream and is collected on bag filters or electrostatic precipitators is mainly impure arsenic oxide, which is refined to commercial arsenic trioxide. ASARCO currently accepts crude arsenic-containing ores and intermediate smelter products on a broad scale. With the possible exception of some problems with its own flue control system, this appears to be a key to adequate management of arsenic wastes from smelters.[610] This is not to say that all smelters have adequate flue-gas control; as reported by Ottinger, some plants refuse to release data on flue-gas composition, and the one plant reporting indicated emission of 1.1 tons (1 tonne) of particulate matter per day with a 34% arsenic content.[610]

The major problem currently associated with arsenic management in the smelter industry, aside from the escape of flue gases from the filters and precipitators, is the fluctuating demand for the arsenic trioxide produced by ASARCO. Large overstocks of arsenic trioxide can and do result, but, fortunately, these are at one site, and controls are fairly easily implemented. Current methods for storage are large siftproof and weatherproof silos at the site of ASARCO's plant in Tacoma, Washington. It has been suggested that, with government subsidy, this system could become a national disposal site for all arsenic trioxide and related arsenic compounds.

Under some conditions of encapsulation, arsenic trioxide might be buried in landfill sites. However, there are insufficient data to determine whether such a system would be adequate. In any event, this method of disposal should be used only if there are large oversupplies of arsenic trioxide and if long-term storage facilities are not available.

The principal concern in metal smelting and arsenic trioxide refining processes is the more complete removal of arsenic from smelter flue gases. The following is a brief description of methods now used to remove dust from exhaust-gas streams:

1. The use of electrostatic precipitators is the most common method, but they are only 70–90% effective and require flushing of grids; smaller, light particles normally escape entrapment; Ottinger *et al.* indicated that the negative responses received from their contacts with smelter operators suggested that this procedure was inadequate.[610]

2. Filter–bag house operations are normally 99% efficient, but they require more power than precipitators and are more expensive to purchase and install; they are expected to be used more extensively when more complete abatement compliance is required.

3. Charged-droplet scrubbers use a stream of electrostatically charged water droplets, which are accelerated through a field between a positive-voltage nozzle and the negative-voltage collector plates on the side of the flue; the water droplets collide with dust particles and carry them to the collector plates, where they drain away; efficiency is estimated at 99%, and power requirements and installation expense are lower than for bag houses and precipitators.

4. Sullivan reported on the use, in the U.S.S.R., of wet-vacuum pumps, instead of fabric bag filters; efficiency was reported to be 100%, although no specific information was made available on the process.[770]

For the treatment of arsenic trioxide wastes, the recommended process is long-term storage. Improved flue-dust abatement equipment is needed. The use of fabric bag filters is currently the preferred method in the industry, but it is not entirely satisfactory.

- *Cacodylic acid:* The Ansul Company of Marinette, Wisconsin, and the Vineland Chemical Company of Vineland, New Jersey, account for about 80 and 20%, respectively, of the U.S. production of cacodylic acid. The commercial production process, according to Ottinger *et al.*, has three steps: Arsenic trioxide reacts with sodium hydroxide to yield sodium arsenite, methanearsonic acid is produced by the addition of methylchloride, and the mixture is reduced with sulfur dioxide and methylated to produce cacodylic acid.[610] There is no liquid waste from this process, because all liquid streams are cycled back into the system. A solid waste is produced; it consists largely of sodium chloride and sodium sulfate with about 1–1.5% cacodylate contaminants. Currently, about 27,200 tonnes of this solid material is stored in concrete vaults in the Marinette, Wisconsin, area. There are no plans for this waste, other than to store it indefinitely. The waste management systems in use are recycle and reuse, long-term storage, and landfill in "class 1" sites. As defined in Ottinger *et al.*,[610] a class 1 site is over either non-water-bearing sediments or unusable water and is protected from surface runoff and flooding. The Ansul Manufacturing Company has indicated that it will accept unused cacodylates that were manufactured by the company and are returned in their original containers.[20] This seems to be an adequate means of waste management, if the materials are in a concentrated form. The long-term storage of cacodylates and the salt wastes appears to be the only system for handling such waste today. Storage containers should be constructed so as to avoid leakage or release of arsenic materials, and they should be inspected routinely. Landfill disposal is generally unacceptable for handling wastes, because of the potential danger to surface or ground water. There are, however, class 1 sites that could be used, but such should be considered only for small quantities of cacodylate wastes and only if no other system is available.

- *DSMA and MSMA:* No information was found on the procedures used for management of wastes of these two compounds, but, inasmuch as the chemistry of their synthesis is similar to that of the cacodylates, the methods for waste management during manufacture should be similar. Ottinger *et al.* indicated that recycling and reuse, storage, and landfill procedures for handling waste products would be similar for MSMA, DSMA, and cacodylates.[610]

- *Calcium arsenate and lead arsenate:* These compounds are manufactured in a completely contained batch process. The only liquid effluents result from cleanup of equipment. The contaminated liquid is

Distribution of Arsenic in the Environment

held in evaporating ponds at the plant site. Water used in the process is removed by drum or spray dryers, whose exhausts are cleaned by scrubbers. The scrubber liquids are then used in the preparation of the next batch of pesticide. Bag filters are used to remove particles that result from grinding and bagging. Any aqueous filtrates from the purification processes are recycled for the makeup of the next batch.

Handling of waste after manufacture requires special consideration, because it is generally a solid material; but, in general, the procedures are similar to those for other arsenic materials. Recycling and reusing excess or unused materials are acceptable practices, and the companies involved have indicated that they would accept their own products in unopened containers. Long-term storage in weatherproof storage bins is considered adequate and is the practical method in use. Land spreading of unwanted stock of the arsenates using light applications on large areas of land is acceptable only if all alternative procedures have been considered. Export of unwanted stock to countries with less restrictive regulations on the use of arsenate has been considered; this procedure would conceivably solve some of our domestic problems, but it would not contribute to the control of global pollution from arsenicals. Another available option is the recovery of other metals, particularly lead; it should be remembered, however, that this would result in the production of arsenic trioxide, which might constitute as much of a disposal problem as the original product. Landfill is generally not acceptable as a disposal technique, because of the potential danger of contamination of ground and surface water; however, the use of class 1 sites is considered adequate for small stocks of arsenates, if all alternative systems have been ruled out.

- *Copper acetoarsenite and sodium arsenite:* As described by Ottinger *et al.*, copper acetoarsenite is believed to be a mixture of cupric arsenite and the copper salt of acetic acid in a ratio of about 3 : 1.[610] Paris green is manufactured by the reaction of sodium arsenite (made from the reaction of arsenic trioxide with sodium hydroxide) with copper carbonate and acetic acid by a batch process. The reaction is considered complete when a green product precipitates from solution, with only a white supernatant fluid remaining. The supernatant solution is said to be arsenic-free. Ottinger *et al.* indicated that only two companies remain as major manufacturers of sodium arsenite: the Chevron Chemical Company and the Los Angeles Chemical Company.[610] The total production from these companies is believed to be about 757–1,514 m^3, containing 479–719 kg of sodium arsenite per cubic meter. The solution is filtered before it is put in drums, and the filter cake is buried. The composition of the filter cake is not known, but it might be expected to contain some arsenic as a contaminant. No other part of the manufacturing process has been identified as a source of arsenic pollution. In general, the sources of arsenic waste and its handling are the same as for the arsenates, except that copper acetoarsenite and sodium arsenite are usually sold and distributed in liquid solutions. The adequate management systems are: recycling and reuse; long-term storage; recovery of such metals as copper and lead and long-term storage of arsenic trioxide; and landfill in class 1 sites. In addition to the arsenic content of these pesticides, as is the case with the arsenates, the metal content should also be considered in the selection of an appropriate disposal system.

• *Miscellaneous industrial sources of arsenic waste:* The glass industry, according to Ottinger *et al.*, consumed about 4,100 tons (3,720 tonnes) of arsenic trioxide in 1968 and 3,000 tons (2,720 tonnes) in 1971.[610] Arsenic trioxide is used as a refining agent and is added in purified form to molten-glass batches in 0.2–0.75% loadings. The arsenic trioxide is volatilized and disperses through the glass. No waste is produced in the process, except for some glass slag, which apparently does not constitute a disposal problem.

The 400 million tons (363 million tonnes) of coal consumed each year produce an estimated 300–6,500 tons (272–5,900 tonnes) of arsenic trioxide per year. Urban areas generally have a slightly higher air arsenic content than rural areas. No particular recommendations have been made for the control of this source of arsenic, and it is unlikely, unless coal consumption increases dramatically, that it constitutes a special pollution hazard. Furthermore, the proper use and design of pollution control devices being incorporated by industries that use coal as an energy source will probably limit arsenic emission.

The recently renewed interest in the land application of municipal sewage sludge for disposal or as a source of plant nutrients has generated concern for the heavy-metal content of these materials and their effects on soil and ground water. Arsenic has not been one of the elements of major concern, and it has been difficult to obtain much information on the arsenic content of effluent wastewater and sewage sludge. In one study, the effluent wastewater and sewage sludge from 58 municipalities in Michigan, including Detroit, were analyzed for a variety of elements, including arsenic.[81] The amounts of arsenic detected ranged from less than 0.005 to 0.023 μg of total arsenic per liter of effluent and from 1.6 to 17 mg/kg of air-dried sludge. However, the content of arsenic and heavy metals probably will keep the use of sewage sludge and wastewater effluents well below the amounts needed to cause toxicity.

Summary

Table 3-18 summarizes the method of disposal of some of the principal arsenic compounds used in the United States. No one disposal system is being used to handle arsenic wastes from the manufacture of the various arsenic compounds; it is unlikely that any system would be wholly satisfactory for the entire arsenic manufacturing industry. In some instances, long-term storage is the only method for disposal until alternative procedures for disposal or recovery of arsenic or metals can be developed. Recycling or reusing arsenic from arsenic manufacture probably solves the greatest number of problems, as far as disposal is concerned. Unfavorable economics is, and will be, the major limiting factor in recycling of waste products. Landfill in general would be a last resort for adequate disposal, primarily because of the scarcity of class 1 sites near manufacturing wastes.

With respect to the disposal of arsenic compounds used in agriculture, few if any well-controlled systems for disposal of crop residues, empty arsenical containers, or other contaminated products are currently used. Most manufacturers will accept unused packages of arsenicals, but the user is generally left to his own devices when disposing of

TABLE 3-18   Method of Disposal of Principal Arsenic Compounds Manufactured in the United States

Compound	Current Disposal System
Arsenic trioxide	1. Entrapment of smelter flue dust and shipment to ASARCO for arsenic trioxide recovery 2. Long-term storage
Cacodylic acid	1. Concrete storage vaults (currently contain 30,000 tons, or 27,200 tonnes, with 1–1.5% cacodylate) 2. Recycling and reuse 3. Landfill in class 1 sites
DSMA and MSMA	1. Recycling and reuse 2. Long-term storage 3. Landfill in class 1 sites
Calcium arsenate	Same as for DSMA
Lead arsenate	Same as for DSMA, plus recovery of metals by ASARCO
Copper acetoarsenite	Same as for DSMA, plus recovery of metals by ASARCO
Sodium arsenite	Same as for DSMA

empty bags, barrels, and bottles. On the basis of the studies that have been conducted, around 2–3% of some arsenical solutions is probably left in containers after use; this represents a considerable potential hazard, as far as the whole environment is concerned. In many areas of the United States, a comprehensive program is needed whereby empty containers can be decontaminated or disposed of in a manner that will not create a hazard to the environment.

THE ARSENIC CYCLE

Frost proposed a closed organic arsenic cycle for the total environment in which some form of arsenic is present in all phases of the ecosystem (Figure 3-2).[268] Very few of the organic arsenicals were identified, but a volatile arsine was suggested as present. Allaway presented overall pathways of environmental movement of trace elements, which included arsenic.[10] Wood also proposed a cycle of toxic-element movement through the "geocycle," with arsenic from natural weathering processes available later to microorganisms, plants, and animals.[871]

Sandberg and Allen proposed a model (Figure 3-3) for the arsenic cycle in an agronomic ecosystem.[701] Their model contained 12 possible

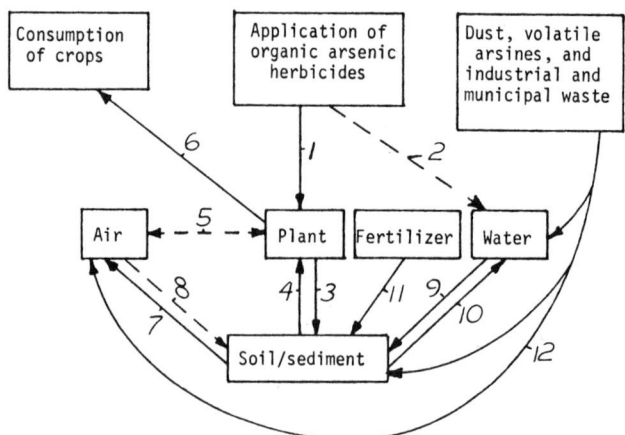

FIGURE 3-3. A proposed model for the arsenic cycle in an agronomic ecosystem. Reprinted with permission from Sandberg and Allen.[701] (Broken lines indicate minor or negligible transfers.)

transfers to and from a field for the organoarsenical herbicides. They concluded that transfers involving reduction to methylarsines, soil erosion, and crop uptake were the primary redistribution mechanisms in this model. Treatment with cacodylic acid resulted in a theoretical buildup of arsenic of 2.6–3.3 ppm/ha per year, whereas MSMA accumulated at only 1.5–1.9 ppm/ha per year. They concluded that "arsenic is mobile and nonaccumulative in the air, plant and water phases of the agronomic ecosystem. Arsenicals do accumulate in soil, but redistribution mechanisms preclude hazardous accumulations at a given site."[701] This model does not include the application of arsenic trioxide to desiccate cotton before harvest.

Inputs into the environment and a redistribution of arsenic in the terrestrial ecosystem are presented in Figure 3-4. Natural inputs are from volcanic action, decay of plant matter, and weathering of minerals within the soil, whereas man-made sources of arsenic are combustion of coal and oil, smelting of ores, and use of fertilizers and pesticides. The largest sink for man-made arsenic in the environment is the soil.

Onishi and Sandell calculated a balance between igneous rocks (arsenic content, 2 ppm) and sedimentary deposits (shale and sediments, 10 ppm; sandstone and limestone, 1.5 ppm).[603] They observed that, if the amounts of sediments equaled that of weathered rocks, then much of the arsenic in sediments must come from volcanism. At present, this input is small, and weathering of continental rocks is in approximate balance with oceanic sediment deposition. Using estimates of arsenic weathering (45,000 tons/year, or 41,000 tonnes/year) and deposition rates, Ferguson and Gavis concluded that "there is no substantial imbalance between natural weathering and deposition of arsenic at present."[249] The amount of arsenic from weathering transported to the oceans as part of the dissolved load of the rivers is 33,000 tons/year (30,000 tonnes/year). Arsenic from man-made sources is redistributed either through industrial processes, such as the burning of coal, or by the refining of oil for gasoline and fuel oil. Man's activity does cause high environmental concentrations at some locations.

Estimates are available for an arsenic balance at a coal-fired steam plant in Memphis, Tennessee.[85] The balance for most trace elements is satisfactory. Elements that can be present in a gaseous form (e.g., arsenic and mercury) are not completely recovered. Most arsenic recovered was in the precipitation inlet fly ash, but 52–64% of the arsenic in coal could not be found. It may have been lost in the gas stream. Coutant et al.[172a] found that "only a small percentage of arsenic is emitted from the stacks" and that it did not pose an important problem from an air-pollution standpoint. "Arsenic tended

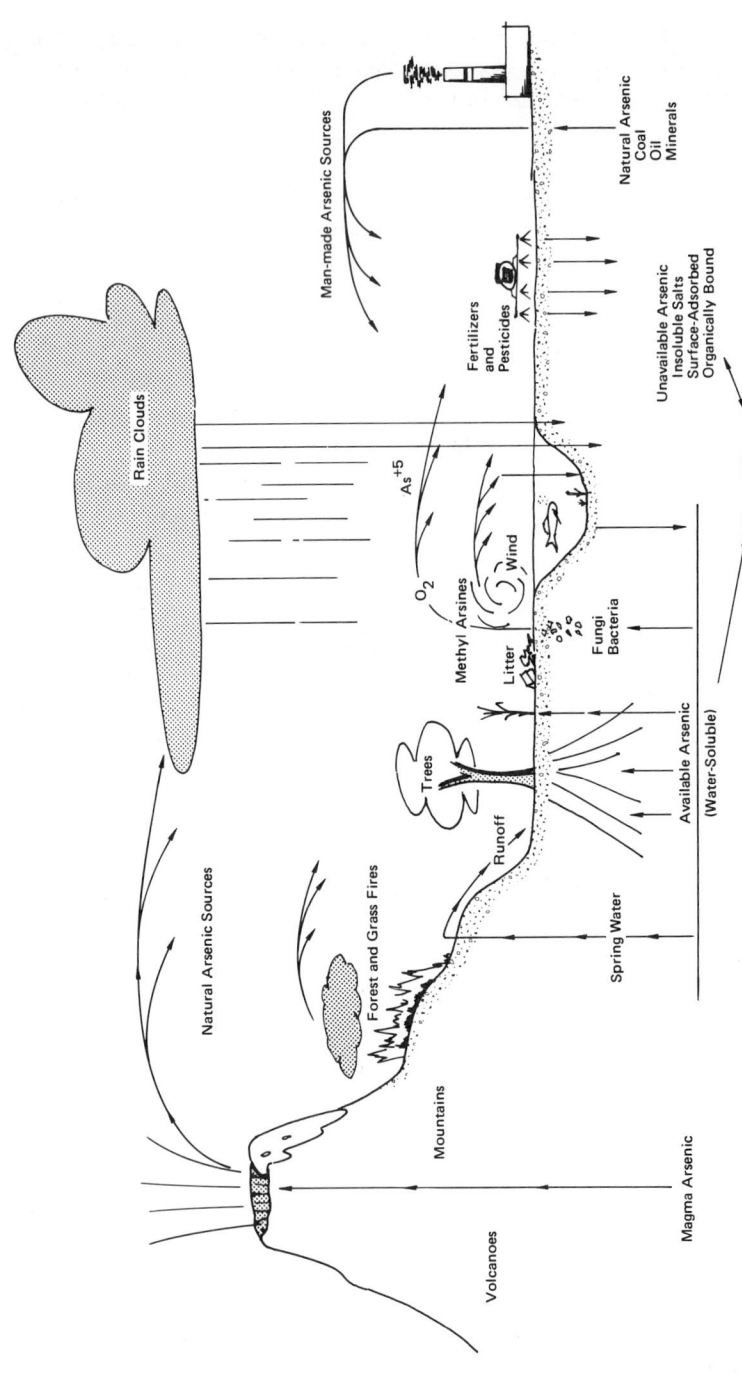

FIGURE 3-4 Environmental transfer of arsenic.

Distribution of Arsenic in the Environment 71

to be distributed continuously through the system as a function of temperature," and "there is a definite tendency for concentration of arsenic in the lower temperature deposits in the combustion system." As coal utilization increases, the amount of arsenic escaping to the environment will increase, unless proper control measures are used.

Smelter activities have traditionally introduced large amounts of arsenic into the environment. The copper smelter at Tacoma, Washington, has been examined for arsenic emission into the environment. Crecelius *et al.* reported that input amounts to 200,000 kg of arsenic trioxide per year into the air via stack dust, 20,000–70,000 kg of arsenic per year into Puget Sound through dissolved arsenicals in its liquid effluent discharge, and 1,500,000 kg of arsenic per year in crystalline slag dumped into the Sound.[186] The installation of more pollution-control equipment at this smelter is planned, so the amount of arsenic released into the air and water will decrease significantly.[186]

Information has been collected, to the extent available, to develop a pattern of arsenic emission into the environment. It included information on the arsenic associated with mineral raw materials and fuels, on the arsenic content of salable mineral products, on solid waste discarded by mineral processors, and on effluent from mineral plants. Complete material-balance reports were obtainable for only a few plants. However, considerable incomplete evidence was accumulated. These data were used to trace the disposition of arsenic—through mineral processing steps and consumption—in commodities containing significant quantities of arsenic. They were also used to determine the distribution of arsenic throughout commercial production and the disposition of arsenic used in agriculture and industry. Arsenic emission to the atmosphere was calculated with the factors listed in Table 3-19.

TABLE 3-19 Arsenic Emission Factors[a]

Arsenic Source	Arsenic Concentration
Mining and milling	0.45 tonne/million tonnes of copper, lead, zinc, silver, gold, or uranium ore
Smelting and refining	955 tonnes/million tonnes of copper produced
	591 tonnes/million tonnes of zinc produced
	364 tonnes/million tonnes of lead produced
Coal	1.4 tonnes/million tonnes of coal burned
Petroleum	5.2 kg/million barrels of petroleum

[a]Calculated on the basis of Davis and Associates[196] and *Minerals Yearbook 1968*.[812]

The principal source of atmospheric arsenic from manufacturing is the processing of nonferrous metals. Gualtieri classified 15% of copper and copper–lead–zinc ores as being arsenical and stated that they have an average arsenic : copper ratio of 1 : 50.[314] Analyses of nonferrous ores considered nonarsenical are not available. However, reference to mineralogic descriptions of other principal nonferrous mining districts indicates that arsenic minerals usually occur in trace quantities, are seldom visible in ore specimens picked at random, and have not caused serious pollution. It is apparent that the arsenic content of nonarsenical ores is less than one-tenth that of arsenical ores. Arsenic concentrations would be equivalent to 160 ppm in arsenical ore containing 0.8% copper and 12 ppm in nonarsenical ore containing 0.6% copper. The arsenic concentrations of rocks in the earth's crust are shown in Tables 3-1 and 3-2 as: granite, 1.5 ppm; other igneous, 2.0–3.0 ppm; limestone, 1.7 ppm; sandstone, 2.0 ppm; and shales and clays, 14.5 ppm. We may assume rock distribution in nonferrous-metal deposits as: granite, 25%; other igneous, 25%; limestone, 25%; sandstone, 15%; and shale, 10%. The average arsenic content of unmineralized rock in mining districts would then be over 3 ppm. The average arsenic content of waste moved in mining is estimated as the average of the values for ore and unmineralized material, or 81 ppm for arsenical districts and 7 ppm for nonarsenical districts.

An estimated 40% of the arsenic in copper or copper–lead–zinc ore is left in the concentrator tailings. Much of the arsenic can be allowed to enter the tailing or can be depressed into an iron sulfide tailing, provided that the arsenic mineral does not contain valuable metals. The tailing is deposited on the surface, and some will be blown away by the wind; however, this quantity should not exceed 1% of the annual output. Arsenic in gold and uranium mill tailings is subject to similar wind losses. Arsenic minerals in tailing dunes may eventually weather to water-soluble compounds that will probably be transported over short distances before reacting with iron, aluminum, calcium, and magnesium in the soil to form largely insoluble substances.

Most of the arsenic emitted to the atmosphere during nonferrous-metal production results from smelting. At the primary smelter, arsenic contained in the ores and concentrates becomes distributed among the metal product, slag, speiss (a heavy metallic mixture of iron and nonferrous arsenides), flue dust, and atmospheric emission. Arsenic in metal is removed by pyrometallurgic or electrolytic refining methods; the arsenic-containing residues are recirculated to the smelting furnaces. After recovery of by-products, primary furnace slag is discarded. Speiss is sent to smelters with facilities for processing high-arsenic ma-

Distribution of Arsenic in the Environment 73

terial. Flue dust contains much of the volatile arsenic that is expelled from the furnace melt and collected in the stack-gas cleaning system. Some finely divided arsenic escapes ordinary dust-precipitating units, but additional cooling and cleaning of the furnace gases, as is done before sulfuric acid recovery, should capture most of the finely divided material. Flue dust is ordinarily recirculated to the furnaces, some of it being removed, if necessary, to keep excessive arsenic from accumulating in the system. The high-arsenic flue dust usually contains considerable metal value and, like the speiss, is shipped to the smelter equipped for processing it. At this smelter, the flue dust and speiss are roasted with fluxes to remove as much arsenic as possible. The arsenic is refined to commercial-grade material, and the calcine is smelted for its metal content.

Atmospheric arsenic emission during smelting was estimated for 1968 conditions by Davis and Associates on the basis of material balances and sampling data obtained from industrial sources.[196] Average arsenic emission was estimated at 4.9 lb/ton (2.5 kg/tonne) of copper produced, 1.3 lb/ton (0.65 kg/tonne) of zinc, and 0.8 lb/ton (0.4 kg/tonne) of lead.

Information obtained in February 1974 showed that arsenic emission at smelters processing arsenical copper ores was much reduced from the 1968 emission and that the average arsenic emission from copper smelting was 2.1 lb/ton (1.05 kg/tonne) of metal. No new data on emission from zinc and lead smelters are available. However, some information was obtained on the arsenic content of ores and concentrates. On the basis of the indicated smelter inputs of arsenical and nonarsenical concentrates and estimated percentage stack losses for smelters treating various types of ore, the recovery factors were estimated. These estimates are similar to those determined by the Davis study for lead and zinc smelters.[196]

Arsenic is in all coal and may be associated with metal sulfides, clay minerals, or organic material in the coalbed. Using data developed by Abernethy,[2] Davis[196] estimated that U.S. coal contains arsenic at an average of 10 ppm in eastern fields, 5 ppm in midwestern fields, and 1 ppm in western fields. A small fraction of the arsenic in coal escapes dust-collecting equipment and reaches the atmosphere. Cuffe and Gerstle estimated the average arsenic discharge to the atmosphere from power plants at 0.000064 grains (0.004 mg) per standard cubic foot, with 1 lb (0.4536 kg) of coal being burned for each 160 scf of flue gas.[190] This is equivalent to 1.4 ppm of the coal burned. This factor should be applicable to industry-wide coal use, inasmuch as nearly all coal consumed is burned in plants with fly-ash control equipment.

TABLE 3-20 Estimated Industrial Materials Balance for Arsenic, 1968[a]

	Arsenic, tons[b]				
Item	Input	Atmospheric Emission	Solid Waste	Intermediate Product	Commercial Product
Coal consumption	4,300	800	3,500	0	0
Fuel-oil consumption	20	20	0	0	0
Nonferrous-metal production:					
Mining and milling	43,100	300	28,000	14,800[c]	0
Smelting and refining	14,800[c]	2,500	2,000	0	10,300[d]
Total	—	3,620	33,500	—	10,300[d]

[a] Calculated on the basis of Davis and Associates, 1968,[196] *Minerals Yearbook 1972*, and *Minerals in the U.S. Economy*, 1975.[811]
[b] To convert to tonnes, multiply values in table by 0.9072.
[c] Includes arsenic in imported concentrates and intermediate smelter products.
[d] From *Minerals in the U.S. Economy*, Bureau of Mines, 1975.[811]

Assuming 600 million tons (544 million tonnes) of coal burned per year in the United States, this would correspond to the emission of 840 tons (762 tonnes) of arsenic.[85]

The arsenic content of petroleum was investigated by Davis and Associates, who obtained analyses of 110 oils.[196] The average content was 0.042 ppm, or about 5.2 kg/million barrels. A future problem may arise from producing oil from shale. Oil from Colorado shale contained arsenic at 82 ppm. This arsenic, however, could be removed by contact with a mixture of nickel sulfide and molybdenum sulfide on alumina under reducing conditions.[572] All arsenic present was removed until there was 7.2% arsenic on the alumina; thereafter, arsenic was found in the effluent gases.

Inconsequential arsenic emission results from mining and processing of phosphate rock. The average arsenic content of mine run rock is estimated at 5.7 ppm; of washed rock, 12.0 ppm; and of discarded material, 2.6 ppm, on the basis of an analysis by Tremearne and Jacob[797] and production data shown in Bureau of Mines *Mineral Yearbooks*.[812] Total arsenic placed in waste impoundments would be about 200 tons (181 tonnes) annually, of which perhaps 1 ton (0.9 tonne) would be expected to enter the atmosphere through weathering. About 17% of phosphate rock is used for electric-furnace manufacture of elemental phosphorus. The total arsenic in the furnace feed is about 60 tons (54 tonnes), of which only a small proportion would reach the atmosphere.

Iron ore contains arsenic, but only insignificant quantities of it are emitted during iron and steel production. Boyle and Jonasson showed arsenic contents of hematite up to 160 ppm and of magnetite up to 3 ppm.[94] Arsenic occurs in part in the form of scorodite, a very stable arsenate of iron. In the blast furnace, the arsenic compounds are reduced to elemental arsenic, which combines with iron to form iron arsenide and dissolves in the metal; very little of the contained arsenic reaches the atmosphere. Table 3-20 shows an industrial balance for arsenic emission into the environment based on the estimated emission factors, the rate of consumption of mineral fuels, and the rate of production of nonferrous metals, including arsenic.

Carton[120] surveyed arsenic input and movement in the United States. He estimated a total movement of about 119,000 tons (108,000 tonnes) of arsenic per year (Table 3-21). He distinguished between arsenic that is found in end products and arsenic that is dissipated onto land, emitted in air and water, or destined for landfills. Of the 108,000 tonnes, most is fixed in products in which the arsenic is immobile or is

TABLE 3-21 Summary of U.S. Arsenic Flow, Dissipation, and Emission, 1974[a]

Location of Arsenic	Arsenic Flow, tons[b]	Ready Environmental Transport
End products:	26,438	
Steel	17,089	No
Cast iron	3,638	No
Other	5,711	No
Dissipation to land:	63,030	
Steel slag	39,690	Unknown
Pesticides	11,565	Yes
Copper leach liquor	9,702	Yes
Other	2,073	Yes
Airborne emission:	9,757	
Losses from copper-smelting	5,292	Yes
Pesticides	2,536	Yes
Coal	717	Yes
Other	1,212	Yes
Waterborne effluent:	165	
Phosphate detergents	121	Yes
Other	44	Yes
Landfill wastes:	19,691	
Copper flue dusts	10,584	No
Copper-smelting slag	3,748	No
Coal fly ash	1,984	No
Other	3,375	No

[a] Derived from Carton.[120]
[b] To convert to tonnes, multiply values in table by 0.9072.

deposited in landfills as waste material. The remainder is in a form that can move readily within the environment.

About half the mobile arsenic comes from the use of pesticides. That which is applied to land becomes predominantly fixed in insoluble compounds and is only minimally available for transport. Arsenic that is emitted into air or water is most mobile and of greatest concern to the general population surrounding the points of emission. It is the airborne arsenic trioxide residues that have been implicated in the arsenic–cancer question. This topic is discussed in Chapter 6.

Arsenic from man-made sources eventually reaches the soil. Processed arsenic is applied by way of pesticides and through natural contamination of fertilizer materials. Arsenic that is gaseous or is adsorbed onto particulate matter is removed from the atmosphere through fallout or in rain. It is deposited on vegetation, on soil, or in

Distribution of Arsenic in the Environment

water. Once in the water, arsenic can be accumulated to some extent by various forms of aquatic life. Arsenate in solution is adsorbed or incorporated into phytoplankton and algae, and an organic compound is synthesized. Fish, when they consume the algae, incorporate this organic arsenic compound. In some cases, the arsenical is further metabolized to yield high-molecular-weight lipid materials, proteins, or easily soluble low-molecular-weight compounds. The arsenical from aquatic life, when consumed, is generally eliminated with very little accumulation.[171]

Pesticidal arsenic that is deposited on the land may have several fates. A portion of methanearsonic acid and cacodylic acid may be reduced to volatile arsines (under both aerobic and anaerobic conditions), but the predominant degradation product is arsenate.[879] Under anaerobic conditions, these two compounds are reduced to volatile arsines. Arsenate and arsenite are also reduced or methylated to volatile arsines under some conditions.[175,499] Braman detected dimethylarsine and trimethylarsine or their oxidation products above grass that had been treated with sodium arsenite, methanearsonic acid, cacodylic acid, and phenylarsonic acid.[97] Volatile arsenicals were detected from soils treated with sodium arsenate, MSMA, and cacodylic acid. Volatilization occurred under both aerobic and anaerobic conditions. Amounts volatilized were 0.64, 8.22, and 14.10% of the applied arsenate, MSMA, and cacodylic acid, respectively, in 150 days under aerobic conditions. Under anaerobic conditions, the amounts produced from arsenate, MSMA, and cacodylic acid were 1.60, 0.84, and 4.48%, respectively. Regardless of initial form or oxidative condition, only dimethylarsine was detected.[875]

Arsenate, from pesticide or from fallout and runoff, is fixed in the soil as slightly soluble salts of iron, aluminum, calcium, and magnesium. These may be true compounds or surface-adsorbed reaction products. In addition, some arsenic is bound in organic forms in the soil. The arsenic that is not in an insoluble form is available for leaching into ground water, is available for uptake by plants and trees, and appears in spring water. As indicated earlier, all vegetation contains arsenic. Burning of agricultural wastes and forest and grass fires redistribute arsenic into the atmosphere, from which it is redeposited on the earth through particulate fallout or rain. Fungi and bacteria in the soil metabolize arsenic and the methylated derivatives to methylarsines. The methylarsines are unstable and are oxidized to As(V). Some of the reactions are shown in Table 3-22. These processes are mediated by microorganisms, as well as by chemical action. The faster reactions are the more environmentally important ones. The stable forms of

TABLE 3-22 Chemical and Biologic Transformation of Arsenicals in Soil[a]

Reactions and Changes	Relative Rate of Change	Products	Biologic Activity	Probability of Occurrence	Conditions for Occurrence	Further Possible Changes
1. Salt formation	High	Insoluble arsenic salts	Insoluble and inactive	Very high	Presence of iron, aluminum, calcium, and magnesium in soil	Formation of an arsenic analogue of fluoroapatite, an extremely insoluble complex mineral
2. Adsorption	High	Soil–arsenic complex	Fixed and inactive	High	Fine soil (colloidal and organic matter)	Formation of sediment in aquatic systems
3. Ion exchange	High	Soil–arsenic complex	Fixed and inactive	High	Soil with high exchange capacity	Exchange release by other salts to react further as 1 or 2
4. Demethylation	Low	Inorganic o-arsenic acid	Reacts as 1, 2, and 3	Low	Microorganisms for demethylation (aerobic)	Same as 1, 2, and 3
5. Reduction	Low	Arsines	Very active	Low	Aerobic and anaerobic conditions or specific microorganisms	React rapidly to form pentavalent arsenicals; then same as 1, 2, and 3
6. Oxidation[b]	Moderate	Pentavalent arsenicals	Reacts as 1, 2, and 3	High	Normal soil conditions (aerobic)	Same as 1, 2, and 3
7. Methylation	Low	Methylarsines	Very active	Low	Presence of specific bacterial microorganisms (anaerobic and aerobic)	React rapidly to form pentavalent arsenicals; then same as 1, 2, and 3

[a]Adapted from the Ansul Company report.[20]
[b]Refers to oxidation of arsenic from trivalent to pentavalent.

Distribution of Arsenic in the Environment

man-made arsenic in the environment are o-arsenic acid and its salts. All other forms of methylated arsenic compounds yield o-arsenic acid in soil as a major sink. This form, however, can be methylated and put back into the cycle in nature. Braman detected arsenic in the III, V, methanearsonic, and cacodylic forms in Florida water.[99] His samples could not have been contaminated by pesticide application, so these forms appear to be part of the natural cycle.

The most important concept with respect to arsenic cycling in the environment is constant change. Arsenic appears everywhere in every living tissue and is constantly being oxidized, reduced, or otherwise metabolized. In the soil environment, insoluble or slightly soluble compounds are constantly being resolubilized and the arsenic presented for plant uptake or reduction by organisms and chemical processes. Man has modified the arsenic cycle only by causing localized high concentrations.

4

Metabolism of Arsenic

PLANTS

Among the many chemical combinations in which arsenic may exist, some readily enter plants and translocate, some in the symplast and some in the apoplast (nonliving cell-wall phase).

Plants take up relatively small amounts of arsenic from soils in their natural state and exhibit no symptoms of arsenic injury. Around smelters, high-arsenic soils may be rendered completely sterile and bare of higher plants.

Natural waters are usually low in arsenic, and plants reflect this in their arsenic contents. However, some natural waters are very high in arsenic and may thus cause problems for plants (as well as animals).

Arsenic in the air in gaseous form has not been known to cause injury to plants. Particles from smelter fumes and smoke may settle out on plants; these may prove toxic to animals or to man, and they may harm plants through the soil.

Absorption of Arsenic Compounds

Arsenic rarely occurs naturally in the topsoil in quantities toxic to plants. Indeed, all soils contain some arsenic, and plants have evolved

Metabolism of Arsenic

in its presence. In outcroppings of ores high in arsenic, small areas may contain arsenic in toxic quantities. Arsenic uptake by plants is of concern principally around smelters, where arsenic trioxide dust has spread over large areas, rendering the topsoil sterile. With the introduction of modern methods of arsenic recovery, cases of soil sterilization by smelter dusts have practically disappeared. Sulfur dioxide, which often accompanies the arsenic trioxide in smelter effluent, has caused more widespread damage.

The uptake of inorganic arsenic by plants affects the arsenic cycle. The arsenic concentrates in leaves, which fall to the ground. It is returned to the surface of the soil—at least in some organic, pentavalent form—after the leaves decay. Arsenic is known to be fixed in soils.[837] Thus, what arsenic occurs in a mobile form is absorbed out of a deep soil profile, is deposited on the surface, is fixed to varying degrees, and, after oxidation, is subject to leaching by rainwater. Eventually, some of the arsenic originally present in the soil is returned by leaching and takes its original position in the soil and ground water. Some of it also moves in the ground water into springs and streams and is eventually carried into the ocean.

Studies of arsenic fixation in soils have indicated that arsenic absorbed by plants must be mainly in the soil solution. Thus, arsenic in water should be available for uptake by microorganisms, algae, and the roots of higher plants. Except for locations around smelters or where the natural arsenic content is unusually high, the arsenic taken up is distributed throughout the plant body in nontoxic amounts, e.g., arsenic trioxide below 0.02% (dry weight) of foliage or 0.0003% (dry weight) of roots in the case of bindweed[179] (see Appendix A). These values are very high, compared with those reported by Woolson for the arsenic contents of a wide variety of plants—0.03–0.5 ppm.

Natural arsenic absorption from the air is negligible. Smelter fumes and dusts may deposit on plant leaves, but there is no evidence that arsenic from this source is taken into plants. Sulfur dioxide in the atmosphere, and more recently constituents of smog, may have deleterious effects on plants, but not arsenic. Although arsenic may be present in volcanic emission and in some soils, it is rapidly oxidized in air to a particulate form that will not penetrate plant cuticle.

Translocation of Arsenic Compounds

The application of dilute sodium arsenite solution to bindweed foliage in 1917 resulted in the killing of root tissues and showed that it was possible for toxic compounds to be translocated in plants.[306]

Two vascular systems in plants are responsible for translocation: the xylem, which transports water and salts absorbed by roots from the soil to the top of a plant; and the phloem, which carries elaborated food materials from green to nongreen parts of the plant.

Under conditions of high transpiration, the rate of intake of water by roots, even from an abundant supply, may fall so far behind the rate of evaporation from leaves that a reduced or subatmospheric pressure is built up not only within the xylem conduits, but within all living cells. Under these conditions, if the xylem is cut or broken under a solution, the liquid will be forced into the conduits until the internal pressure equals that of the atmosphere. If the plant is growing in soil in which the moisture is below field capacity, solution will be forced into the cut stem and move throughout the roots, the liquid originally present in them moving osmotically back into the soil. This is a reversal of the normal flow of the transpiration stream. If a solution of a strong acid is applied to the leaves so that they die rapidly, the sap that the cells contain can be forced into the xylem and down into the roots. If arsenic in sufficient quantity is included in such a solution, it too will be injected into the roots, where its toxic action is expressed, and the roots will die. This is the mechanism responsible for translocation of arsenic in the acid–arsenical method.

When the tops of plants were cut off at the ground level under sodium arsenite solution, the roots were killed to depths of 7 ft (2.1 m) and even more. And if normal plants were sprayed with the acid–arsenical solution and resprayed with water often enough to keep the foliage wet for an hour, depth of penetration of the arsenic was increased. On the basis of the anatomy and physiology of bindweed plants and their distribution in soils, it was explained that the translocated acid–arsenical spray could not be used for eradication, because roots at the edges of infestations have available water and hence do not absorb arsenic solution.[179] The authors stressed the influence of temperature, incident radiation, humidity, and air velocity on evaporation from leaves. They recommended delaying application until after dark.

In years of deficient rainfall, when the soil is moistened to only 3 ft (0.9 m) or less, the acid–arsenical method is not effective for killing bindweed, because arsenic does not penetrate below the current season's roots, which are confined to the moist soil layer. The acid–arsenical method might prove useful in eliminating old deep-rooted perennial weeds before the application of a soil sterilization treatment.

Sodium arsenite, long used as a general contact herbicide, was not considered to be translocated, probably because, as a contact treatment, it was used at a concentration that rapidly destroyed the foliage.

This prevented food movement with which arsenic movement is associated. At lower concentrations, it was combined with acid to hasten penetration; this also rapidly killed the foliage. Rumberg et al.[693] compared DSMA at 100 mg/ml with sodium arsenite (4 parts arsenic trioxide to 3 parts sodium hydroxide) at 50 mg/ml; both DSMA and sodium arsenite were labeled with arsenic-76. With soybean plants, they found evidence of translocation of sodium arsenite, but the organic form of arsenic, DSMA, proved to be more mobile. Sodium arsenite injury appears first as loss of turgidity, indicating possible effects on membrane integrity, whereas the organic arsenicals usually cause slowly developing chlorosis with little or no wilting; different enzyme systems may be affected. Rumberg et al.[693] suggested that the rapid injury from sodium arsenite treatment may be responsible for the lesser transport; the arsenite usually produces injury symptoms within a few hours of treatment, whereas DSMA requires many hours or even days to produce chlorosis.

Cacodylic acid is considered to be a general contact toxicant. It is applied in solution to cuts around the base of trees or on foliage. Apparently, its only translocation is apoplastic. DSMA and dodecyl (octyl)ammonium methanearsonate (amine methanearsonate, AMA—equal parts of tetraoctylammonium and tetradodecylammonium methanearsonates) were both shown by Long and Holt to be effective for controlling purple nutsedge *(Cyperus rotundus)* in Bermuda grass *(Cynodon dactylon)* turf.[483] This result can be explained only by translocation from foliage to tubers, a movement that occurs via the phloem. In a later paper, Long, Allen, and Holt showed that those organic arsenicals kill nutsedge tubers if they are applied several times over a 2-year period.[482] Long and Holt[483] showed amine methanearsonate to be somewhat superior to DSMA at equivalent rates of application—a result that seems logical in view of the mechanism of herbicide activation described by Crafts and Reiber.[180]

In further studies on purple nutsedge, Holt et al.,[366] using single and repeated applications of amine methanearsonate to shoots of single tubers and shoots of terminal tubers on chains of tubers, found that arsenic was translocated laterally into tubers separated from the treated shoots by up to four tubers. The tuber at the opposite end of the chain from the treated shoots tended to have a higher arsenic content than the tubers between; translocated arsenic tended to be higher in tubers in which active growth was taking place. This is in accord with the source-to-sink nature of food movement; actively growing tubers are active sinks. There was no apparent relationship between the arsenic content of tubers and their ability to produce new shoots, and there was a tendency for tubers to produce more than one shoot in the regrowth after treatment. Evidently, arsenic treatment altered the apical dominance in tubers that received arsenic. The writers concluded that death of tubers after repeated treatments was due to depletion of food reserves, rather than to the concentration of arsenic in the tubers. The variability in arsenic content in killed tubers and the variability in the number of treatments required to kill tubers suggested that failure to sprout is not related to the overall arsenic content of the tuber; some viable tubers contained more arsenic than some dead ones. Interruption of normal oxidative phosphorylation and exhaustion of the food supply resulting from increased sprouting may also have been involved in the ultimate death of tubers. In the repeated-application tests, the arsenic content decreased in tubers from which new rhizomes, tubers, and shoots developed. This indicated retranslocation, a property common to phosphate, amitrole (3-amino-1,2,4-triazole), and dalapon (a sodium salt of 2,2-dichloropropionic acid) in plants. The high arsenic content of terminal tubers and the appearance of chlorosis in untreated shoots confirm this interpretation. Roots and newly developing shoots were not analyzed, and these might account for the loss of arsenic after the initial influx into a sprouting tuber.

Translocation of the methanearsonates is indicated in many field studies. For example, Johnsongrass greenhouse studies by Sckerl et al.[719] showed rhizome deterioration when 12-in. (30.5-cm) plants were sprayed with DSMA. Kempen et al.[419] showed that a single 6-lb/acre (6.7-kg/ha) treatment gave better rhizome and regrowth control than 3 lb/acre (3.4 kg/ha). However, McWhorter found no evidence of rhizome deterioration in his many trials; he ascribed control to top-kill only.[535]

On *Paspalum conjugatum* (sourgrass), Headford suggested that failure of sequential treatments of DSMA to give good results may have been due to relatively inferior transport to the shoot apices.[340] On purple nutsedge, Holt et al.[366] showed arsenic accumulation in tubers after foliar sprays. On hardstem bulrush, Hempen indicated that rhizomes showed symptoms.[418] Lange's trials on deciduous trees indicated translocation, in that symptoms appeared in new growth and in untreated growth on the trees (personal communication, 1968). Studies on cotton by Ehman and Baket et al. indicated that arsenic derived from methanearsonates applied to the foliage may ultimately be present in cottonseed.[46,229]

Rumberg et al. did comparative translocation studies with [^{76}As] DSMA and [^{76}As]sodium arsenite on soybean at 85 F (29.4 C) and found translocation to be greater with DSMA.[693] But he was able to recover only 30–40% of the radioactivity from the DSMA in the foliage, whereas 85% of the arsenite was recovered. He assumed that the DSMA not recovered may have gone into the roots, which he did not measure.

With crabgrass, Rumberg et al.[693] found translocation and toxicity with DSMA greater at 85 F (29.4 C) than at 60 F (15.6 C) on crabgrass and soybean; on the latter plant, movement was more basipetal (to the basal stem) than acropetal (to the opposite primary leaf and trifoliate leaf). The toxicity of sodium arsenite and cacodylic acid was not affected by the temperature difference.

Sckerl and Frans indicated that [^{14}C]methanearsonic acid ([^{14}C]MAA) was absorbed by Johnsongrass roots in significant amounts in 1 h and moved throughout the plant in 8 h.[717] Spot applications of the acid formulation to foliage resulted in acropetal movement within 8 h and movement throughout the plant within 24 h.

Duble et al. studied the translocation of two organic arsenicals in purple nutsedge.[216] DSMA and AMA were the forms used, and tracers containing carbon-14 were applied to greenhouse plants. Chromatographic tests on extracts from [^{14}C]DSMA-treated plants indicated that the compound was not readily degraded; the ^{14}C–As bond appeared to remain intact, although some [^{14}C]carbon dioxide was found several days after treatment. Comparison of the retardation factors (R_f) of plant extract–DSMA with that of standard [^{14}C]DSMA suggested that a plant extract–DSMA conjugate might have been formed; the values for extract and standard solution were 0.59 and 0.66, respectively; only one spot was found in each case. Over 85% of the material applied to the plant remained in the treated shoots. DSMA moved both acropetally and basipetally in single leaves, and such movement was not influenced by relative age of the leaf. The writers reported that both DSMA and AMA are moved symplastically and apoplastically—a property that they share with amitrole. Carbon-14 distribution in an untreated shoot appeared to be very similar to that reported by Andersen[15] for amitrole distribution in the same plant.

It seems apparent from those results that translocation in nutsedge follows a source-to-sink pattern and that the amount of arsenic moved into a tuber depends very much on the sink activity of that tuber. Duble et al. found that actively growing terminal tubers in a chain accumulated arsenic, whereas intermediate and dormant tubers did not.[216] Thus, the arsenic content of a tuber may not serve as an index of the lethality of a treatment; the effects of the initial impact of arsenic on later growth activity may be the critical factor in lethality and continuing transport of arsenic to growing roots. Other tubers and shoots may mask the effects of the arsenic content, as determined by analysis at any time.

McWhorter found no evidence of translocation of DSMA in Johnsongrass in field and greenhouse tests.[535] Sckerl and Frans, by contrast, found that [^{14}C]MAA was both xylem- and phloem-mobile in Johnsongrass and cotton.[718] Root uptake of this labeled arsenical by Johnsongrass from nutrient solution was rapid, and translocation into all portions of the plant took place within 4 h. Apoplastic movement in both plants was more rapid than symplastic movement; symplastic movement was more rapid in Johnsongrass than in cotton.[716] As Duble et al. found, chromatography of extracts from Johnsongrass revealed values that differed from those of treated plants and standard [^{14}C]MAA solutions; Sckerl and Frans suggested complexing with sugars, organic acids, or both. When amino acid fractions were prepared from methanol extracts of both plants, an MAA metabolite with a positive ninhydrin reaction was found in the Johnsongrass fraction. Comparing R_f values, the authors suggested a complex with histidine or one of its analogues. Amino acid accumulation was noted in Johnsongrass as a result of MAA treatment, and the authors suggested that the MAA metabolite may block protein synthesis or some other biosynthetic pathway.

Wilkinson and Hardcastle produced radioactive arsenic (arsenic-76) by neutron activation and determined concentrations of this radioisotope in new (unsprayed) and old (MSMA-sprayed) cotton leaves and in the soil from beneath the plants; MSMA treatment rate was 2.24 kg/ha.[861] By using long counting periods, they were able to extend the lower limit of detection to 5 ng of arsenic. Table 4-1 presents the results

TABLE 4-1 Arsenic Content of Leaf and Soil Samples Taken from Field-Grown Cotton Treated with MSMA at 2.24 kg/ha[a]

	Arsenic Content, μg/g		
No. Treatments	New Leaves (Unsprayed)	Old Leaves (Sprayed)	Soil
0	0.05	0.17	3.75
1	0.13	0.45	8.25
2	0.95	1.05	8.35
3	0.23	0.90	7.50
4	3.15	17.30	10.15
5	4.80	41.10	4.00
6	10.30	30.25	11.20

[a] Derived from Wilkinson and Hardcastle.[861]

of the analyses. Differences in arsenic content of young untreated leaves from the two increments of MSMA application (i.e., one to three and four to six applications) may be due to dilution of arsenic content by continued growth. The increasing arsenic content in new unsprayed leaves also indicates the presence of translocatable arsenic from MSMA-treated leaves.

Kempen has made a study of MSMA in plants, principally Johnsongrass, using both detached leaves and whole plants.[417] He found that relatively high temperature, 35 C, and light, 2,800 ft-c (30,128 lx), produced 50% necrosis of rhizomatous Johnsongrass foliage in less than a day, whereas lower temperature, 15 C, and light, 320 ft-c (3,443.2 lx), required 12 days to give the same results. Regrowth from rhizomes showed similar trends, indicating that the arsenic had translocated into the rhizomes. Translocation of the label from leaf-applied [^{14}C]MSMA was primarily acropetal in the xylem, but small amounts also moved basipetally, proving that this organic arsenical is phloem-mobile. Within a week, the arsenic was transported from a treated mature leaf into the leaf base and sheath, to meristematic regions, and to roots and rhizomes; this indicates symplastic movement. Presence of the methanearsonate was detected by autoradiography and by counting.

Sachs and Michael found cacodylic acid and MSMA to be transported about equally from the leaves to the terminal buds and expanding leaves of bean plants.[695] There was no indication that either was demethylated or reduced to a trivalent compound. With [^{14}C]MSMA, Sachs and Michael found that about 40% of the carbon-14 and arsenic recovered was bound to another molecule to form a ninhydrin-positive complex.[695] Sckerl and Frans[718] reported this ninhydrin-positive complex, as well as a sugar complex, and postulated that such a complex may block a specific biosynthetic pathway and that this blockage may account for the herbicidal activity. Duble et al. noted that DSMA was almost completely complexed with some plant component and that the complex was the mobile form of the herbicide.[217] They also found that less than 0.1% of the carbon-14 applied as DSMA was metabolized and given off as volatile carbon-14 10 days after treatment. They concluded that the carbon–arsenic bond was stable in plants. However, von Endt et al.[827] found this carbon-arsenic bond to be rapidly broken in soils, which suggested that the bond is subject to attack by some biologic systems.

In studies with ^{14}C-labeled MSMA, MAA, and DSMA, Keeley and Thullen found little translocation of these herbicides from cotyledons to developing leaves of cotton seedlings.[414] An exception was noted where [^{14}C]MSMA was applied at 13 C; there was little contact injury of the treated cotyledons, and the terminal leaves were well labeled.

With the same three herbicides in studies on purple and yellow nutsedge, Keeley and Thullen found the yellow species to be more susceptible; the yellow species absorbed and translocated more of the ^{14}C-labeled tracers than did the purple.[413,415] In chromatography of plant extracts and standards, there was less than 5% variation; nutsedge plants did not readily metabolize these arsenicals in 72 h.

Surfactants have been found to increase the penetration and translocation of the organic arsenical herbicides. The principal manufacturer of the methanearsonates formulates mixtures containing tested surfactants. Apparently, anionic and nonionic surfactants are satisfactory with these materials.

A summary of the above discussion is presented in Table 4-2. In almost all cases, the arsenicals are translocated either upward or downward. The rate and direction of movement vary according to plant species and chemical. The degree of response may be temperature-dependent. A metabolite may be formed in susceptible species, but the formation is apparently not necessary for efficacy.

MICROORGANISMS

The sources of arsenic available to animals and man are natural[295] (such as water, plants, and animal tissue) and synthetic[527] (such as agricultural chemicals, industrial wastes, and drugs). The natural sources of arsenic are modified by bacteria, molds, and algae, and they will be discussed from this point of view.

Bacteria

It has recently been shown[527] that *Methanobacterium* (MoH strain) can reduce and methylate arsenate to dimethylarsine (cacodyl hydride). The medium must contain methylcobalamin as a methyl donor and adenosine triphosphate in a hydrogen atmosphere. The formation of the alkylarsine was detected by its odor and by aerating into 2 N nitric acid to oxidize it to cacodylic acid. With [^{14}CH$_3$]cobalamin and [^{74}As]sodium arsenite, a double-tagged compound was isolated whose ratio of [^{14}C]methyl to arsenic-74 was 2.0:1. When cacodylic acid was used as a substrate, the alkylarsine was formed without the need of a methyl donor. The presence of an excess of sodium arsenite inhibited the production of the alkylarsine, the reaction producing methanearsonic acid. The use of formal oxidation numbers for arsenic in Figure 3 of Wood's article[796] can be misleading, in that there is no actual change in the valence of arsenic, as explained by Zingaro.[892] It should be noted that dimethylarsine was not positively identified, because both cacodyl (tetramethyldiarsine) and cacodyl oxide, which have a strong garlic odor, could have been formed and would have the same methyl: arsenic ratio. The recent suggestion[796] that such a reaction in stream sediments could be hazardous to fish is without foundation; methylarsine decomposes to methanearsonic acid in the presence of oxygen,[658] and the latter compound is less toxic than sodium arsenite.

The necessity for an anaerobic atmosphere greatly limits the possibility of this reaction in soil. Such conditions may be present in the rumen of the cow, and there is evidence that both arsenate and arsenite can be methylated by rumen flora.

The reverse procedure, the demethylation of MSMA in soil, has been reported.[827] When [^{14}C]MSMA was added to loam, 1.7–10% of the compound was degraded, yielding [^{14}C]carbon dioxide and arsenates. This did not occur in soil sterilized by heat. A fungus and two actinomycetes isolated from the soil degraded 3, 13, and 9% of MSMA added to a substrate. The bacterial species similarly isolated degraded 20% of the MSMA to arsenate; this changes the arsenical to a more toxic form.

Fungi and Molds

As early as 1815, cases of arsenic poisoning were reported to have been caused by wallpaper containing such arsenic compounds as Scheele's green (cupric arsenite) and Schweinfurt green (copper acetoarsenite, Paris green). The mechanism was first thought to be the ingestion of particulate material from the paper; but, when poisoning occurred with fresh paper, that theory was abandoned. Gmelin (cited in Challenger *et al.*[139]) was the first to report that rooms where symptoms occurred had a garlic odor, and he ascribed it to a volatile arsenic compound produced by molds on damp arsenic-pigmented wallpaper. Numerous investigations attempting to identify the chemical nature of this volatile arsenical have been reviewed by Challenger,[135,136] whose own research established the chemical structure of the compound.

Gosio used pure cultures of bacteria and fungi on a potato medium and found that, although no bacteria produced a garlic odor, a mold, *Penicillium brevicaule* (formerly *Scopulariopsis brevicaulis*), was very active. He analyzed the gas formed and concluded that it was an alkyl

TABLE 4-2 Summary of Arsenical Herbicide Translocation

Compound Applied	Species	Trans-location	Mode of Movement[a]	Temp.-Dep.[b]	Metabo-lite[b]	Notes	Ref.
Arsenous acid	Soybean	Yes	X,P	NT	ND	Base added, ^{76}As	693
	Bindweed	Yes	X	Yes	ND	Acid added to force xylem movement, improves with low moisture	
	Crabgrass	ND	ND	NT	ND	ND	306
	Green beans	Yes	X,P	ND	ND	ND	693
MAA	Johnsongrass	Yes	X,P	ND	Yes	^{14}C throughout, 24 h	695
	Cotton	Yes	X,P	ND	No	^{14}C, 4 h	716–718
	Cotton seedlings	Yes	X	ND	No	Did not check roots	718
	Yellow nutsedge	Yes	X,P	ND	No	^{14}C	414
	Purple nutsedge	Yes	X,P	Yes	No	^{14}C in daughter plants	413
MSMA	Johnsongrass	Yes	X,P	Yes	ND	Control improves with high light	413
	Cotton	Yes	X,P	ND	ND	^{76}As	417
	Cotton seedlings	Yes	X	No	No	Did not check ^{14}C in roots	861
	Yellow nutsedge	Yes	X,P	Yes	No	^{14}C in daughter plants	414
	Purple nutsedge	Yes	X,P	Yes	No	^{14}C in daughter plants	413
	Green beans	Yes	X,P	ND	Yes	^{14}C	695

Herbicide	Plant					Comments	Ref
DSMA	Johnsongrass	Yes	P	ND	ND	Rhizome deterioration	719
		No	ND	NT	ND	Based on regrowth data	535
	Cotton	Yes	X	ND	ND	Based on total residues	46,229
	Cotton seedlings	Yes	X	No	No	Did not check ^{14}C in roots	414
	Yellow nutsedge	Yes	X,P	Yes	No	^{14}C in daughter plants	413
	Purple nutsedge	Yes	X,P	Yes	No	Repeat application; ^{14}C in daughter plants	216,366, 413,482, 483
	Soybean	Yes	X,P	Yes	ND	^{76}As	693
	Crabgrass	Yes	ND	Yes	ND	^{76}As	693
	Hilograss	No	ND	ND	ND	Poor transport to shoot apices	340
	Coastal Bermuda grass	Yes	X,P	ND	Yes	^{14}C	217
	Hardstem bulrush	Yes	P	ND	ND	Rhizome symptoms	418
AMA	Purple nutsedge	Yes	X,P	ND	No	^{14}C to shoots from tubers	216,366, 483
Cacodylic acid	Green beans	Yes	X,P	ND	No	^{14}C	695
	Crabgrass	ND	ND	NT	ND	^{76}As	693

[a] X = movement in xylem is apoplastic (i.e., upward); P = movement in phloem is basipetal (i.e., downward).
[b] NT = no trend; yes = increased movement or injury with increased temperature; no = decreased movement or injury with increased temperature; ND = no data.

arsine (actually, trimethylarsine, called Gosio gas).[300] Sodium cacodylate also produced garlic odor in cultures of *S. brevicaulis*[134] and *Monilia sitophila* Saccardo.[650]

In a series of studies begun in 1931, Challenger *et al.* identified the volatile substance produced from breadcrumb cultures of four strains of *S. brevicaulis* as trimethylarsine.[139] Bird *et al.* reported that trimethylarsine was produced from sodium arsenite, sodium methanearsonate, and sodium cacodylate.[77]

In 1932, Thom and Raper[784] isolated from soil several strains of fungi that were active in producing trimethylarsine, including strains of *Aspergillus, Fusarium,* and *Penicillia*. They also found that the strains were active with a wide variety of arsenicals used commercially and suggested that any arsenical could probably be acted on by fungi.

Several fungi isolated from sewage[174,175] can reduce arsenic compounds to trimethylarsine (TMA), as identified by gas chromatography and mass spectroscopy. *Candida humicola* was the only organism producing TMA from arsenate and arsenite. *C. humicola, Penicillium,* and *Gliocladium* produced TMA from arsonates.

It is apparent that a wide variety of fungi, particularly those found in soil, can methylate both organic and inorganic arsenic compounds to the highly volatile TMA, which could thereby be lost to the air. The environmental fate of TMA is unknown, because there have been no studies to place this process in the normal arsenic cycle; it may play an important role where arsenic concentrations are high as a result of the use of arsenical pesticides.

Algae

The review of Vinogradov[823] on marine organisms includes a table of the arsenic contents of the principal varieties of marine algae reported by workers from 1902 to 1948. The values vary from 0.1 to 95.0 ppm, without apparent relation between a species and its arsenic content. The marine algae had higher contents than freshwater species. This difference may be due to the lower concentration of arsenic in fresh water; it was found in New Zealand that algae grown in lakes fed by hot springs with arsenic contents as high as 0.1 ppm had arsenic concentrations between 20 and 1,450 ppm on a dry-matter basis.[448] These concentrations prevented the use of the dried algae for animal food, because the arsenic concentrations produced in edible organs were above tolerance.

The relationship between the water concentration and the uptake of arsenic by algae has been studied experimentally in aquariums containing several species of algae, fish, and soil. The addition of [^{74}As]sodium arsenite to such a system resulted in high concentrations of arsenic in all species of algae within 2 h. The arsenic was easily washed off with dilute hydrochloric acid and was considered to be loosely held on the surface, rather than absorbed into the tissues.[47]

Isensee et al.[383] studied the distribution of cacodylic acid and dimethylarsine in nontoxic concentrations in an ecosystem including algae, *Daphnia magna,* snails, and fish. They found (Tables 4-3 and 4-4) that the lower food-chain organisms, algae and *Daphnia,* accumulated more cacodylic acid and dimethylarsine than the snails and fish and that there was no buildup throughout the food chain. The gradual loss of cacodylic acid and dimethylarsine from the water phase of the ecosystem could be accounted for by the increasing mass of the growing algae. It was suggested that adsorption, and not biomagnification, was important in the distribution pattern, inasmuch as algae and *Daphnia* have larger surface : area ratios than snails and fish.

Lunde[498] has shown that absorption takes place when marine and fresh-water algae are grown in aquariums in the presence of trivalent and pentavalent inorganic arsenic. Algae of both marine and freshwater origin can synthesize both fat-soluble and water-soluble organic arsenic compounds, as shown in Table 4-5. It was suggested that algae

TABLE 4-3* Tissue Content (Ppm) of ^{14}C-Cacodylic Acid in Algae, *Daphnia,* Fish, and Snails after Various Exposure Times, Rates, and Treatments[a]

Treatment ppm[b]	Algae[c]	*Daphnia*[c]	Fish w *Daphnia*[d]	Fish w/o *Daphnia*[d]	Snails w algae[e]	Snails w/o algae[e]
0.1	4.5 (45)[f]	3.9 (39)	0.09 (0.9)	0.14 (1.4)	0.9 (9)	2.0 (20)
1.0	17.0 (17)	41.6 (42)	0.36 (0.4)	0.92 (0.9)	2.3 (2.3)	8.5 (68.5)†
10.0	71.4 (7)	254.0 (25)	6.71 (0.7)	11.20 (1.1)	7.3 (0.7)	68.3 (6.8)

[a] Average of 3 replications.
[b] Solution concentrations of ^{14}C-labeled cacodylic acid.
[c] Samples taken after two-day exposure.
[d] w *Daphnia*—fish placed in untreated solution containing CA-treated *Daphnia*. Without *Daphnia,* fish placed in CA-treated solution not containing *Daphnia*. All fish harvested after two days.
[e] w *Algae*—snails placed in untreated solution containing CA-treated algae. Without algae, snails placed in CA-treated solution not containing algae. All snails harvested after 7 days.
[f] Bioaccumulation ratios given in parentheses.

*Reprinted with permission from Isensee et al.[383]
† A typographic error in the original publication; should be 8.5 (8.5).

TABLE 4-4[*] Accumulation of ^{14}C-Labeled Cacodylic Acid and Dimethylarsine (Generated in Oxygen or Nitrogen) by Algae, Snails, *Daphnia*, and Fish

Treatment		Solution Concentration, ppb[a]		Algae	Snails[b]		*Daphnia*	Fish
		1 day	32 days		1st harvest	2nd harvest		
Cacodylic acid	BR[c]	10.6	6.1	1635 ± 358[d]	419 ± 21	110 ± 16	1658 ± 463	21 ± 6
	Ppm[a]			9.82 ± 1.18	2.60 ± 0.04	0.69 ± 0.13	16.40 ± 10.00	0.32 ± 0.07
Dimethylarsine (oxygen)	BR[c]	7.0	3.9	1605 ± 155	446 ± 21	176 ± 23	2175 ± 290	19 ± 7
	Ppm[a]			6.26 ± 0.60	1.74 ± 0.08	0.69 ± 0.09	10.35 ± 3.11	0.07 ± 0.02
Dimethylarsine (nitrogen)	BR[c]	7.0	4.7	1248 ± 140	299 ± 12	129 ± 13	736 ± 104	49 ± 24
	Ppm[a]			5.92 ± 0.66	1.41 ± 0.06	0.61 ± 0.08	5.23 ± 0.68	0.17 ± 0.05

[a]Based on total ^{14}C activity, expressed as parent compound, at 32 days. Fish exposed for 3 days.
[b]First harvest, half of snails harvested at 32 days. Second harvest, half of snails placed in untreated solution and harvested 16 days later.
[c]Bioaccumulation (ratio) calculated by dividing cpm/mg tissue by cpm/mg of solution.
[d]Standard error of the mean for 2 replications.

[*]Reprinted with permission from Isensee *et al.*[383]

Metabolism of Arsenic

TABLE 4-5* Accumulation of Arsenic[a] in Algae as Arseno Organic Compounds in the Lipid Phase and in the Aqueous Phase, Respectively

	Culturing Media			
	Salt Water		Fresh Water	
	Lipid Phase	Aqueous Phase	Lipid Phase	Aqueous Phase
Phaeodactylum tricornutum	2900	2000	2800	1800
Chlorella ovalis	1600	1300		
Chlorella pyrenoidosa			400	190
Oscillatoria rubescens			540	240
Skeletonema costatum	1100	710		

[a]The calculation is based on the ratio between organic bound As-74 in the lipid phase and inorganic As-74 in the medium, and correspondingly in the aqueous phase and in the medium.

*Reprinted with permission from Lunde.[498]

are an important source of the organic arsenic compounds found in organisms higher in the food chain.

The total arsenic in seaweed collected from the fjords of Norway, where there is minimal pollution, varies with the species from 0.15 to 109 ppm on a dry-matter basis,[495] as shown in Tables 4-6 and 4-7. If the oil from seaweed is saponified, the major part of the arsenic is found in the unsaponified lipid, rather than in the fatty-acid fraction, as shown in Table 4-8.[491]

TABLE 4-6 Arsenic in Seaweed (Reine in Lofoten)[a]

Sample and Location	Date of Collection	Ash, % of dry matter	Arsenic Content, ppm
Pelvetia canaliculata, Reine	March 1951	23.6	22
Pelvetia canaliculata, Reine	June 1951	17.6	21
Fucus serratus, Reine	March 1951	27.6	47
Fucus serratus, Reine	June 1951	23.8	40
Fucus spiralis, Reine	March 1951	25.3	34
Fucus spiralis, Reine	June 1951	21.6	26
Fucus vesiculosus, ovre Reine	March 1951	23.2	65
Fucus vesiculosus, ovre Reine	June 1951	20.6	26
Laminaria digitata lamina, Reine	April 1952	36.2	73

[a]Derived from Lunde.[495]

TABLE 4-7 Arsenic in Seaweed (Trondheimsfjord)[a]

Sample and Location	Date of Collection	Ash, % of dry matter	Arsenic, Content, ppm
Laminaria digitata lamina, Munkholmen	October 1956	27.6	109
Laminaria digitata lamina, Flakk	April 1957	38.0	107
Laminaria hyperborea lamina, Munkholmen	February 1957	37.0	69
Laminaria hyperborea lamina, Munkholmen	January 1962	36.9	55
Laminaria hyperborea stipes, Munkholmen	June 1957	36.8	94
Ascophyllum modosum, Flakk	September 1968	19.9	22
Gigartina mamillosa, Flakk	April 1952	30.5	10
Rhodymenia palmata, Flakk	March 1952	31.5	13
Fucus vesiculosus, Flakk	March 1952	20.0	39
Fucus vesiculosus, Flakk	September 1968	17.9	24
Fucus serratus, Flakk	September 1968	21.9	28
Fucus spiralis, Flakk	September 1968	24.8	15
Pelvetia canaliculata, Flakk	September 1968	23.7	15

[a]Derived from Lunde.[495]

Plankton

The term "plankton" includes both phytoplankton and zooplankton. Both are primary sources of food for marine and freshwater animals and are the starting point for the biologic phase of the recycling of arsenic. In spite of its primary importance, there is little specific information about the metabolism of arsenic by marine or freshwater plankton.

In 1942, Ellis *et al.*,[233] who were interested in the source of arsenic in the oil of fresh-water fish, analyzed the zooplankton of a pond and found that the ether-extracted remainders contained arsenic at 3.0–51 ppm, and the oil fraction, 4.0–25.7 ppm. Dupree,[223] in 1960, treated ponds with sufficient sodium arsenite to give a water concentration of 4.2 ppm. This concentration decreased slowly, to 2.0 ppm at 30 days and 0.2–1.7 ppm at 78 days. The arsenic in the plankton rose from an initial value of 5.9–10.6 ppm to a peak of 6,955 ppm at 27 days and then fell to 2,172 ppm at 78 days. Ball and Hooper[47] used sufficient [^{74}As]sodium arsenite on a pond and in aquariums to be able to follow

TABLE 4-8 Arsenic in Oil and Fatty Acids
Extracted from Seaweed[a]

Sample[b]	Arsenic Content, ppm	
	Oil	Fatty acid
Laminaria digitata	221	36
Laminaria saccharina	155	7.5
Laminaria hyperborea	197	16
Ascophyllum nodosum (1968)	7.8	5.2
Ascophyllum nodosum (1969)	49	21
Fucus vesiculosus	35	5.1
Fucus serratus	27	6.1
Fucus spiralis	5.7	5.0
Pelvetia canaliculata	10.8	7.3

[a]Derived from Lunde.[495]
[b]Samples collected off the west coast of Norway.

its concentration in a complete ecosystem of fish, water plants, plankton, and soil over an extended period. The initial water concentration, 200 pCi/ml, declined at an exponential rate to 50 pCi/ml during a 60-day period. The bottom soil concentration increased during this period from 0 to 1,900 pCi/g. The plants reached 1,100 pCi/g in 2 h. Leaves that dropped off early in the death of the plants retained their shape, but showed counts as high as 15,000 pCi/g. The low-arsenic tissue was probably lost early, leaving tissue having the highest retentivity for arsenic. The early rapid uptake by the leaves at a time when the soil concentration was low indicates that the leaves, not the roots, are the primary path of arsenic uptake. The plant chara was not killed, but did accumulate high concentrations of arsenic. Phytoplankton were reduced by 50% in a day and recovered slowly over 4 days. Zooplankton were greatly reduced and recovered even more slowly. The fish showed little or no radioactivity, indicating that they take up arsenic from the water not directly, but mainly from arsenic-containing food.

These results indicate that water plants take up arsenic from the water rapidly and that, when they die, their arsenic is recycled, except for that eaten by animals. It would be interesting to determine the chemical composition of the arsenic compounds involved at each step of this ecosystem.

MOLLUSKS AND CRUSTACEANS

There are no reliable data on the arsenic content of freshwater mollusks and crustaceans, but it is generally considered to be much lower (by a factor of 10) than that in marine species, as stated by Vinogradov.[823]

It is interesting to compare the work reported between 1919 and 1933, as compiled by Vinogradov in Table 4-9, and later work of Costa and Da Fonseca,[167] Del Vecchio et al.,[202] Coulson et al.,[171] and Lunde,[492] as shown in Table 4-10. Although there are wide variations between studies and within the same species in a single series, there is no evidence of a trend in arsenic concentration with time, nor are there significant geographic differences.

The arsenic compounds present in mollusks and crustaceans have never been characterized chemically, but studies in which shrimp were fed to rats and humans clearly indicated that the compounds are less toxic than arsenic trioxide and, although absorbed from the gastrointestinal tract, rapidly excreted in the urine in both rats and humans. Coulson et al.[171] were probably correct in postulating that the arsenic was found in a complex organic molecule, whose characteristics deserve study by modern biochemical methods. Concern over the high arsenic content of seafood makes such study imperative.

TABLE 4-9 Arsenic in Shelled Mollusks[a]

Organism	Arsenic Concentration, ppm (wet wt)	Reference	Date
Oyster	4.1	143	1926
Oyster	3.7	176	1925
Oyster	2.0	853	1933
Oyster	1.1	356	1919
Oyster	34.0	143	1926
Mussel	68.0	143	1926
Cockle	19.0	143	1926
Whelk	18.0	143	1926
Sea snail	21.0	143	1926
Land snail	0.3	143	1926
Softshell clam	2.0	853	1933

[a] Data from Vinogradov.[823]

TABLE 4-10 Arsenic in Mollusks and Crustaceans

Organism	Arsenic Concentration, ppm (wet wt)	Reference and Date	Location
Gulf shrimp	1.94	171, 1935	Texas
Bay shrimp	2.44	171, 1935	Texas
Bay shrimp	15.10	171, 1935	Georgia
Bay shrimp	9.10	171, 1935	Georgia
Bay shrimp	1.27	171, 1935	Alabama
Bay shrimp	18.80	171, 1935	Louisiana
Bay shrimp	3.83	171, 1935	S. Carolina
Deep-sea shrimp	17.30	171, 1935	S. Carolina
Deep-sea shrimp	36.60	171, 1935	S. Carolina
Deep-sea shrimp	41.60	171, 1935	S. Carolina
Deep-sea shrimp	5.94	171, 1935	S. Carolina
Deep-sea shrimp	15.40	171, 1935	S. Carolina
Deep-sea shrimp	30.70	171, 1935	S. Carolina
Cockle	3.7–6.6	167, 1967	Portugal
Cockle	1.3–2.4	167, 1967	Portugal
Sea snail	3.6–63	167, 1967	Portugal
Rockshell	14.6–26.4	167, 1967	Portugal
Rockshell	1.8–3.7	167, 1967	Portugal
Cuttlefish	6.2–11.5	167, 1967	Portugal
Mussel	0.7–2.8	167, 1967	Portugal
Oyster	1.2–3.6	167, 1967	Portugal
Octopus	2.6–40.3	167, 1967	Portugal
Shrimp	4.4–19.6	167, 1967	Portugal
Shrimp	1.3–38.2	167, 1967	Portugal
Crab	2.7–7.0	167, 1967	Portugal
Crab	2.1–33.4	167, 1967	Portugal
Lobster	12.0–54.5	167, 1967	Portugal
Lobster	7.9–19.4	167, 1967	Portugal
Lobster	10.8–17.2	167, 1967	Portugal
Mussel	3.0–3.3	202, 1962	Fiume, Italy
Mussel	2.6–2.9	202, 1962	Civitavecchia, Italy
Mussel	3.5–3.7	202, 1962	Taranto, Italy
Lobster	2.2	492, 1970	Norway
Mussel	8.0	492, 1970	Norway
Clam	11.6	492, 1970	Norway
Oyster	7.6	492, 1970	Norway
Squid	6.5	492, 1970	Norway

FISH

The presence of relatively high arsenic concentrations in marine fish has been known since 1875, and commissions were set up in England and Sweden in 1900 to study reported cases of arsenic poisoning due to the eating of fish. Vinogradov[823] summarized the early reports and included data on both marine and freshwater species. There was no clear difference between marine and freshwater species, with respect to arsenic concentration in the entire fish—it varied between 0.2 and 3.6 ppm. However, the arsenic content of the liver oils was much higher in freshwater than in marine fish. Ellis et al.[233] analyzed 15 species of freshwater fish and found that the arsenic concentration of the whole fish varied from 0.30 to 1.3 ppm, whereas that of the liver oils was 0.9–101.0 ppm. He attributed these concentrations to the arsenic in the diet of these fish, inasmuch as he found that the livers of amphipods, isopods, and crustaceans had total arsenic concentrations of 3.0–5.0 ppm and arsenic at 4.5–26.0 ppm in their oils. Lovern[486] had shown that the oil of freshwater fish had a composition that resembled the lipid fraction of the zooplankton on which the fish fed.

Sadolin[697] in 1928 found total arsenic concentrations in codfish and herring of 1.3 and 0.4–0.8 ppm, respectively. He found liver to have a higher arsenic concentration than muscle, owing to its larger oil content. The oil that had an arsenic content of 3.0–4.0 ppm was studied extensively by him, but he was unable to isolate the compound to which the arsenic was bound.

Although fish-oil concentrations are high, most of the total arsenic in fish is in the muscle. Lunde[492] has studied the water extract (N-liquor) and pressed cake of fish muscle and found that the water fraction had most of the arsenic and selenium (Table 4-11). Attempts to fractionate the N-liquor with Sephadex did not yield conclusive results, but indicated that more than one organic arsenic compound was present with a molecular weight below 5,000. He had previously shown that the arsenic was tightly bound and did not exchange with either [^{74}As]arsenate or [^{74}As]arsenite.[500]

Lunde[491] has attempted to isolate the lipid fraction containing the lipid-soluble organic arsenic compound in the oil of fish and other marine animals. He found that there are two types of compounds, an arsenic-containing acid that follows the fatty acids during saponification and a type that is converted to a water-soluble compound by this process. More recently, Lunde[496] has analyzed fish from various seas around Norway for organic and inorganic arsenic. He distilled the

TABLE 4-11 Arsenic and Selenium in Dehydrated Raw Material and N-Liquor of Marine Organisms

Sample	Raw Material		N-Liquor	
	Arsenic, ppm	Selenium, ppm	Arsenic, ppm	Selenium, ppm
Cod fillet	2.2	1.2	13	2.6
Cod bone	0.9	0.7	11	1.6
Cod liver	9.8	3.7	37	4.6
Cod skin	3.5	8.6	6.1	1.4
Herring fillet	3.8	1.0	24	2.4
Herring bone	1.9	0.8	n.d.	n.d.
Herring skin	7.2	0.8	n.d.	n.d.
Mackerel fillet (mature)	3.5	1.3	n.d.	2.9
Mackerel fillet (immature)	3.0	1.4	17	3.9
Norway haddock fillet	3.3	1.5	23	4.5
Lobster fillet	5.3	1.5	14	2.9
Mussel	8.0	3.9	9.7	1.1
Clam	11.6	2.6	18	1.0
Oyster	7.6	n.d.	9.8	0.9
Squid	6.5	3.0	17	0.6
Whale meat	0.36	0.5	0.9	0.4

aDerived from Lunde.[492]
n.d. = no detectable amount.

inorganic arsenic from 6.6 N hydrochloric acid as arsenic trichloride and considered the remainder to be bound to organic molecules. He also recognized that the arsenic trichloride could in part have come from the breakdown of easily decomposed organic arsenic compounds. As shown in Table 4-12, most of the arsenic in marine fish is present in the organic form.

When freshwater ponds are treated with sodium arsenite to control water weeds, the arsenic concentrations in the water are reflected in the fish. Gilderhus[289] compared water and fish concentrations; the results are shown in Table 4-13.

BIRDS

The diet of birds, excluding predators, is composed of seeds, grass, fruit, and insects. The concentration of arsenic in the diet is quite low—around 0.1 ppm, according to Schroeder and Balassa.[709] With a

TABLE 4-12 Organic Bound and Inorganic Arsenic in Marine Samples[a]

Sample	Locality	Arsenic Concentration, ppm (dry wt)			By X-Ray Fluorescence
		By Neutron Activation			
		Inorganic[b]	Organic	Total	
Mackerel	Southern Norway	1.8	4.0	4.7	6
Mackerel	Southern Norway	1.1	8.9	9.2	5
Haddock	More	0.9	12.0	10.8	17
Cod	More	1.3	23.0	n.d.	20
Capelin	Northern Norway	1.3	10.9	6.1	7
Tunny	West of Slotteroy	1.2	8.4	n.d.	5
Coalfish	Trondelag	1.0	7.8	7.2	9
Herring	Western Norway	1.7	3.4	4.2	5
Herring	Western Norway	1.0	5.2	n.d.	7
Herring	Northern Norway	1.3	5.7	n.d.	4
Defatted enzyme hydrolyzed cod liver	Lofoten	1.4	53.6	56.6	59
Defatted enzyme hydrolyzed cod liver	Northern Norway	3.2	17.9	23	n.d.
Seaweed	Trondheimfjord	0.9	139	142	n.d.
Extract of herring	Western Norway	0.8	28.4	27	29
Extract of coalfish	Western Norway	0.7	35.6	37	37
Herring meal[c]	Western Norway	1.0	5.2	6.5	5
Herring meal	North Sea	1.3	5.7	6.9	4

[a] Derived from Lunde.[496]
[b] Includes organic bound arsenic degradable by 6.6 N hydrochloric acid.
[c] Factory-produced.
n.d. = not determined.

Metabolism of Arsenic

TABLE 4-13 Arsenic Residues in Water, Bottom Soils, and Fish from Pools Treated for 8 Weeks in 1962[a]

Pool	Arsenic Application Rate in Herbicide, ppm	Arsenic Residue after 8 Weeks, ppm		
		Water	Fish Flesh	Soil
1	2.31 yearly	1.01	0.38	92.1
2	0.69 yearly	0.056	0.35	37.3
3	0.23 yearly	0.024	1.02[b]	10.7
4	0.69 monthly	0.43	0.17	38.1
5	0.23 monthly	0.12	0.02	22.5
6	control	n.d.	n.d.	n.d.
7	0.69 weekly	4.81	3.88[b]	44.9
8	0.23 weekly	0.98	0.78[b]	36.7
9	0.023 weekly	0.12	0.09	6.5

[a]Derived from Gilderhus.[289]
[b]Small fish.
n.d. = no detectable amount.

method that determines organic (methanearsonate) and inorganic arsenic simultaneously, Lakso et al.[447] found both Johnsongrass and cottonseed to contain methanearsonic acid at 0.05–0.10 ppm and only traces of inorganic arsenic. The tissues and excreta of birds should reflect this intake, but no such studies have been made.

Quantitative studies have been made to determine the arsenic residues in birds that were fed growth-promoting drugs. In 1948, Ducoff[220] injected [^{76}As]sodium arsenite into chickens and other animals and found that it was excreted faster by the chicken than by any other animal. The chicken retained only 2% at 60 h, compared with 90% for the rat.

The chemical nature of the arsenic normally found in bird tissues is not known, but analyses of eggshells with the helium-arc method suggest that the high concentrations of methanearsonic acid and cacodylic acid present must have been derived from the bird's tissues (R. S. Braman, personal communication, 1974) (Table 4-14).

MAMMALS

Forms of Arsenic in the Diet and Water

Normally, the intake of arsenic from water is not significant, except in areas of abnormally high concentration, such as Fallon, Nevada, and

TABLE 4-14 Analysis of Various Samples for Methylarsenic Compounds[a]

Sample	Arsenic Concentration, ppb	
	Methanearsonic Acid	Cacodylic Acid
Chicken eggshell	1.3	4.8
Bobwhite eggshell[b,c]	7.3	14.3
Scrub jay eggshell[b]	1.7	7.9
	1.3	5.2
Seashell (unidentified)[d]	1,300	7,000
Phosphate rock (local source)	0.005	0.005

[a]Data from R. S. Braman (personal communication. Accuracy is within 10%.
[b]Eggshells collected at the Archbold Research Station, Florida.
[c]Phenlarsonic acid tentatively identified in this sample.
[d]Also contained As(III) at < 20 ppb and As(V) at 3,140 ppb.

Lane County, Oregon.[294] The arsenic compounds present presumably are pentavalent inorganic, but proof has not been reported. It would be interesting to determine the selenium : arsenic ratio in areas where the high arsenic concentrations appear to be innocuous to animals, because these elements are known antagonists.

Plants

Arsenic concentrations in plant foods are presented in Chapter 3 and Appendix A. The finding that the arsenic in Johnsongrass and cottonseed is almost entirely in the form of methanearsonate,[447] a compound of low toxicity, should be considered in evaluating the importance of arsenic derived from plant sources.

Animal Tissues

The work of Coulson et al.[171] was discussed earlier. "Shrimp arsenic" is probably an organic compound of low molecular weight that is easily absorbed and rapidly excreted by rats and humans. A compound with similar properties is found in the liver of swine that are fed arsanilic acid.[615] When the dried liver was fed to rats, 97% of the arsenic was excreted in 7 days, whereas only 30% of the equivalent amount of arsenic fed as arsenic trioxide was excreted in the same time.

Metabolism of Arsenic

The normal sources of arsenic available to man and animals are probably complex organic molecules, whose nature offers a necessary and interesting field of research.

The abnormal sources of arsenic that can enter the diet from plants or animals include arsenical pesticides, such as lead arsenate, arsenic acid, and sodium arsenite.

Physiologic Aspects of Arsenic Absorption from the Gastrointestinal Tract

Compounds that enter the gastrointestinal tract are subjected to the action of bacteria and enzymes and, after absorption into the portal venous system, must pass through the liver before reaching the general circulation. This process could alter the chemical form of such compounds before they reach other organs.

It has recently been shown that arsenates and arsenites are altered in cows and dogs.[446] After a control period, cows were fed sodium arsenate and potassium arsenite daily for 5 days and then fed the control diet for 7 days. Urine samples were collected twice a day and analyzed for inorganic arsenic and methanearsonates.[629] As shown in Figure 4-1, the concentrations were low in the control period, increased during the feeding of the arsenicals, and returned to normal within 5-7 days after return to control feed. It is clear that more than 50% of both the trivalent and pentavalent inorganic arsenic was methylated. Because the rumen is anaerobic and is a site of great bacterial activity, it was thought that the action was similar to that of methanobacteria. However, when the experiment was repeated on dogs (Figure 4-2), a similar degree of methylation occurred, which cast doubt on bacterial action as the sole mechanism. Inasmuch as the process results in a less toxic compound of arsenic, it is truly detoxifying. The rapid excretion of the relatively large doses of arsenic suggests that no substantial portion of the added arsenic is retained.

The mechanism of intestinal absorption of organic arsenicals in rats has been studied.[378] Solutions of carbarsone, tryparsamide, and sodium cacodylate were injected into isolated loops of small intestine in anesthetized rats, and the arsenic remaining in the loops was determined periodically. The results indicated that the process was simple diffusion and was not an active transport mechanism. The rate of diffusion was not related to the molecular size of those compounds, and, inasmuch as the compounds had a high trichloromethane : water ratio, they probably passed through the lipid portion of the cellular membranes.

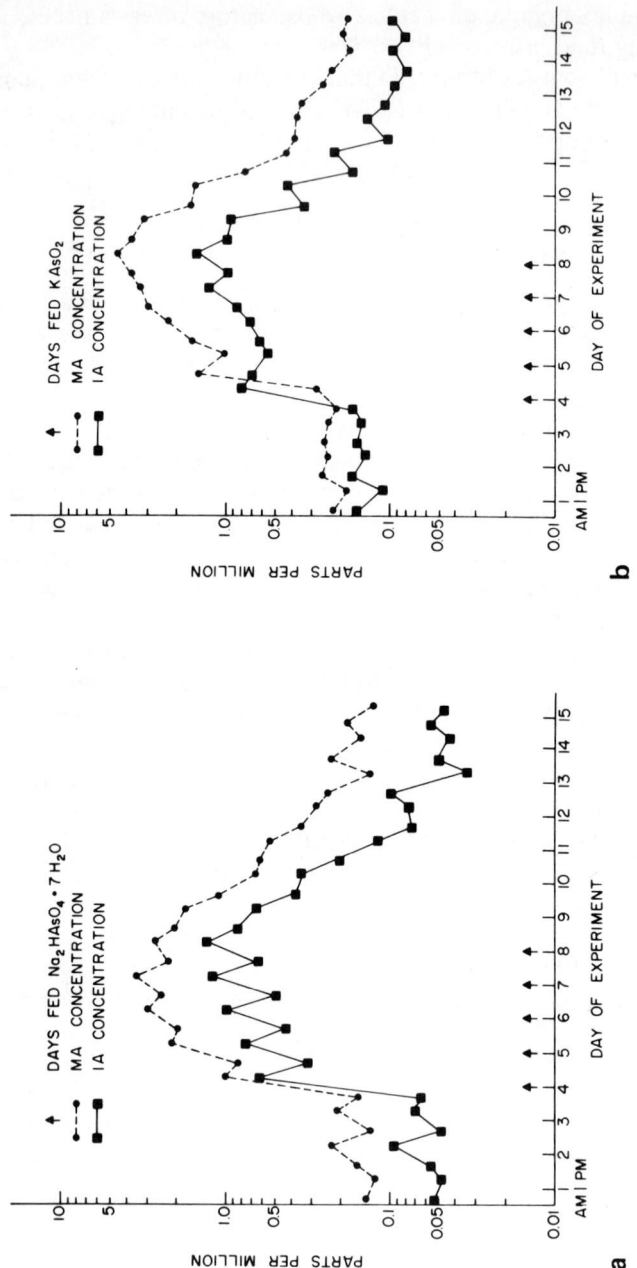

FIGURE 4-1 (a) Average concentrations of methanearsonic acid (MA) and inorganic arsenate (IA) in the urine of four cows fed sodium arsenate (2.75 mg/kg). (b) Average concentrations of methanearsonic acid (MA) and inorganic arsenate (IA) in the urine of four cows fed potassium arsenite (1.30 mg/kg). Reprinted with permission from Lakso and Peoples.[446]

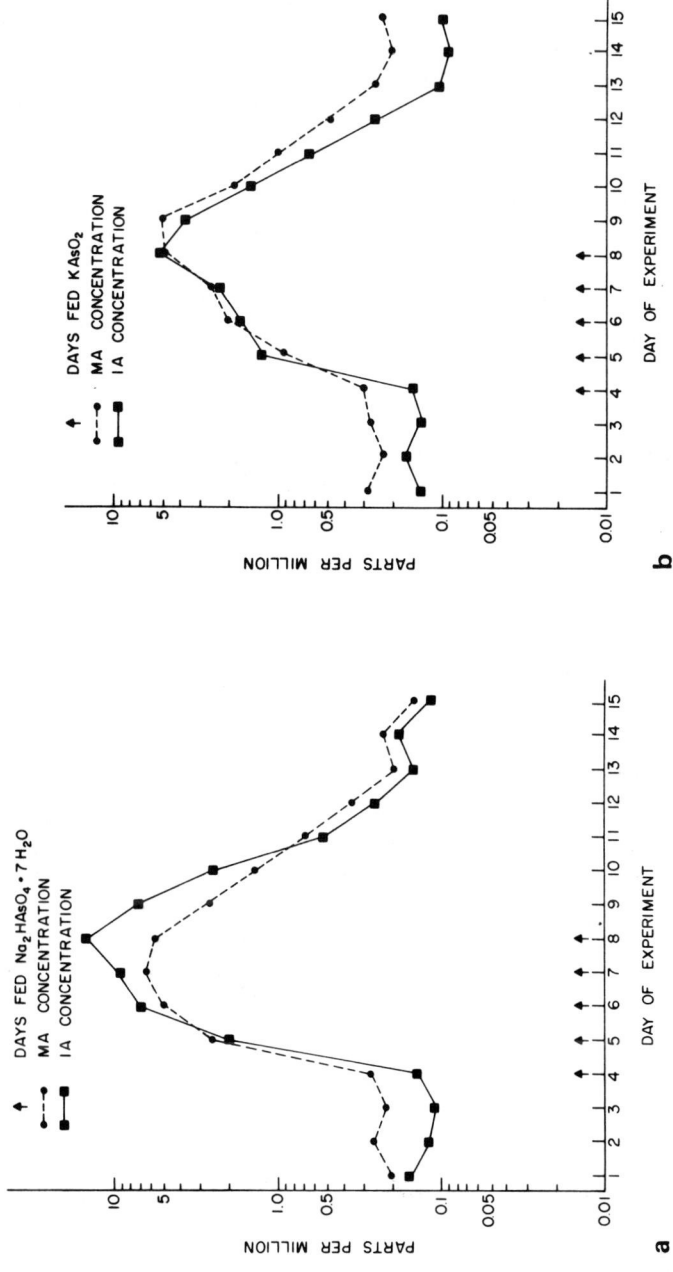

FIGURE 4-2 (a) Average concentrations of methanearsonic acid (MA) and inorganic arsenate (IA) in the urine of four dogs fed sodium arsenate (4.13 mg/kg). (b) Average concentrations of methanearsonic acid (MA) and inorganic arsenate (IA) in the urine of four dogs fed potassium arsenite (1.94 mg/kg). Reprinted with permission from Lakso and Peoples.[446]

Distribution of Arsenic in the Body

The most complete study of the distribution of arsenic in animals and man resulted from studies with radioactive isotopes of arsenic.

In 1942 Hunter et al.[376] injected [^{74}As]potassium arsenite subcutaneously into rats, guinea pigs, rabbits, chimpanzees, a baboon, and leukemic humans and analyzed their tissues and body fluids. With the exception of the rat, in which the arsenic concentrates in the red blood cells, the arsenic is generally distributed to all tissues, with the largest total amount going to the muscles. Most of the arsenic was excreted by the kidneys; excretion was essentially complete in 6 days, with only a trace appearing in the feces. Arsenic does not pass into the spinal fluid of humans, but small amounts were found in apes.

Lowry et al.[488] fractionated various tissues from this experiment and studied the acid-soluble lipid and protein fractions for arsenic and phosphorus content. They also separated liver protein into different fractions, including nucleoprotein. Most of the arsenic was in the protein fraction, a small amount in the acid-soluble portion, and a trace in the lipid fraction. The nucleoproteins did not take up more arsenic than other proteins, and there was no evidence that phosphorus was displaced by arsenic in tissues.

Ducoff et al.[220] used [^{76}As]sodium arsenite on rats, rabbits, mice, and man, studying their excretion rates and tissue distribution patterns. The rat retained most of the arsenic in the red blood cells, with smaller concentrations in the spleen, heart, lungs, kidneys, and liver. In rabbits, the arsenic was lowest in the blood and highest in liver, kidneys, and lungs. The most interesting results are shown in Figures 4-3 and 4-4, which compare the relative excretion rates in rat, man, and rabbit and the blood concentrations of arsenic in rat, man, rabbit, and chicken.

Lanz et al.[452] studied the absorption, distribution, and excretion of arsenic-74 injected intramuscularly in the rat, dog, cat, chick, guinea pig, and rabbit. The accumulation of arsenic in the tissues after 48 h showed that less than 0.27% was stored in the organs studied in all species except the rat and cat, which stored 79% and 5.6%, respectively, in the blood. They studied the distribution of arsenic in rat blood and found that none was bound in the plasma proteins, a trace in cellular "ghosts," and most of it in hemoglobin from which it could not be removed by dialysis. Arsenic was rapidly excreted in the urine as inorganic compounds, with 10–15% of the arsenate being reduced to the trivalent form. Their analytic method required the precipitation of

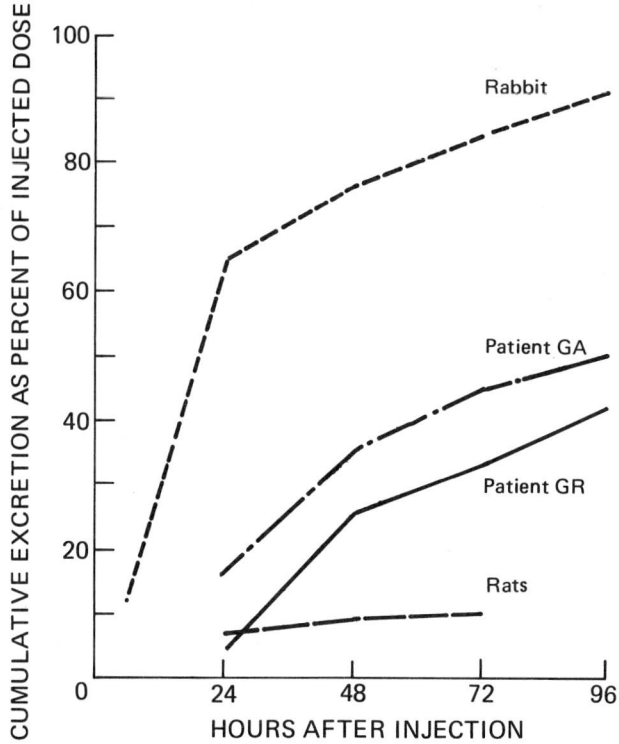

FIGURE 4-3 Excretion of arsenic-76. Cumulative excretion from the time of injection is expressed as percentage of the administered dose. Reprinted with permission from Ducoff et al.[220]

the arsenate as magnesium ammonium arsenate; the filtrate was assumed to be trivalent arsenic (which is highly questionable).

Mealey et al.[536] studied the distribution and turnover of radioactive arsenic after intravenous injection into man. The isotope used, arsenic-74, was 90% in the trivalent form and was given as the sodium salt in a dosage of 2.3 mCi/70 kg. The different rates of urinary excretion indicated that the arsenic was distributed into three compartments, as shown in Figure 4-5. Clearance rates for each were calculated as the percentage of the total dose per hour, giving 25%/h for compartment I, 2.5%/h for II, and 0.3%/h for III. The proportion of pentavalent arsenic in the urine showed a steady increase until the fourth day, when it remained constant at 75%.

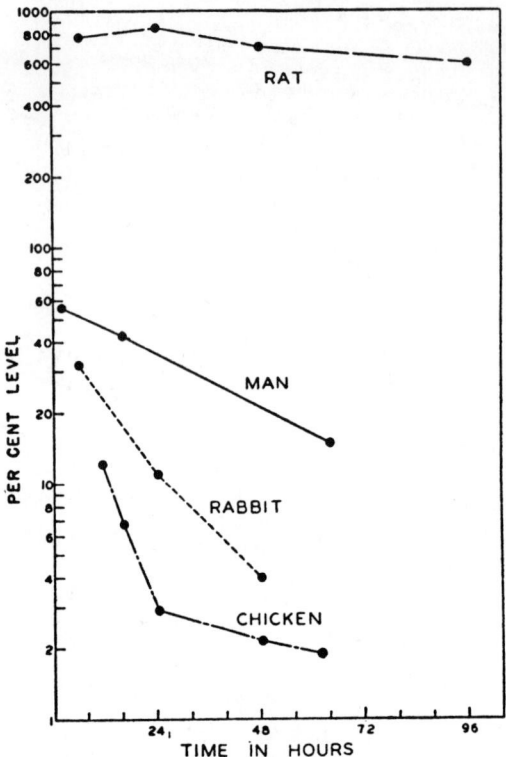

FIGURE 4-4 Arsenic-76 in whole blood. Concentration of arsenic-76 per gram of blood at a particular time is expressed as percentage of the administered dose per gram of body weight. Reprinted with permission from Ducoff et al.[220]

The low rate of excretion of arsenic in the rat is probably due to fixation of 80–90% of it in the hemoglobin of the red cell, which must break down before the arsenic can be released. The high content in blood also makes it difficult to get true tissue values in such organs as the spleen and liver. In an attempt to find another small-animal model for man, Peoples[625] studied the distribution of arsenic in rats, guinea pigs, rabbits, and hamsters that were fed arsenic trioxide; the results are shown in Table 4-15. The hamster appears the animal of choice, with the rabbit also a good possibility.

The relationship between arsenic ingestion and urinary arsenic has led to its use in measuring industrial exposure. The importance of

Metabolism of Arsenic

checking the diet for the intake of seafood has been reported.[708] It is interesting that a wide variety of fish, crustaceans, and mollusks caused increases of up to 10 times the normal content lasting for over 20 h. No symptoms were reported at concentrations that would have caused serious poisoning if the substance ingested had been sodium arsenite. The chemical nature of the arsenic compound is unknown, but it is probably organic.

With the helium-arc method,[99] the urine of four subjects was analyzed for As(III), As(V), methanearsonic acid, and cacodylic acid; the results are shown in Table 4-16. The average excretion of 66% of the arsenic as DMA is striking, especially because the subjects were from Florida and likely to eat seafood. The relationship of industrial exposure to seafood intake should be analyzed with this method.

The distribution of arsenic in the cow has been studied with a variety of compounds in nontoxic doses.[625] The feeding of arsenic acid to cows at 0.05–1.25 mg/kg of body weight for 8 weeks did not increase the arsenic content of the milk, but it did increase the arsenic in the tissues. Urine was the main pathway of excretion, which was very rapid—the urine was free of arsenic 2 days after arsenic administration was

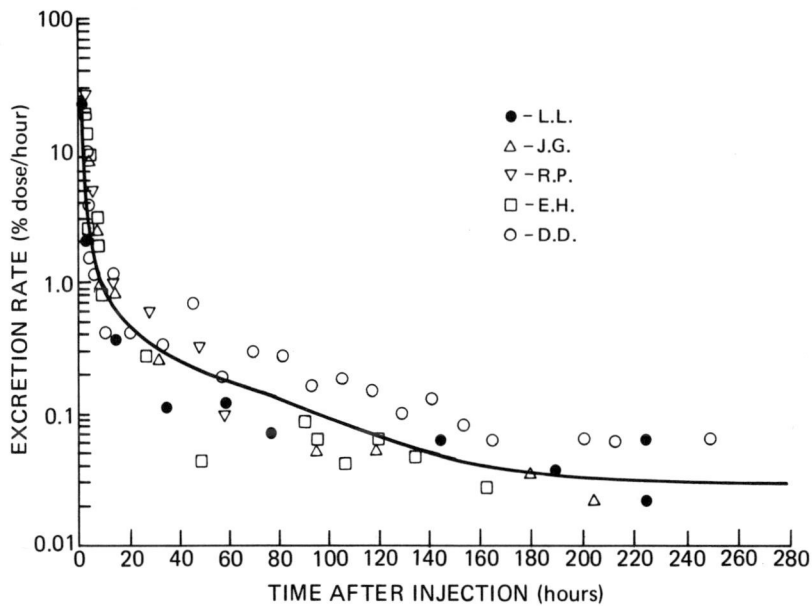

FIGURE 4-5 Rate of urinary excretion of radioarsenic in five subjects. Reprinted with permission from Mealey et al.[536]

TABLE 4-15 Arsenic in Tissues after 21 Days of Feeding a Diet Containing Arsenic Trioxide at 50 ppm[a]

		Arsenic Concentration, ppm									
Animal[b]		Liver	Heart	Kidney	Spleen	Fat	Muscle	Brain	G.I. Tract	Skin	Blood
Rat	Control	0.0	3.3	1.5	0.6	0.6	0.7	0.5	0.6	0.6	15.0
	Fed	20.0	43.0	25.0	60.0	12.0	3.0	3.8	15.0	27.0	125.0
Guinea pig	Control	0.0	0.0	0.0	0.0	0.0	0.0	0.0	1.0	0.0	0.0
	Fed	1.0	20.0	1.0	15.0	0.8	2.0	0.0	2.0	—	4.0
Rabbit	Control	0.0	0.0	0.0	0.0	0.0	0.0	0.0	0.1	0.0	0.1
	Fed	1.0	0.2	1.5	0.2	0.2	0.2	0.0	1.5	2.5	1.5
Hamster	Control	0.0	0.0	0.0	0.0	0.0	1.8	0.0	1.5	0.0	0.0
	Fed	15.0	7.0	5.0	2.0	0.7	2.5	1.0	30.0	38.0	2.5

[a]Derived from Peoples.[625]
[b]Four in each group.

TABLE 4-16 Analysis of Human Urine Samples for Arsenic Compounds[a]

Subject	As(III) ppb	%	As(V) ppb	%	Methane-arsonic Acid ppb	%	Cacodylic Acid ppb	%	Total, ppb
M, age 28	<0.1	—	0.84	8.1	0.61	5.9	8.9	86.5	10.4
M, age 27	5.1	20	7.9	30	2.5	9.7	10.4	40.2	25.9
M, age 42	<0.5	—	2.4	7.8	2.4	8.1	25.2	84.0	30.0
F, age 40	2.4	10	4.3	18	1.8	7.6	15.5	64.5	24.0
Average	1.9	—	3.9	—	1.8	—	15.0	—	22.6

[a] Derived from Braman.[99] The results are given in parts per billion (ppb) as arsenic. The precision of individual runs is ±10% relative, or ±0.1 ppb for small sample sizes. Four other samples not completely analyzed gave: methanearsonic acid, 3.6 ± 2.4 (S.D.) ppb; and cacodylic acid, 15.5 ± 6.8 (S.D.) ppb.

discontinued. The valence of urinary arsenic was determined; pentavalent arsenic was the only form found. A similar study with sodium arsenite and cacodylic acid yielded essentially the same results (Peoples, unpublished data). When MSMA was fed to lactating cows, the blood concentration of arsenic rose, but the milk concentration remained low.[627]

These results support the conclusion that there is a blood–mammary barrier to arsenic. The most likely explanation is that an active transport mechanism is saturated at normal plasma concentrations. Aliphatic organic and inorganic arsenic must use the same transport mechanism. Toxic doses of arsenic do not break down the barrier to arsenic. Marshall[521] gave Jersey heifers lead arsenate in their feed at 12.95 mg/100 lb (0.285 mg/kg) of body weight for 126 days and noted no values in the milk above the control value of 0.05 ppm. The same results were obtained by Fitch,[254] who fed a heifer 0.3428 g of arsenic trioxide daily for 3 days without increasing the arsenic content of the milk. In these acute studies, the skin and hair were found to have low concentrations, indicating slow uptake. Dubois et al.[219] showed that exposure to arsenic in atmospheric dust can give fallacious results—up to 243 ppm. Washing in detergent reduced all values to 3.0 ± 1.0 ppm.

Lander et al.[449] examined hair in arsenic poisoning cases and found a wide range of concentrations, 3.0–26.0 ppm. These values were reached a short time after exposure, and the concentration in hair near the scalp was often no higher than that in hair near the tip. The difference was thought to be due to contamination from sweat. The same situation was found in the nails.

Perkons and Jervis[632] used neutron-activation analysis on human hair and reported the frequency distribution of 12 elements, including arsenic, as shown in Figure 4-6. The range of arsenic concentration of 1–5.5 ppm is in accord with the concentrations in washed hair found by Dubois et al.[219] Apparently, the value of hair as a reliable indicator of chronic arsenic poisoning is open to serious question (see Chapter 6).

The valence of arsenic in water, food, and body tissues is largely unknown, not because of its lack of importance, but because of the technical difficulties involved. The method of Crawford and Storey,[184] in which ethyl xanthate is used to extract trivalent arsenic, has worked well in the hands of Ginsburg,[291] who used it in renal clearance studies of arsenite and arsenate in dogs. Ginsburg found that arsenate is reabsorbed in the proximal renal tubule and is reduced in part to arsenite, which then appears in both urine and blood. This is the only evidence of a reduction in valence in a living animal. Winkler[868] analyzed the livers of rats that had been fed sodium arsenite and found that most of the arsenic was pentavalent. Livers of rats fed sodium arsenate and sodium arsanilate contained only pentavalent arsenic. With Winkler's method, Peoples[625] found only pentavalent arsenic in the urine of cows fed arsenic acid.

The arsenic content of neoplasms has received scant attention, although arsenic is often listed as a carcinogen, particularly in books on dermatology (see Chapter 6). Domonkos[209] reviewed studies on the arsenic content of normal skin, skin that was pigmented by exposure to arsenic, and keratoses. Most of the reports indicated normal or low concentrations of arsenic in the lesions, compared with nearby normal skin. He used neutron activation to determine the arsenic in skin and epitheliomas in humans with and without a history of arsenic ingestion. The arsenic content of skin samples varied from 0.15 to 95 ppm when taken from the same patient, and that of four epitheliomas in one patient, from 0.22 to 4.1 ppm. The values for skin vary from 0.1 to 5.0 ppm, regardless of a history of arsenic ingestion. He concluded that arsenic determination in skin lesions was of no value.

There are some data on other types of tumors. Ducoff et al.[220] administered sodium arsenite to a person with a parotid tumor; the tumor took up less arsenic than the liver and kidney and the same amount as most of the other organs. Ducoff et al. also studied the uptake in mice inoculated with Jackson-Brues embryoma and lymphoma. The concentrations in the tumors and organs were too variable

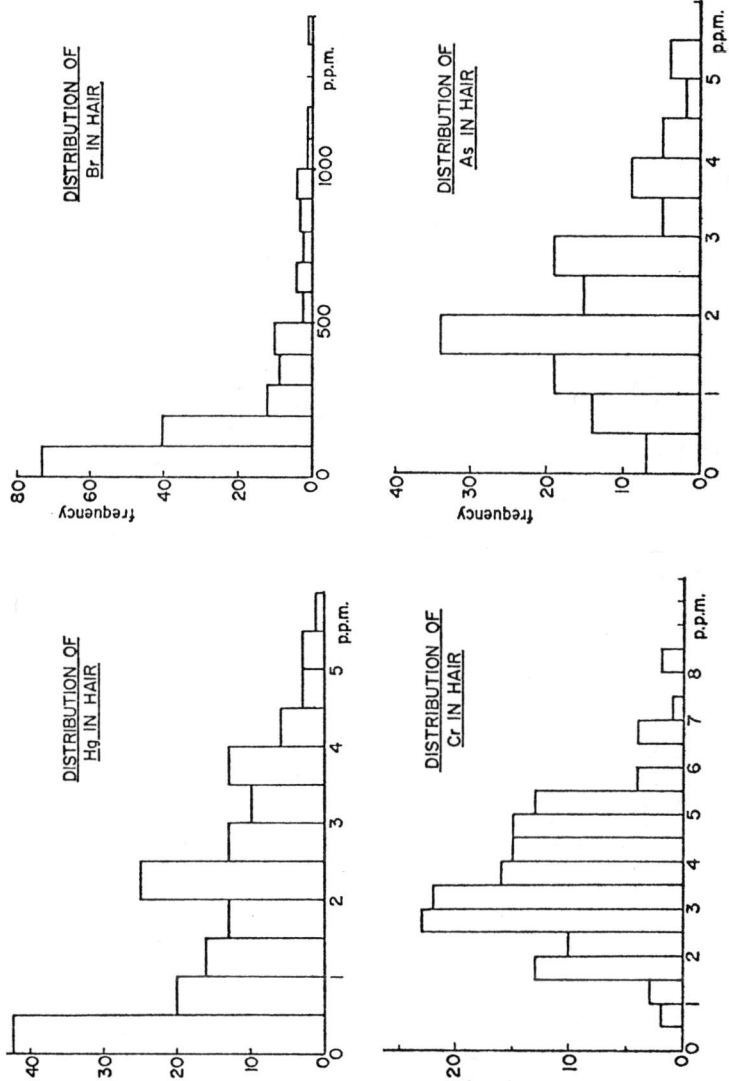

FIGURE 4-6 Frequency distribution of various elements in human hair samples. Reprinted with permission from Perkons and Jervis.[632]

to show a significant trend. The liver : spleen : kidney arsenic ratios were different in normal and tumorous mice.

Hunter et al.[385] injected [^{74}As]potassium arsenite into two leukemic humans and found that the tissue distribution resembled that in the guinea pig.

There is no evidence from these data that neoplasms have any peculiar ability to store arsenic.

Dermal Absorption of Cacodylic Acid in Man

In 1972, the forestry workers in north central Washington applied MSMA and cacodylic acid into the cambium layers of trees.[781] The purpose was to thin the trees and thereby ensure a better stand. The technique resulted in wetting of the workers' clothing, and many developed a garlic breath odor. Urinary arsenic studies were made on a six-man crew over a period of 9 weeks, samples being taken on Monday and Friday of each week. Each man used a different procedure, as follows: (1) a control, hack squirt tool with (2) MSMA or (3) cacodylic acid, injection hatchet with (4) MSMA or (5) cacodylic acid, and (6) MSMA with injector tool. The difference between the two chemical means and the method means was not significant at the 5% level. The control was significantly lower than all chemical treatments, with Monday values being significantly lower than Friday values. The values plateaued or dropped during the study, indicating that the chemicals did not accumulate. There were no health problems related to the compounds used.

Further studies were made by Wagner and Weswig on forestry workers who were exposed to cacodylic acid over a 2-month period.[832] An attempt was made to correlate blood and urinary arsenic concentrations with degree of exposure—without much success. The urinary values were markedly increased, but did not reach the heights of the previously mentioned study. They attributed the odor to arsine; it is highly unlikely that arsine caused the odor, because it is so toxic. When cacodylic acid was commonly used as a tonic, the odor on the breath was reported to be caused by tetramethyldiarsine (cacodyl).[750] Sufficient amounts of arsine to give the breath an odor would be lethal. As would be expected, none of the workers complained of ill health, because the amounts of cacodylic acid absorbed were less than the dose formerly prescribed as a drug, or 30 mg/day.

5

Biologic Effects of Arsenic on Plants and Animals

Arsenic has long held a position of ambiguity with regard to its activity in biologic systems. In spite of the recognized toxicity of many forms of arsenic, various arsenicals have been used in the practice of medicine. A specific nutritional role for inorganic arsenic has been uncovered only recently, but animal feeds have been supplemented with "growth-promoting" organic arsenical additives for many years. Another curious feature of arsenic biochemistry is the ability of the element partially to counteract the ill effects of yet another toxic substance, selenium. This chapter summarizes what is known about the detrimental and beneficial effects of arsenic on living systems other than man and discusses in as much detail as appropriate the molecular mechanisms responsible for these effects. Previous reviews have dealt with the toxicology,[109] general biochemistry,[814,815] and pharmacology[783] of arsenic.

MICROORGANISMS

Toxicity

The state of knowledge regarding the effects of arsenic on microorganisms was summarized very well in a study by Mandel et al.[517] on the action of arsenic on *Bacillus cereus*. Trivalent sodium arsenite was found to inhibit growth at a lower concentration (0.4 mM) than pentavalent sodium arsenate (10 mM). The toxicity of the arsenate could be increased by lowering the phosphate concentration of the growth medium, whereas the inhibitory effect of arsenite was independent of phosphate concentration. This inverse relationship between the toxicity of arsenate and the concentration of phosphate might be related to the fact that arsenate can compete with phosphate for transport.[681] However, Da Costa[193] found that phosphate could suppress the inhibitory effects of arsenite, as well as arsenate, on the growth of fungi. Mandel *et al.*[517] showed that neither arsenate nor arsenite produced any specific effects in *B. cereus* on the incorporation of radioactive precursors into ribonucleic and deoxyribonucleic acids, proteins, or cell wall. Radioarsenite was bound by the microorganism much more strongly than radioarsenate, in agreement with the hypothesis that the toxicity of a particular arsenical was related to the binding of it to the tissues.[358] Because no instance of interconversion between As(V) and As(III) could be established, it was concluded that the two compounds inhibited the growth of *B. cereus* by separate mechanisms. The mechanisms of toxicity of arsenicals for this organism seem to be similar to those proposed for mammalian systems, which are discussed later.

Adaptation

The adaptation of microorganisms to arsenic compounds was of great practical interest during the earlier part of this century, because organic arsenicals were used extensively as trypanocides at that time. The resistance to organic arsenicals was found to depend on the nature of the chemical substituents on the phenyl ring:[5] water-attracting groups (such as $-OH$ and $-NH_2$), less hydrophilic groups (such as $-CH_3$ and $-NO_2$), and groups highly ionized at a pH of 7 (such as $-COOH$). The state of oxidation of the arsenic is of little consequence in inducing resistance to any of these compounds. The mechanism of drug resistance in trypanosomes is usually a decreased permeability to the drug, and the nonarsenical portion of the molecule largely determines the uptake of the drug by the parasite.

A decreased permeability to arsenic appears to be a rather widespread adaptational mechanism, in that a decreased arsenic uptake was observed in *Escherichia coli* mutants that were resistant to arsenate[70] and in *Pseudomonas pseudomallei* that had adapted to arsenite.[25] In the latter case, no increase in the content of α-ketoglutarate dehydrogenase, total sulfhydryl compounds, or lipoic acid was observed in the resistant bacteria.[72] That the total quantity of free thiol groups may be important in some cases of arsenic tolerance, however, was suggested by the work of Harington,[327] who found that resistant strains of the blue tick contained more total sulfhydryl than sensitive strains.

Novick and Roth[591] showed that the penicillinase plasmids, a series of extrachromosomal resistance factors in *Staphylococcus aureus*, carry determinants of resistance to several inorganic ions, as well as resistance to penicillin. Among the inorganic ions were arsenite, arsenate, lead, cadmium, and mercury. Resistance to arsenate was found to be induced in cultures of plasmid-positive strains by prior growth with an uninhibitory concentration of the anion. Dyke *et al.*[225] observed that strains resistant to arsenate, mercury, and cadmium were nearly always resistant to multiple antibiotics and produced large amounts of penicillinase. Although the general genetic and physiologic properties of these ion-resistance markers have been studied, hardly any work has been done on the biochemical mechanisms of this sensitivity and resistance.

PLANTS

Arsenic occurs in all soils and natural waters; thus, plants have obviously evolved in the presence of arsenic ions. It could therefore well be that arsenic is an essential element for plant growth, but it has not been proved. There are no well-authenticated beneficial effects of arsenic on plants. Arsenic is chemically similar to phosphorus, an essential plant nutrient. That it can substitute for phosphorus in plant nutrition, however, is doubtful; in some soils, the application of phosphate fertilizer increases arsenic toxicity (through the release of fixed arsenic).[715] Other interactions between arsenic and plant nutrients are treated later.

Biochemical Response to Arsenic Compounds

When arsenic in solution penetrates the cuticle and enters the apoplast system (the nonliving cell-wall phase), it bathes the external surface of the plasmolemma of the symplast. This is the location of at least some of the enzymes of the living plant. One of the first symptoms of injury by sodium arsenite is wilting, caused by loss of turgor, and this immediately suggests an alteration in membrane integrity. Reaction of trivalent arsenic with sulfhydryl enzymes could well explain the effects of membrane degradation—injury and eventually death.

In general, arsenates are less toxic than arsenites. The arsenate symptoms involve chlorosis, but not rapid loss of turgor (at least in the early expression of toxicity), and the contact action of the arsenates is more subtle. Arsenate is known to uncouple phosphorylation. Thus, the coupled phosphorylation of adenosine diphosphate (ADP) is abolished, the energy of adenosine triphosphate (ATP) is not available, and the plant must slowly succumb.[207]

Arsenate has other profound effects on plant systems. For example, Figure 5-1 shows the relative effects of arsenite and arsenate on the activation of the enzyme fumarase. Fumaric acid is a constituent of all plants and is involved in the citric acid cycle. Fumarase carries out the conversion of fumarate to L-malate.

The above examples typify the role played by the organic arsenical herbicides in plant metabolism. When one considers the number of reactions in plants that involve sulfhydryl groups and phosphorus, it is easy to appreciate the ways in which arsenites and arsenates may upset plant metabolism and interfere with normal growth. The ability of arsenate to enter into reactions in place of phosphate is probably the most important way in which arsenic acts as a toxicant. Not only does it substitute for phosphate in a number of ways, but work with labeled arsenates and arsonates has indicated that these compounds are absorbed and translocated much as phosphates are. It is difficult to visualize a more effective way in which an herbicide might kill a plant.

Phytotoxicity of Organic Arsenicals

Injury symptoms on crop plants resulting from toxic quantities of arsenic in soils were noted in the 1930's, when it was found that young trees planted in old orchard soils grew slowly and were stunted.[748] Young apple trees, in addition to being stunted, had leaf symptoms that indicated water-deficiency stress, which implied injury to the roots; pears showed similar symptoms.[785]

Peach trees planted on these old orchard soils that have accumulated lead arsenate exhibit by midsummer a red or brown discoloration along the leaf margins and then throughout the leaves. The discolored tissues die and drop out, giving the leaves a shot-hole appearance. Defoliation also occurs and may be complete by late summer. The injury appears first in the older leaves; young leaves on shoot tips may remain normal. Yields of fruit may be reduced, and the trees are usually stunted. Thompson and Batjer[785] performed experiments aimed at correcting arsenic injury to peach trees. They found correlations between shot-holing and defoliation and between leaf arsenic content and defoliation;

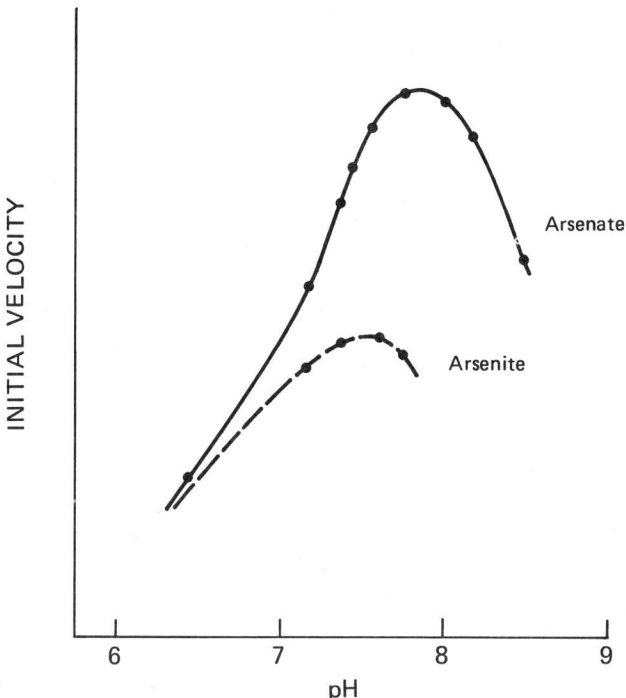

FIGURE 5-1 Velocity of activation of fumarase by arsenate and arsenite ions as a function of pH. Adapted from Dixon and Webb.[207 (p. 473)]

arsenic content varied between 1 and 4 ppm. They found that zinc sulfate applied at 10 lb (4.5 kg) per tree reduced defoliation; nitrogen application at 1.4 lb (0.6 kg) per tree also reduced defoliation; a combination of these two treatments reduced defoliation that had been as high as 81% to around 2–3%, and even eliminated it in some orchards. Repeat treatments with zinc in later years had little or no effect, but maintaining a high nitrogen content reduced defoliation at later years.

Lindner and Reeves[473] explained that arsenic injury was confused with western X-disease, which is caused by a virus. They described the symptoms of the viral disease and arsenic toxicity; both cause shot-holing and defoliation, but arsenic-affected trees have greener leaves, and X-disease causes some chlorosis. Leaves that showed arsenic injury symptoms contained arsenic at 2.1–8.2 ppm; normal leaves, 0.9–1.7 ppm. Viral-diseased trees may produce deformed fruits, which drop prematurely; fruits of arsenic-affected trees are of normal form and remain on the tree for the normal period. Arsenic analyses of leaves provide the most accurate diagnosis.

Woolson[873] studied the uptake and phytotoxicity of arsenic in six vegetable crops grown in a greenhouse. Sodium arsenate was mixed into three soil types; after moistening, the cultures were left for a month for the arsenic to come to equilibrium. Sensitivity to the arsenic decreased in the following order: green beans, lima beans, spinach, cabbages, tomatoes, and radishes. All crops were fertilized at ra es indicated by standardized soil tests and crop needs. The yields indicated that arsenic was generally most phytotoxic in the Lakeland soil; no plants grew when the arsenic concentration was 500 ppm. At 10, 50, and 100 ppm, crops survived; growth was proportional to arsenic concentration. The amount of available arsenic in some treatments continued to change throughout the 19-month experimental period; some of the change may have been the result of the addition of phosphate fertilizers, particularly where available arsenic reached a minimum and then increased. Plant growth at any particular degree of available arsenic in the soil may be affected by the amount of available phosphorus in the soil solution.[878]

The organoarsenical herbicides are not growth-regulators in the way that plant hormones are; they apparently act through or on enzyme systems to inhibit growth. They kill relatively slowly; the first symptoms are usually chlorosis, cessation of growth, and gradual browning, and dehydration and death follow. Rhizomes and tubers may show browning of the storage tissues; buds fail to sprout, and the whole structure eventually decomposes. Cotton plants treated by directed spraying with MSMA show retarded growth from which they may recover.[447]

When resprouting of tubers or rhizomes does occur, treatment should be repeated when some of the leaves have reached full size; treatment before then will not result in translocation, because movement of the assimilate stream into the underground organs is necessary to carry the toxicant to the proper sites of action.

Rumberg et al.[692] reported DSMA-induced loss of chlorophyll in crabgrass within 2–3 days of treatment at 75 or 85 F (24 or 29 C), but it was hardly noticeable after 5 days at 60 F (16 C); the results are summarized in Table 5-1.

Others have observed symptoms on various annual plants, but few detailed descriptions are noted in the literature. Many annual weeds are ultimately desiccated and become necrotic after treatment. Regrowth from axillary buds is usually chlorotic. Cotton and other plants

TABLE 5-1 Effect of Temperature after Treatment on the Degree of Chlorosis Induced by DSMA in Crabgrass[a]

DSMA		Chlorosis Rating[b]					
		60 F (16 C)		75 F (24 C)		85 F (29 C)	
lb/acre	kg/ha	5 Days	10 Days	5 Days	10 Days	5 Days	10 Days
2	2.2	0.2	2.7	3.2	2.2	1.8	2.0
6	6.7	0.2	3.3	6.8	6.0	5.1	7.1
18	20.2	0.3	2.7	7.1	7.1	5.4	7.6
Mean		0.2	2.9	5.7	5.1	4.1	5.6

[a] Derived from Rumberg et al.[693]
[b] A scale of 0–10: 0 = no chlorosis; 10 = complete chlorosis.

become deeply pigmented (red) in the stem and petiole and even the leaves, if the arsenicals are applied in sublethal dosages.

On perennials, such as Johnsongrass, chlorosis does not develop before necrosis on sprayed foliage, but regrowth usually is chlorotic for some period.[419] On purple nutsedge (*Cyperus rotundus*), Holt et al.[366] described symptoms as "a chlorotic appearance which starts at the leaf base and progresses toward the leaf tip until the entire leaf is chlorotic" and as "first visible four days after the initial applications of AMA."

On hardstem bulrush (*Scirpus acutus*), an aquatic species, stems became chlorotic; necrosis proceeded from the tip concurrently with development of a tan discoloration over the length of the stem; after a month, the entire stem became brown and collapsed.[418] Stems regrowing from the bulrush rhizome were chlorotic with necrotic tips and usually died.

Lange[450] studied MSMA toxicity symptoms on stone fruits by spraying MSMA at 4 and 16 lb/acre (4.5 and 17.9 kg/ha) on the bottom one-third of the foliage. He observed a spotty chlorosis of the leaf, followed by necrosis of all or part of the leaf and often defoliation. Untreated upper leaves and new growth showed symptoms of injury that indicated movement of the toxic material to the untreated area.

Many factors could affect response; they include herbicide application rate and formulation, surfactant, timing, volume of carrier, quality of diluent, pH, timing of evaluation, ecotypes, senescence, stage of growth, dormant-season disturbance of root systems before treatment, fertility, moisture availability and continuity, plant competition, temperature, light intensity, and insect and mechanical wounding of foliage before treatment. Any of these can have a dominant effect on the response.

Several researchers who have studied methanearsonates have reported temperature-influenced results. Sckerl et al.,[719] Kempen et al.,[419] Laurin and Dever,[454] Riepma,[669] and Bounds[90] all mentioned that toxicity was greater at higher temperatures. Toxicity was less on Johnsongrass in regions of California influenced by cool marine air, and higher rates of application were required than in hotter regions. One controlled-environment study of Rumberg et al.[693] indicated that chlorosis occurred considerably earlier in crabgrass at higher temperature (24 or 29 C, versus 16 C), and injury, as measured by dry weight after 10 days, was greater at higher temperature. With sodium arsenite and cacodylic acid, temperature had no effect.

Kempen[417] found that relatively high temperature (35 C) and light [2,800 ft-c (30,140 lx)] increased the necrosis of Johnsongrass foliage and the kill of the rhizomes, compared with low temperature (15 C) and light [320 ft-c (3,445 lx)]. He found that only 1 day was required for 50% necrosis of the foliage at the higher temperature and light, but 12 days at the lower temperature and light. McWhorter[535] and Kempen et al.[419] suggested that droughtiness after application increased weed control.

In studies on the effects of AMA on food reserves in purple nutsedge, Duble and Holt[215] found, by tracer experiments and chemical analysis, that starch disappeared and arsenic increased in tubers of plants that were given repeated applications of the herbicide. In general, AMA-treated plants had a higher rate of utilization of the products of photosynthesis than untreated plants. Apparently, carbohydrates were utilized in preference to fats and proteins.

From the results of Woolson et al., it is evident that total arsenic in a soil is not correlated with phytotoxicity; correlation between plant growth and available arsenic is better.[876] Some soils can remove arsenic from the soil solution more rapidly and more completely than other soils by fixation on soil colloids. In these experiments, Hagerstown soil removed 2–5 times more arsenic than did the other two soils. Woolson et al. concluded that the large amount of available arsenic in the Christiana soil may have resulted from the high phosphorus content, which prevented formation of insoluble iron arsenates through competition for reaction sites on the surface of soil particles. Also involved is the larger amount of available aluminum in the Hagerstown soil. Woolson, Axley, and Kearney[877] have shown that, at high arsenic concentration in some soils, aluminum is more important than iron in removing arsenic from the soil solution.

Arle and Hamilton[26] found that topical applications of MSMA affected growth of cotton more than applications of DSMA. There were usually no deleterious effects of single treatments with DSMA; single applications of MSMA later and at higher rates reduced yields. Repeated treatments with MSMA reduced yields more than DSMA treatments.

Keeley and Thullen[414] studied the responses of cotton plants to topical applications of MSMA, DSMA, and MAA at 13, 20, and 31 C. DSMA proved to be less injurious to young cotton plants than MSMA. Injury by MSMA was severe at 13 C, intermediate at 20 C, and low at 31 C, and inclusion of 0.4% surfactant with the MSMA increased the injury. Injury by DSMA was intermediate at 13 C, low at 20 C, and lacking at 31 C, and inclusion of surfactant in the spray solution increased injury only slightly.

Cotyledons of cotton seedlings absorbed [^{14}C]MAA and [^{14}C]DSMA. The MSMA solution in these experiments was adjusted to a pH of 6.4, and the DSMA to a pH of 10.4. Autoradiographs of cotton plants treated with ^{14}C-labeled MSMA, MAA, and DSMA showed evidence of greatest absorption and translocation of MSMA at 13 C, slight translocation at 20 C, and no translocation at 29 C. Very little [^{14}C]MAA or [^{14}C]DSMA was translocated. These results are contrary to the generalization for translocation of assimilates and other tracers, which normally penetrate and move more readily at high temperatures. (Rumberg et al.[693] found chlorosis from DSMA treatment and the translocation of DSMA to increase with temperature.)

Interactions between Arsenicals and Nutrients

Several studies have been conducted on interactions between phosphorus and arsenic in soils and nutrient solutions. Because these two elements have somewhat similar chemical characteristics, substitution of arsenic for phosphorus might occur in plant metabolic products. Rate trials in soil and nutrient solutions, however, have yielded conflicting results, partially because available phosphorus and arsenic concentrations have not generally been determined.

Schweizer[715] showed that high phosphorus content increased the toxicity of DSMA to cotton, but there was considerable variation between the two soil types tested.

Little is known of interactions between arsenic and phosphorus in plants. Everett[239] indicated that phosphorus increased the arsenic content of bluegrass in a turf treated with tricalcium arsenate. However, he found that phosphorus reduced absorption of tricalcium arsenate (measured as arsenic) from nutrient solutions from 246 to 29 ppm. He stated that phosphorus at 100 ppm reduced the soluble arsenic in the nutrient solution from 15.8 ppm to 2.6 ppm. This might account for the lack of increase in arsenic uptake with high phosphorus in nutrient solutions. Everett also indicated that crabgrass absorbed twice as much tricalcium arsenate as did bluegrass; this suggests a species difference. Sckerl,[716] in his review of the literature, indicated that phosphorus reduced arsenic toxicity.

Webb[843] suggested that arsenates inhibit various phosphatase enzymes about as potently as phosphate and probably combine with the enzymes in a similar manner. Sckerl[716] related that arsenate competes with phosphorus for uptake and transport in the cell.

That arsenicals might interact with zinc was indicated by work of Batjer and Benson[55] and Martin (personal communication, 1968). Batjer and Benson showed that toxicity in peaches (but not apples) grown in arsenic-contaminated soils could be reduced by foliar applications of zinc or iron chelates or soil applications of zinc or iron sulfates.[55] Zinc chelates worked best and reduced the symptoms and the arsenic content of peach leaves. Martin related that orchardists in the northwestern United States use zinc sulfate at 5 lb (2.3 kg) per tree plus generous amounts of ammonium sulfate when starting peach trees in high-arsenic soils.

Burleson and Page[119] did root studies with flax that indicated that, with absorption of more than optimal phosphorus, phosphorus and zinc reacted together in a manner that reduced either their mobility or their solubility. Sharma et al.[722] showed that translocation of zinc to shoots was inhibited by high soil phosphorus.

Krantz and Brown[438] published a list of zinc- and iron-sensitive plants; there was no obvious correlation between symptoms of deficiency and susceptibility to methanearsonate sprays.

Mode of Action

Considering the overall action of arsenites as herbicides, it seems important that they are able to penetrate the cuticle and enter into the apoplast phase of the plant system. Here, they may move with transpiration water and bathe the cells of the foliar organs to which they have been applied. At low concentration, it seems possible that arsenites are absorbed into the symplast and then translocated for at least short distances. Under most conditions in which these compounds have been used in the field, their concentrations have been such that rapid contact injury has precluded extensive translocation. This is related at least partly to their rapid effect in membrane degradation.

The arsonates, in contrast, have much lower contact toxicity; they are absorbed and translocated, at least in species that have succumbed to treatment, such as Johnsongrass and nutsedge. In susceptible perennial weeds, the great virtue of MSMA and DSMA has been their ability to penetrate into and destroy underground tubers and rhizomes. Thus, with a few repeated applications, these arsenicals have controlled two of the most serious perennial weed species—species that have resisted control by any other means.

As topical sprays, these compounds are inactivated almost instantaneously on contact with the soil and therefore may be used with impunity in many row crops; cotton is one of the more important of these. Although arsenicals in ordinary herbicidal dosages are rapidly rendered unavailable to plants in the soil, and although most soils have a very great capacity to inactivate and hold arsenic, arsenic residues in soils may eventually become troublesome. For this reason, in any weed control activity involving arsenical herbicides, integrated programs of herbicide rotation should be used. If such programs are used, occasional application of the organic arsenicals in the particular roles in which they are highly effective may not result in soil residues of any significance.

As for the chemical mechanisms by which the organic arsonates kill plants, their relatively slow action involving translocation and producing chlorosis as a primary symptom seems to implicate disturbance of phosphorus metabolism. Not only are they absorbed and translocated in plants much as are phosphates, but also they affect many organelles in the cells, including the chloroplasts, in all of which phosphorus plays important roles.[35]

This interpretation is further strengthened by evidence of Schweizer[715] that the addition of phosphorus to two silt-loam soils increased the toxicity of DSMA to cotton, possibly by saturating sites in these soils on which both arsenate and phosphate are fixed. As early as 1934, Albert[6] reported that residues of calcium arsenate became more toxic to several crops where phosphate fertilizer was applied heavily. There is substantial evidence that phosphates and arsonates tend to replace each other chemically, but that arsenic cannot serve the many essential roles of phosphorus in plants.

The uncoupling of oxidative phosphorylation and the formation of complexes with sulfhydryl-containing enzymes may also enter the picture of arsenic phytotoxicity. However, trivalent arsenic is the form commonly associated with these effects, and this would implicate arsenites, rather than arsenates or arsonates.

LABORATORY ANIMALS

Factors That Can Influence the Toxicity of Arsenic Compounds

Table 5-2 summarizes information on the toxic and no-effect doses of several arsenic compounds. The variety of systems described in the table suggests some of the factors that can influence the toxicity of arsenic. For example, the studies of Harrison et al.[329] illustrated effects that the chemical and physical properties of arsenic trioxide can have on its acute toxicity. The toxicity of arsenic trioxide depended on the purity of the substance used; the crude commercial material was less toxic than the purified material. Although the impure arsenic trioxide was less toxic, it caused much more gastric and intestinal hemorrhage than the purified arsenic trioxide. This study and many of those discussed below were carried out in rats, which have a highly peculiar metabolism of arsenic (see Chapter 4). The reader should be aware of this problem and understand that the rat is an animal to be avoided in arsenic research.

In addition to testing the oral toxicity of aqueous solutions of the "crude" and "pure" arsenic trioxide, Harrison et al.[329] investigated the acute toxic effects of both preparations when given in the dry state mixed in feed. When arsenic trioxide was administered in this manner, the toxic dosage was almost 10 times as high as when it was given in aqueous solution, regardless of whether the crude or the pure material was tested. These results are in accord with those of Schwartze,[713] who found that a solution of arsenic trioxide was more toxic than the undissolved compound and that the toxicity of different preparations of solid arsenic trioxide administered orally varied markedly, depending on their coarseness or fineness. The dependence of the toxicity of arsenic trioxide on the physical form in which it is given is probably a result of its rather poor solubility; e.g., Harrison et al.[329] commented that heating was required to solubilize arsenic trioxide. The practical consequences of the great variation in toxicity of arsenicals due to their different solubilities were recently emphasized by Done and Peart,[210] who criticized government regulations that equated the poison hazard of the highly soluble sodium arsenite with that of the less soluble (and thereby less toxic) arsenic trioxide (although the latter does have a toxic potential).

Harrison et al. also demonstrated a species difference in the resistance to acute poisoning with arsenic trioxide: mice were less affected by the arsenic compound than were rats. Similar species differences were shown by Kerr et al.,[422] who noted that turkeys and dogs were more susceptible to the toxic effects of the organic arsenical 3-nitro-4-hydroxyphenylarsonic acid than were chickens and rats. McChesney et al.[528] reported that sodium p-N-glycoloylarsanilate was about 20 times as toxic to cats as to mice. The work of Harrison et al.[329] revealed that even different strains of mice had very different abilities to tolerate arsenic trioxide. These species and strain differences in the toxicity of arsenic could have important implications regarding the use of laboratory animals as predictive models for human response. The average estimated fatal dose of arsenic trioxide for humans is 125 mg.[815] For a 70-kg man, this is equivalent to about 1.4 mg of arsenic per kilogram of body weight. Thus, a human is much more sensitive to the toxic effects of arsenic on a weight basis than a rat, and it is obviously dangerous to extrapolate results from rodents to humans.

Another factor that can influence the toxicity of arsenic is the valence of the element. Direct comparison of the intraperitoneal LD_{75} of sodium arsenite and sodium arsenate in the rat shows that the trivalent form of arsenic is about 4 times as toxic as the pentavalent form.[263] This difference due to valence is also seen in tissue-culture studies in which many confounding metabolic effects are avoided.[704] Differences related to valence apply to the organic arsenicals, as well as to the inorganic. In fact, the greater toxicity of the trivalent form versus the pentavalent is such a good generalization that a microbiologic assay for distinguishing As(III) and As(V) on the basis of their different toxicities has been suggested.[489]

The toxicity of a number of synthetic aromatic organic arsenicals has been the subject of several investigations, because of the value of these compounds for improving weight gain and feed efficiency in swine and poultry. Generally speaking, the organic forms of arsenic are considered less hazardous than the inorganic forms, and this is shown by the tissue-culture work of Savchuck et al.[704] Arsenic concentrations of 84 and 65 ppm in the form of 3-nitro-4-hydroxyphenylarsonic acid and sodium arsanilate, respectively, were needed to cause a 50% growth inhibition of HeLa cells, whereas a concentration of only 2 ppm in the form of sodium arsenate was required to inhibit growth by the same amount. However, feeding arsenic at 114 ppm in the diet of rats as 3-nitro-4-hydroxyphenylarsonic acid caused an 83% mortality in 4 days,[422] whereas arsenic at 125 ppm in the diet as sodium arsenate caused only a mild growth depression after 12 weeks. Furthermore, the intraperitoneal LD_{50} of arsenic as 3-nitro-4-hydroxyphenylarsonic acid is 18.8 mg/kg in rats,[422] whereas the LD_{75} of arsenic as sodium arsenate is given as 14–18 mg/kg.[263] To put the above studies in the proper perspective, it should be pointed out that the recommended concentra-

TABLE 5-2 Toxic and No-Effect Doses of Some Arsenic Compounds

Compound	Toxic Dose of Arsenic	Criterion of Toxicity	No-Effect Dose	Criterion of No Effect	Mode of Administration	Animal	Reference
Arsenic trioxide, "crude"	23.6 mg/kg	96-h LD_{50}	10 mg/kg	Survival	Oral intubation of aqueous solution	Rat	329
	214 mg/kg	96-h LD_{50}	124 mg/kg	Survival	Dry, mixed in feed	Rat	329
Arsenic trioxide, "pure"	15.1 mg/kg	96-h LD_{50}	<10 mg/kg	Survival	Oral intubation of aqueous solution	Rat	329
	145 mg/kg	96-h LD_{50}	30 mg/kg	Survival	Dry, mixed in feed	Rat	329
	39.4 mg/kg	96-h LD_{50}	10.4 mg/kg	Survival	Oral intubation of aqueous solution	Swiss mouse	329
	25.8 mg/kg	96-h LD_{50}	19.9 mg/kg	Survival	Oral intubation of aqueous solution	C_3H mouse	329
Arsenic trioxide	—	Liver respiration	108 ppm	General appearance	Dry, mixed in feed	Dog	127
	—	—	215 ppm	Fertility and fecundity	Dry, mixed in feed	Rat	561
Sodium arsenite	5 ppm	Liver respiration	—	—	Drinking water	Mouse	66
	4.5 mg/kg	48-h LD_{75}	<4 mg/kg	Survival	Intraperitoneal	Rat	263
	62.5 ppm	Growth inhibition	31 ppm	Growth	Dry, mixed in feed	Rat	123
	125 ppm	Bile duct enlargement	—	—	Dry, mixed in feed	Rat	123
	—	—	5 ppm	Growth and life span	Drinking water	Rat	711
	5 ppm	Shortened life span	—	—	Drinking water	Mouse	710
	5 ppm	Alteration of sex ratio	—	—	Drinking water	Mouse	712

Compound	Dose	Effect	Route	Species	Ref
	14–16 mg/kg	40% LD75	Intraperitoneal	Rat	263
	125 ppm	Growth inhibition	Dry, mixed in feed	Rat	123
	250 ppm	Bile duct enlargement	Dry, mixed in feed	Rat	
	0.1 ppm	Behavioral impairment	Water environment	Goldfish	846
3-Nitro-4-hydroxyphenyl-arsonic acid	2.0 ppm	50% growth inhibition	Added *in vitro*	HeLa cells	704
	33 mg/kg	LD$_{50}$	Oral	Chicken	422
	9.7 mg/kg	LD$_{50}$	Intraperitoneal	Chicken	422
	17.4 mg/kg	LD$_{50}$	Oral	Turkey	422
	44 mg/kg	LD$_{50}$	Oral	Rat	422
	18.8 mg/kg	LD$_{50}$	Intraperitoneal	Rat	422
	114 ppm	Growth, survival	Dry, mixed in feed	Chicken	422
	114 ppm	Growth, survival	Dry, mixed in feed	Rat	422
	96 ppm	50% growth inhibition	Added *in vitro*	HeLa cells	704
	84 ppm	50% growth inhibition	Added *in vitro*	Skin cells	704
Sodium-*P-N*-glycoloylarsanilate	1,195 mg/kg	24-h LD$_{50}$	Intravenous	Mouse	414
	4,600 mg/kg	24-h LD$_{50}$	Oral	Mouse	414
Sodium arsanilate	125 mg/kg	LD	Subcutaneous	Mouse	756
	65 ppm	50% growth inhibition	Added *in vitro*	HeLa cells	704
Arsanilic acid		<10% mortality	Oral	Rat	272
	138 ppm	Incoordinated gait	Dry, mixed in feed	Swine	590
	138 ppm	Growth inhibition	Dry, mixed in feed	Turkey	12
"Shrimp" arsenic		Reproduction		Rat	273
		Growth, histology	Added to food as shrimp	Rat	172

tion of 3-nitro-4-hydroxyphenylarsonic acid for feed-additive use is only 25–50 ppm in the diet, or arsenic at 7–14 ppm.

Arsanilic acid is another aromatic organic arsenical that is widely used as a growth-promoter, and Frost et al.[273] reported that it had no harmful effects on rats over several generations when fed at 500 ppm in the diet. However, Notzold et al.[590] noted an incoordinated gait in swine, and Al-Timimi and Sullivan[12] saw a growth inhibition in turkeys when arsanilic acid was fed at an arsenic concentration of 400 ppm. Again, to put these studies in perspective, it should be emphasized that the recommended concentration of arsanilic acid for feed-additive use is only 50–100 ppm.

Perhaps of more direct concern to consumers is the toxicity of arsenic that occurs naturally in seafood, such as shrimp (such arsenic compounds are commonly referred to as "shrimp arsenic"). Public awareness of this potential hazard was heightened by an article in *Consumer Reports*.[275] However, many of the allegations in the article were disputed in a press report.[548] The work of Coulson et al.[171] showed that rats (and humans) do indeed absorb shrimp arsenic from the gastrointestinal tract readily, but this form of arsenic is excreted rapidly in the urine. These authors also found no evidence of toxic effects of feeding "shrimp arsenic" at 17.7 ppm in the diet of rats for 52 weeks. Criteria of toxicity included growth, physical appearance, activity, and histologic appearance of the liver, spleen, and kidneys.

No toxic symptoms were reported by Morgareidge,[560] who supplemented rat diets at 16 ppm with protein-bound arsenic derived from the livers of turkeys whose diets had contained 0.56% *p*-ureidobenzenearsonic acid (carbarsone). Welch and Landau[848] observed no toxic reactions in rats fed a diet containing 1% arsenocholine (the arsenic analogue of choline) for a week. The apparent lack of toxicity of this arsenic compound may be of considerable interest, in light of the work of Lunde,[493] who discovered in fish oils two arsenolipids with chemical properties that resemble those of phospholipids.

Still another class of organic arsenical compounds is the aliphatic arsenicals, such as cacodylic acid and the sodium salts of methanearsonic acid, which are discussed later. Although these compounds are used widely as herbicides, their toxicity is less than that of inorganic arsenical herbicides.

The Problem of Toxic versus "No-Effect" Dosages

In addition to the complexities just discussed, there is a factor that confounds the interpretation of toxicologic data—namely, the criterion used to judge whether a given dosage is toxic. For example, arsenic at 5 ppm in the drinking water as sodium arsenite from weaning until death is not toxic to rats, with respect to growth or life span,[711] and is only slightly toxic to mice.[710] An identical experiment, however, carried out through three generations of mice revealed that the ratio of males to females born increased in mice exposed to arsenic, compared with controls.[712] It was concluded that exposure to some trace elements in dosages that do not interfere with growth or survival may affect reproduction. Thus, a more sensitive indicator of toxicity showed the detrimental effects of a dosage that had previously been regarded as "safe." With sophisticated assessment techniques, such as biochemical and enzyme measurements, even more subtle effects of poisons can be detected. For example, Bencko and Simane[66] found that the respiration rate of liver homogenates prepared from mice that had received arsenic at 5 ppm as arsenic trioxide in their drinking water was only 61% of that of the normal controls. However, the dosage of arsenic used by Bencko and Simane was 100 times higher than the currently recommended maximal concentration (0.05 ppm) of arsenic in drinking water.[578]

An even more sensitive method for determining the toxic effect of arsenic compounds was used by Weir and Hine:[846] a conditioned-avoidance technique to assess the deleterious effects of various ions in the aquatic environment of fish. In this study, arsenic (as arsenate) was found to impair conditioned-avoidance behavior of trained goldfish after 48 h of exposure to a concentration of only 0.1 ppm, which is only 1/320 of the lethal concentration for 50% and only 1/15 of the lethal concentration for 1% of the fish. The relevance of this work to mammalian systems is far from clear, but the data suggest at least that similar behavioral experiments should be carried out with animals exposed to various substances suspected of being environmental hazards.

Mechanisms of Toxicity of Arsenic Compounds

The difference in toxicity between trivalent and pentavalent arsenic compounds can best be understood by considering the biochemical mechanisms of action of these two distinct families of compounds. This aspect of arsenic toxicology has been the subject of numerous reviews.[17,397,634,762,815] The early work of Ehrlich, Voegtlin, and others suggested that organic arsenicals exert their toxic effects *in vivo* by first being metabolized to the trivalent arsenoxide form and then reacting with sulfhydryl groups of tissue proteins and enzymes to form an arylbis(organylthio)arsine:

$$R-As=O + 2R'SH \longrightarrow R-As\begin{matrix} SR' \\ \\ SR' \end{matrix} + H_2O.$$

Later work showed that several enzyme systems containing thiol groups could be poisoned in this way and that in most cases the activity of the enzyme could be restored by adding an excess of monothiol.

An important exception to this generalization, however, proved to be the pyruvate oxidase system, which could not be protected against trivalent arsenicals by even a 200% excess of monothiol. Such an apparent anomaly was clarified when it was shown that, under some circumstances, arsenicals can complex with two sulfhydryl groups in the same protein molecule, thereby forming a stable ring structure that is not easily ruptured by monothiols. This finding stimulated the testing of various dithiol compounds for their ability to block the action of arsenicals on pyruvate oxidase and led to the discovery of British antilewisite (BAL), which eventually became a widely used antidote for arsenic poisoning. The simultaneous interaction of arsenic with two thiol groups led Peters and associates[594] to postulate the existence of a dithiol-containing cofactor in the pyruvate oxidase system. This idea was later verified experimentally when lipoic acid was identified as a component of pyruvate oxidase. The reaction of an arsenoso compound with lipoic acid to yield a ring structure that can be cleaved by BAL is illustrated in Figure 5-2. This reaction summarizes what is currently felt to be the mode of action of trivalent monosubstituted arsenicals in exerting their toxic effects in biologic systems and illustrates the biochemical rationale for the use of BAL to counteract arsenic poisoning.

It should be pointed out, however, that the toxic effects of inorganic trivalent arsenic (arsenite) can often be potentiated by BAL *in vitro*. Fluharty and Sanadi,[257] for example, showed that an equimolar mixture of arsenite and BAL uncouples oxidative phosphorylation in rat liver mitochondria and drew the conclusion that arsenite is the true active inhibitory species and that the BAL served only as a vehicle for transporting arsenite to a dithiol enzyme site. Siegal and Albers[729] found that addition of equimolar BAL decreased the arsenite concentration necessary to produce 50% inhibition of *Electrophorus* (electric eel)

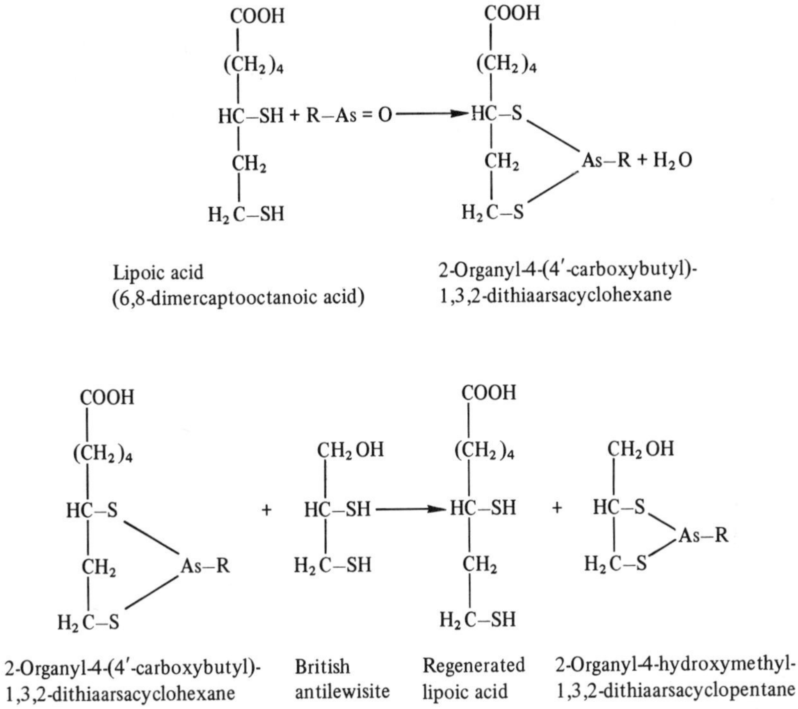

Biologic Effects of Arsenic on Plants and Animals

$$
\begin{array}{c}
\text{COOH} \\
|\\
(CH_2)_4 \\
|\\
HC-SH \\
|\\
CH_2 \\
|\\
H_2C-SH
\end{array}
+ R-As=O \longrightarrow
\begin{array}{c}
\text{COOH} \\
|\\
(CH_2)_4 \\
|\\
HC-S\\
|\quad\quad\diagdown\\
CH_2\quad\quad As-R \\
|\quad\quad\diagup\\
H_2C-S
\end{array}
+ H_2O
$$

Lipoic acid
(6,8-dimercaptooctanoic acid)

2-Organyl-4-(4'-carboxybutyl)-
1,3,2-dithiaarsacyclohexane

$$
\begin{array}{c}
\text{COOH}\\
|\\
(CH_2)_4\\
|\\
HC-S\\
|\quad\diagdown\\
CH_2\quad As-R\\
|\quad\diagup\\
H_2C-S
\end{array}
+
\begin{array}{c}
CH_2OH\\
|\\
HC-SH\\
|\\
H_2C-SH
\end{array}
\longrightarrow
\begin{array}{c}
\text{COOH}\\
|\\
(CH_2)_4\\
|\\
HC-SH\\
|\\
CH_2\\
|\\
H_2C-SH
\end{array}
+
\begin{array}{c}
CH_2OH\\
|\\
HC-S\\
|\quad\diagdown\\
H_2C-S\quad As-R
\end{array}
$$

2-Organyl-4-(4'-carboxybutyl)-   British   Regenerated   2-Organyl-4-hydroxymethyl-
1,3,2-dithiaarsacyclohexane   antilewisite   lipoic acid   1,3,2-dithiaarsacyclopentane

FIGURE 5-2 Reaction of lipoic acid with a trivalent monosubstituted arsenical, and regeneration of lipoic acid by addition of BAL.[635]

microsomal (Na^+/K^+)-ATPase from 6 mM to 0.1 mM. The authors suggested that the BAL–arsenite complex reacted directly with the enzyme. Wu[882] performed a careful kinetic analysis of the dithiol-dependent inhibition of rat liver glutamine synthetase by arsenite and proposed the scheme shown in Figure 5-3. This scheme was thought to account for several facts regarding the dithiol-dependent inhibition by arsenite, including the ready dissociation of the enzyme–arsenite complex and the reversal of the inhibition by cysteine. McDonough[529] suggested that the BAL-arsenite complex can act as an inhibitor of germination, inasmuch as lettuce seeds soaked in mixed solutions of sodium arsenite and BAL yielded lower germination ratios than did seeds soaked in either compound alone.

The mechanism of action of the toxic effects of inorganic pentavalent arsenicals is less clearly understood than that of the trivalent arsenic compounds. It is possible that pentavalent arsenic is reduced to trivalent arsenic before exerting its toxic effects,[87,292] but whether that

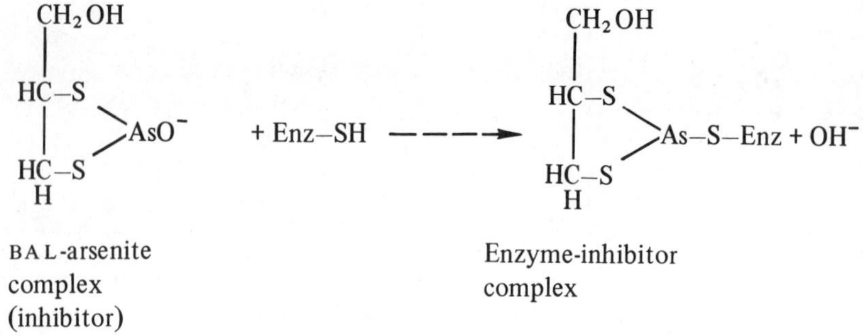

```
   CH₂OH                              CH₂OH
    |                                  |
   HC-S                               HC-S
    |   >AsO⁻   + Enz-SH  ———→         |   >As-S-Enz + OH⁻
   HC-S                               HC-S
    H                                  H
```

BAL-arsenite   Enzyme-inhibitor
complex   complex
(inhibitor)

FIGURE 5-3 Reaction of glutamine synthetase with BAL–arsenite complex.[882]

happens *in vivo* is controversial.[709,868] Unlike the trivalent arsenicals, the pentavalent forms do not appear to react directly with the active sites of enzymes.[397] Rather, arsenate can compete with inorganic phosphate in phosphorylation reactions to form unstable arsenyl esters, which then decompose spontaneously.[211] Arsenate has also been shown to uncouple oxidative phosphorylation,[182] presumably by competing with inorganic phosphate at one of the energy-conserving steps. Chan et al.[142] have isolated an arsenylated component of rat liver mitochondria that they feel may represent the arsenic analogue of a low-molecular-weight phosphorylated mitochondrial constituent that plays a role in oxidative phosphorylation. A nonhydrolytic mode of action of arsenate in inhibiting mitochondrial energy-linked functions has recently been proposed.[549]

Adaptation to Toxicity of Arsenic Compounds

Most early investigators reported that animals were unable to adapt to the toxic effects of inorganic arsenic compounds,[713] although adaptation to some organic arsenicals was readily achieved.[441] In spite of the early failures to demonstrate adaptation to inorganic arsenic, Bencko and Symon[68] have recently shown that the LD_{50} for arsenic as arsenic trioxide administered subcutaneously could be increased from 10.96 to 13.98 mg/kg in hairless mice as a result of giving arsenic at 50 ppm as arsenic trioxide in the drinking water for 3 months. Additional evidence that suggested an adaptive response to arsenic was the finding that the decreased metabolic oxygen consumption observed with the liver homogenates from mice given arsenic at 50 ppm in the water for 32 days returned to normal after 64 days in the experiment.[63] However, no

Biologic Effects of Arsenic on Plants and Animals

such adaptation was seen in mice given arsenic at either 5 or 250 ppm in the water. Moreover, this experiment seems somewhat inconsistent with an earlier report from the same laboratory, which showed that liver homogenates from mice given arsenic at 50 ppm in the water for 256 days exhibited a decreased consumption of oxygen.[66] Apparently, the range of experimental conditions under which adaptation to arsenic can be obtained is quite limited.

The mechanisms of these adaptive responses to arsenic are not known, but Bencko and Symon[67] found that mice given arsenic at 50–250 ppm in the water accumulated arsenic in the liver and skin until the sixteenth day of the experiment, after which retention decreased. The authors suggested that either decreased absorption or increased excretion of arsenic could account for their results. Studies with [^{74}As]arsenate revealed that mice previously exposed to arsenic at 50 ppm as arsenite in the water for 64 days displayed a significant decrease in the retention of a later dose of radioarsenate administered parenterally.[65] Although the authors interpreted their results as evidence of an increase in capacity of the excretory mechanism for arsenic due to arsenic exposure, this experiment could also perhaps be explained by a saturation of the tissue binding sites for arsenic by previous arsenic intake, which could then cause an "apparent" increase in the excretion of the element. Clearly, more research is needed to determine whether animals are able to adapt to the toxic effects of inorganic arsenicals.

Experimental Inhalation Toxicity

Air pollution due to arsenic is a particular problem in some parts of Czechoslovakia, because of the high arsenic content of some coal burned in power plants there. Consequently, Bencko and associates of the Institute of Hygiene in Prague have carried out a number of studies concerned with the experimental inhalation toxicity of arsenic.[62,69] These workers pioneered the use of the hairless mouse for such investigations, because other animal models had several disadvantages for research in arsenic toxicology.[68] The rat, whose arsenic metabolism is peculiar (arsenic tends to accumulate in the blood), was ruled out as a test animal. The rabbit and guinea pig were also considered unsuitable for these studies, because in some of the work arsenic was to be administered via the drinking water, and the variable consumption of fresh vegetables by the animals would contribute to an irregular water intake. However, the hairless mouse had a number of experimental advantages for inhalation toxicity determination. First, it could not put its nose into its fur to "filter" the air being breathed. Moreover, there was no hair to trap the arsenic-containing dust; such dust could otherwise be ingested later as a result of cleaning or grooming. Finally, the lack of hair on the mouse enabled the investigators more readily to determine any dermatologic changes caused by the arsenic.

Hairless mice were exposed to fly ash whose particle size was less than 10 µm and that contained 1% arsenic in the form of arsenic trioxide. The exposures were carried out on 5 days/week for 6 h/day in dust chambers specially designed for the application of solid aerosols. The mean arsenic concentration in the dust chamber was 179.4 ± 35.6 µg/m^3 of air, which was about 3 times higher than the maximal concentration of arsenic found in the vicinity of the offending power plants. During the first 2 weeks of the experiment, there was a considerable increase in the concentration of arsenic in the livers, kidneys, or skin of the exposed mice. However, there was a significant decrease in the arsenic content of the liver and kidney samples during the fourth week of exposure, although no such decrease was observed in the skin. This decline in the arsenic content of tissues was similar to that seen in animals given arsenic orally and suggested an adaptation to arsenic. Unfortunately, these workers did not carry out physiologic measurements to evaluate effects of the arsenic exposure on the metabolism of the experimental animals.

Zharkova[890] studied the effect of continuous 24-h exposures to arsenic trioxide at 25–37 µg/m^3 of air on various physiologic characteristics in rats. He found that such treatment resulted in a lag in weight gain, disordered chronaxy ratios of antagonist muscles, suppression of cholinesterase activity, a reduction in concentration of sulfhydryl groups in blood proteins, an increase in the number of reticulocytes, a decrease in blood hemoglobin, porphyrinuria, a reduction in ascorbic acid in all organs and tissues, and accumulation of arsenic in the organs and tissues. Few experimental details were presented in the translated paper, so it is difficult to assess the biologic significance of these results. Although the physiologic importance of disordered chronaxy ratios, suppressed enzyme activities, and reduction in sulfhydryl groups in proteins might be questioned, weight lag, anemia, and porphyrinuria are more difficult to ignore. Moreover, the concentrations of arsenic used in the investigation were very low, although they still exceeded the occupational exposure standard for inorganic arsenic recently recommended by the National Institute for Occupational Safety and Health (NIOSH).[809]

Rozenshtein[688] investigated the effect of continuous exposure to arsenic trioxide aerosols on albino rats. He found that round-the-clock exposure to arsenic trioxide at 60.7 $\mu g/m^3$ produced inhibition in the central nervous system, reduced the content of sulfhydryl groups, inhibited cholinesterase activity, and raised the concentration of pyruvate in the blood. Similar continuous exposure to a concentration of 4.9 $\mu g/m^3$ caused disturbances of conditioned reflexes and of the chronaxy ratio of antagonistic muscles and a reduction in the content of sulfhydryl groups in the blood. Exposure to both concentrations resulted in a marked accumulation of arsenic in the body and morphologic alterations in the organs and tissues. Inasmuch as no functional, biochemical, or morphologic alterations were observed when the animals were exposed to arsenic trioxide at 1.3 $\mu g/m^3$, Rozenshtein recommended 1 $\mu g/m^3$ as the maximal mean diurnal permissible concentration of this compound in the atmosphere.[688] Again, the physiologic implications of these results are not clear.

The main drawback in the research of both Zharkova and Rozenshtein was that the test animal used was the rat, which has a peculiar arsenic metabolism. Also, the rats had considerable body hair, which could trap the arsenic aerosol. The arsenic trapped in this way could then be ingested by the animal as a result of cleaning and grooming. Finally, the rats used in both studies were exposed to arsenic trioxide on a continuous 24-h/day basis, whereas the NIOSH standard was meant to apply only in situations of intermittent exposure. Nonetheless, further research should be carried out to evaluate both experiments.[806]

Arsenicals and Resistance to Infection

Gainer and Pry[278] showed that virus-infected mice treated with large doses of arsenicals had higher mortality rates than untreated controls. Viral diseases so affected by arsenic included pseudorabies, encephalomyocarditis, and St. Louis encephalitis. Although several experimental protocols were used, arsenical treatment generally consisted of injecting subacute doses of sodium arsenite at the time of inoculation with virus or administering sodium arsenite or 3-nitro-4-hydroxyphenylarsonic acid at rather high concentrations of arsenic (75–150 ppm) in the drinking water for various periods before or after inoculation. In one case (western encephalitis virus), mortality was significantly reduced if the mice were given sodium arsenite at the time of inoculation with virus, but mice treated with 3-nitro-4-hydroxyphenylarsonic acid in the drinking water after inoculation had higher mortality than did controls. British antilewisite did not inhibit, but appeared to stimulate, the mortality-increasing activity of sodium arsenite in pseudorabies infection. This observation is consistent with other reports that under some circumstances BAL may potentiate the toxicity of arsenicals.

The protective effect of a synthetic double-stranded homopolynucleotide complex of polyinosinic acid and polycytidylic acid (poly I/poly C) against mortality in mice due to western encephalitis virus was inhibited by sodium arsenite treatment. Because the protective role of poly I/poly C against viral disease has been associated with the action of interferon, Gainer and Pry[278] hypothesized that the arsenical stimulation of mortality after inoculation with viruses was at least partially explainable by interferon dysfunction. Indeed, a later paper by Gainer[277] showed that the induction of interferon by poly I/poly C in rabbit kidney cell cultures could be inhibited by sodium arsenite. It was found somewhat unexpectedly, however, that, although high concentrations of arsenite inhibited the action of exogenous mouse interferon added to cultures of mouse embryo cells, low concentrations of arsenite increased the antiviral activity of low concentrations of interferon.

The research of Gainer and Pry[278] seems to have two major ecologic consequences. First, exposure to large doses of arsenic clearly impairs a mouse's ability to resist viral disease. However, the doses of arsenic used in these studies were such that any relevance of these data to human pollution problems would have to be limited to outbreaks of massive arsenical toxicosis, such as the Morinaga dry milk incident[575] and the Ube soy sauce episode.[711] In this regard, the follow-up study revealed that children poisoned in the Morinaga incident, among other problems, also had a decreased resistance to infection. The mechanism of action of arsenic in decreasing resistance to infection is not known with precision, but the results of Gainer indicate that decreased interferon production or action may be involved. A nonspecific effect of heavy-metal poisoning cannot be ruled out, inasmuch as Hemphill *et al.*[343] have shown that mice treated with lead had a greater susceptibility to challenge with *Salmonella typhimurium* than controls that received no lead. A decrease in resistance to infection might very well be expected in any group of animals additionally stressed by exposure to a metabolic poison. Although Koller and Kovacic[433] recently found that exposure to lead decreased antibody formation in mice, Gainer and Pry were able to rule out alterations in antibody formation or action as the primary factors accounting for the stimulating effects of arsenicals on the mortality of their virus-infected mice.

A second ecologic consequence of Gainer's experiments is related to the remarkable observation that low concentrations of arsenic appeared to increase the ability of exogenously added mouse interferon to block the infection of cultured mouse embryo cells with vesicular stomatitis virus.[277] Although the author himself had some reservations concerning the proper interpretation of his data, the stimulation of interferon action by arsenic seemed to be real. Gainer suggested that an increased antiviral activity of interferon could provide a rationale for the beneficial "growth-promoting" effects of arsenical feed additives in livestock through reduction in disease incidence or severity.[277] Any conclusions regarding the possible effects of low concentrations of arsenicals in the environment on the ability of humans to resist disease must await further research.

Arsenic as Antagonist to Selenium Poisoning

Moxon[565] first demonstrated the protective effect of arsenic against selenium poisoning when he found that arsenic at 5 ppm as sodium arsenite in the drinking water largely prevented liver damage in rats whose diet contained selenium at 15 ppm as seleniferous wheat. Moxon and DuBois[566] then showed that arsenic was unique in its ability to prevent selenium toxicity; all other elements tested were unable to protect against all manifestations of chronic selenosis. Sodium arsenite and sodium arsenate were equally effective against seleniferous grain, but the arsenic sulfides were ineffective.[218] Arsanilic acid and 3-nitro-4-hydroxyphenylarsonic acid, two organic arsenicals used as "growth-promoters" for livestock, also exhibited a beneficial action against selenium poisoning in rats when given in the drinking water.[344] There is evidence that it would be practical to use these two agents to protect swine and poultry in high-selenium regions.[130,834] Amor and Pringle[13] even suggested the use of an arsenic-containing tonic as a prophylactic agent against selenium poisoning in exposed industrial workers.

The metabolic basis for the beneficial effect of arsenic in selenium poisoning remained confused for some time, because arsenic was known to block the biosynthesis of dimethylselenide, a detoxification product in animals that received subacute doses of selenium by injection.[599] Moreover, the protective effect of arsenic against dietary selenium was not seen if the arsenic was given in the diet, instead of the drinking water,[280] and Frost[271] has shown that the toxicities of arsenic and selenium are additive if both elements are given in the drinking water. These results agree with those of Obermeyer et al.,[593] who recently observed an additive toxicity between arsenite and trimethylselenonium chloride or dimethylselenide.

Ganther and Baumann[279] studied the influence of arsenic on the metabolism of selenium when both elements are injected in subacute doses and found that the excretion of selenium into the gastrointestinal tract was markedly stimulated by arsenic. Levander and Baumann[463] observed an inverse relationship in arsenic-treated rats between the amount of selenium retained in the liver and the amount excreted into the gut; and they concluded that the bile might be the route by which selenium was appearing in the gastrointestinal tract. This hypothesis proved correct when it was discovered that in 3 h over 40% of the selenium injected could be recovered in the bile of rats that also received arsenic, whereas only 4% of the selenium was excreted into the bile of rats not given arsenic.[464] This effect of arsenic on the biliary excretion of selenium was not confined to subacute-toxicity experiments: A response of selenium to arsenic was seen at dosages approaching a rat's daily intake of selenium when fed some crude commercial diets. Sodium arsenite was the most effective form of arsenic in enhancing the biliary excretion of selenium, but arsenate and 3-nitro-4-hydroxyphenylarsonate were also active to some extent. In experiments with radioactive arsenic, it was found that selenium stimulated the biliary excretion of arsenic, just as arsenic stimulated the excretion of selenium. Initial attempts to characterize the forms of selenium in rat bile suggested that the element is probably present in several forms, including some macromolecularly bound selenium.

Although these studies provide an understanding on a physiologic basis of how arsenic counteracts selenium toxicity, the chemical mechanism of the process is still far from clear. The most logical hypothesis to account for the arsenic–selenium antagonism from the molecular point of view assumes that arsenic combines with selenium—perhaps, in analogy with sulfur chemistry, by reacting with selenol ($-SeH$) groups—to form a detoxification conjugate that passes readily into the bile.

Nutritional Essentiality of Arsenic

A number of older reports suggested that arsenic in small amounts may play a useful metabolic role in tissues, rather than being merely an accidental contaminant. Underwood[801] has cited several of these early references that claimed beneficial effects of arsenic, including stimulation of growth in tissue cultures and enhancement of growth and metamorphosis of tadpoles. More recently, Askerov et al.[36] have found that spraying leaves with a 0.002% arsenic solution leads to a 10% increase in viability of silkworm caterpillars and a 29% increase in cocoon yield.

Despite several subjective reports on the effects of arsenic on the appearance of the haircoat or in the prevention or cure of anemia, numerous attempts to induce an experimental dietary deficiency have failed, probably because of the ubiquity of the element. Hove et al.[371] fed rats a milk diet fortified with iron, copper, and manganese and found that arsenic caused a slight initial delay in the decrease of hemoglobin when the minerals were withdrawn from the milk. However, these authors concluded that, if arsenic is essential for rats, the requirement must be somewhere below the 2 µg daily that was provided by the milk alone. Schroeder and Balassa[709] reported that rats and mice grew well and survived normally when they received only 0.26 µg of arsenic per 100 g of body weight per day in food. Skinner and McHargue[736] found that rats responded to arsenic supplements with increased hemoglobin when fed a ration composed mainly of skim milk powder and sucrose and adequately supplemented with iron and copper.

Sharpless and Metzger[723] have presented some evidence that arsenate can act as a mild goitrogen when fed in the diet at 5 ppm. To get a significant goitrogenic effect, however, such high concentrations of arsenic were needed that these workers concluded that there was only a remote possibility that arsenic could act as a positive goitrogenic agent in man.

A report by Muth et al.[570] suggested that arsenic may have some activity in preventing selenium-deficiency diseases, inasmuch as addition of arsenic at 1 ppm as sodium arsenate to selenium-deficient ration significantly reduced the incidence of myopathy in lambs. This observation has not been confirmed, however (Westwig and Whanger, unpublished data). Attempts to demonstrate a beneficial effect of arsenic in other selenium deficiency diseases, such as liver necrosis in rats[714] and exudative diathesis in chickens,[621] have been unsuccessful.

Using purely theoretical arguments based on the tissue distribution of various trace elements, Liebscher and Smith[469] decided that arsenic behaves more like an environmental contaminant than a nutritionally essential mineral. However, a recent preliminary communication has presented evidence of a requirement for arsenic by the rat.[586] To demonstrate an arsenic deficiency, the experimental animals had to be housed in plastic cages placed in laminar flow racks. The rats were fed a specially formulated purified diet that contained arsenic at only 30 ppb. The deficiency signs were most striking in male rats and included rough haircoat, low growth rate, splenomegaly, decreased hematocrit, and increased osmotic fragility of red cells. These preliminary results appear to have been verified by recent work describing an arsenic deficiency in goats and minipigs fed semisynthetic rations containing arsenic at less than 50 ppb.[19] Deficiency signs included impaired reproductive performance, decreased birth weights, increased neonatal mortality, and lower weight gains in second-generation animals. None of these deficiency signs were observed in control animals fed the semisynthetic diet supplemented with arsenic at 350 ppb.

DOMESTIC ANIMALS

Inorganic and Aliphatic Organic Arsenicals

Arsenic appears to be second only to lead in importance as a toxicant in farm and household animals.[115,335] Toxicoses caused by inorganic and aliphatic organic arsenicals are generally manifested by a syndrome entirely different from that caused by the phenylarsonic feed additives and therapeutic agents; therefore, the phenylarsonic compounds will be discussed separately.

Some of the more common sources of arsenic poisoning include grass clippings from lawns that have been treated with arsenical crabgrass-control preparations; grass, weeds, shrubbery, and other foliage that have been sprayed with arsenical herbicides;[113,114] dipping of animals in vats that years before had been charged with arsenic trioxide; and soils heavily contaminated with arsenic, either through the burning of arsenic formulations in rubbish piles or through the application of arsenical pesticides to orchards and truck gardens.[153,656] The more common sources of arsenic for small animals, especially cats, include ant and snail baits, which usually contain 1–2% arsenic.[115]

Man and all lower animals are susceptible to inorganic arsenic poisoning, but poisoning is most often encountered in the bovine and feline species and results from the contamination of their food supply. The incidence of arsenic poisoning in these two species is closely followed in other forage-eating animals, such as sheep and horses.[564] Poisoning by inorganic arsenicals occurs only occasionally in dogs and rarely in swine and poultry.

The toxicity of inorganic arsenicals varies with the species of animal exposed, the formulation (e.g., trivalent arsenicals are more toxic than pentavalent), the solubility, the route of exposure, the rate of absorption from the gastrointestinal tract, and the rates of metabolism and excretion.[153,656] In practice, the most dangerous arsenic preparations are dips, herbicides, and defoliants in which the arsenic is in a highly soluble form. Unfortunately, animals often seek out and eat such materials as insulation, rodent baits, and dirt and foliage that have been contaminated with an inorganic arsenical.

Because so many factors influence the toxicity of arsenic, there is little point in attempting to state its toxicity in terms of milligrams per kilogram of body weight. The lethal oral dose for most species, however, appears to be 1–25 mg/kg of body weight as sodium arsenite, and 3–10 times that range as arsenic trioxide.

That the toxicity of an arsenical is greatly influenced by its solubility and particle size and thus by the extent of its absorption from the intestinal tract or skin is illustrated by an experiment conducted with swine.[115] Sodium arsenite was given in the feed at up to 500 ppm continuously for 2 weeks. The pigs readily ate the contaminated feed, but manifested no signs of acute arsenic poisoning. When the concentration was increased to 1,000 ppm, the pigs refused to eat the feed. When sodium arsenite was added to their drinking water at 500 ppm, severe poisoning and death occurred within a few hours. It was concluded that the lethal dose of sodium arsenite via drinking water was 100–200 mg/kg of body weight.

Experience with field cases of arsenic poisoning has indicated that animals that are weak, debilitated, and dehydrated are much more susceptible to arsenic poisoning than normal animals, probably because renal excretion is reduced.

Arsenic poisoning in most animals is usually manifested by an acute or subacute syndrome. Chronic poisoning, although it has been reported, is seldom seen and has not been clearly documented.

Arsenic affects tissues that are rich in oxidative systems, primarily the alimentary tract, kidneys, liver, lungs, and epidermis. It is a potent capillary poison; although all capillary beds may be involved, the splanchnic area is the most commonly affected. Capillary damage and dilatation result in transudation of plasma into the intestinal tract and sharply reduced blood volume. Blood pressure usually falls to the point of shock, and cardiac muscle becomes weakened; this contributes to circulatory failure. The capillary transudation of plasma results in the formation of vesicles and edema of the gastrointestinal mucosa, which eventually lead to epithelial sloughing and discharge of the plasma into the gastrointestinal tract.[656]

Toxic arsenic nephrosis is more commonly seen in small animals and man than in farm animals.[115,148] Glomerular capillaries dilate, allowing the escape of plasma; this results in swelling and tubular degeneration. The anhydremia that results from the loss of fluid through other capillary beds and the low blood pressure contribute to the oliguria that is characteristic of arsenic poisoning. The urine usually contains protein, red blood cells, and casts.[115]

After percutaneous exposure, capillary dilatation and degeneration may result in blistering and edema, after which the skin may become dry and papery. The skin may then crack and bleed, providing a choice site for secondary invaders.[656]

Most textbooks report that arsenic is accumulated in the tissues and slowly excreted, but this appears to be true only in rats. Most species of livestock and pet animals apparently excrete arsenic rapidly. This phenomenon is very important when one considers arsenic content of tissues as a means of confirming suspected poisoning. Experience with field cases in the Veterinary Diagnostic Laboratory, Iowa State University, has indicated that, if an animal lives several days after consuming a "toxic" amount of arsenic, the liver and kidney tissues may contain less arsenic than is ordinarily considered diagnostic of arsenic poisoning.[110,112] Other authors have reported similar findings.[564]

Signs and Lesions of Toxicosis

Peracute and acute episodes of poisoning by inorganic and aliphatic organic arsenicals are usually explosive, with high morbidity and mortality over a 2- to 3-day period. The poisoning produces intense abdominal pain, staggering gait, extreme weakness, trembling, salivation, vomiting (in dogs, cats, pigs, and perhaps even cattle), diarrhea, fast feeble pulse, prostration, ruminal atony, normal to subnormal temperature, collapse, and death.[115,656]

In subacute arsenic poisoning, animals may live for several days and show depression, anorexia, watery diarrhea, increased urination followed by anuria, dehydration, thirst, partial paralysis of the rear limbs, trembling, stupor, coldness of extremities, and subnormal temperature. The stools may contain shreds of intestinal mucosa and blood. Convulsive seizures are not usual. Poisoning resulting from arsenical dips usually results in some of the signs noted previously, in addition to blistering and edema of the skin, followed by cracking and bleeding with associated secondary infection.[656]

Characteristic gross lesions associated with inorganic and aliphatic organic arsenic poisoning include localized or general reddening of the gastric mucosa (abomasum in ruminants), reddening of the small intestinal mucosa (often limited to the first few feet of the duodenum), fluid gastrointestinal contents (sometimes foul-smelling), a soft yellow liver, and red edematous lungs. Occasionally, in peracute poisoning, no gross changes are noted postmortem. The inflammation is usually followed by edema, rupture of the blood vessels, and necrosis of the mucosa and submucosa. The necrosis sometimes progresses to perforation of the stomach or intestine. The gastrointestinal contents may include blood and shreds of mucosa. There may occasionally be hemorrhages on all surfaces of the heart and on the peritoneum.[153]

Histopathologic changes include edema of the gastrointestinal mucosa and submucosa, necrosis and sloughing of mucosal epithelium, renal tubular degeneration, hepatic fatty changes and necrosis, and capillary degeneration in vascular beds of the gastrointestinal tract, skin, and other organs. In cases involving cutaneous exposure, a dry, cracked, leathery, peeling skin may be prominent.[656]

Diagnostic Criteria

In peracute, acute, and subacute poisoning, arsenic tends to be concentrated in the liver and kidneys. Normal animals usually have a concentration of arsenic in these tissues of less than 0.5 ppm (wet-weight basis). In animals that are dying of acute or subacute arsenic poisoning, the concentration may be 2–100 ppm in these organs, usually higher in the kidneys than the liver. A concentration above 10 ppm would confirm arsenic poisoning.[115] The urine of poisoned animals often contains protein, red blood cells, and casts. The arsenic content of the urine varies with the form of arsenic, the route of exposure, and the species and usually ranges from 2 to 100 mg/liter.[115]

Whenever an episode of illness is characterized by rapid onset and gastroenteritis, with only minor signs of central nervous system involvement, and results in weakness, prostration, and rapid death, inorganic or aliphatic organic arsenic poisoning should be considered. The diagnosis is substantiated by the finding of excessive fluid in the gastrointestinal tract with inflammation and necrosis of the gastrointestinal mucosa. Liver, kidney, stomach and intestinal contents, and urine should be obtained for arsenic analysis. A modified Gutzeit method has worked well in one laboratory;[112] it involves the digestion of 5 g of wet tissue in nitric–perchloric–sulfuric acid or air oxidation in the presence of magnesium oxide in a muffle oven and the use of an arsine generator and a silver diethyldithiocarbamate arsenic-sensitive color reagent.

In acute poisoning, renal tissue and often hepatic tissue may contain arsenic at more than 10 ppm (wet-weight basis). If several days have elapsed since exposure, however, the liver tissue may contain only 2–4 ppm, whereas the kidney tissue may have a diagnostically significant concentration.[115,335] The concentration of arsenic in gastrointestinal contents and urine will also aid in determining the route and degree of exposure.

Diseases often confused with arsenic poisoning, especially in ruminants, include hypomagnesemia (grass tetany), urea poisoning, organophosphorus-insecticide poisoning, bovine viral diarrhea (mucosal disease complex), and poisoning from plants containing nitrates, cyanide, oxalates, selenium, or alkaloids. Lead poisoning in bovines sometimes results in sudden death and could be confused with arsenic poisoning. However, central nervous system signs—such as blindness, circling, depression, and convulsive seizures—are more prominent in lead poisoning.[115]

Conditions that may be easily confused with arsenic poisoning in dogs and cats include heavy-metal intoxications (thallium, mercury, and lead) and ethylene glycol poisoning. Arsenic poisoning is considerably more acute than the syndromes associated with heavy metals. Enteric infections that cause vomiting, diarrhea, and collapse can also resemble arsenic poisoning.

Therapeutic Measures

The key to successful treatment of inorganic and aliphatic organic arsenic poisoning is early diagnosis. Even so, the prognosis should be heavily guarded.

In ruminants and horses, which do not vomit readily, large doses of saline purgative may be given in an attempt to remove the unabsorbed material from the gastrointestinal tract. Demulcents may be given to coat the irritated gastrointestinal mucous membrane. Sodium thiosulfate should be given orally and intravenously: adult horses and cattle, 20–30 g orally in approximately 300 ml of water and 8–10 g in the form of a 10–20% solution intravenously; and sheep and goats, about one-fourth of those amounts. British antilewisite is a sulfhydryl-containing specific antidote for trivalent arsenic. Its value as a therapeutic agent for arsenic poisoning in large animals is questionable. Therapeutic results with this compound in large animals have been disappointing, perhaps because veterinarians have not repeated the treatment every 4 h for the first 2 days, four times on the third day, and twice a day for the next 10 days until recovery is complete, as has been recommended. Five-percent BAL is added to a 10% solution of benzyl-benzoate in arachis oil and given at 3 mg/kg of body weight.[153] It is important to give supportive therapy, such as electrolytes to replace body fluids, and to provide plenty of drinking water.

In small animals, if there is an opportunity for early treatment, the stomach should be emptied before the arsenic can pass into the intestine and be absorbed. Gastric lavage with warm water or a 1% solution of sodium bicarbonate is preferred, although such emetics as apomorphine may be used early in the treatment. When signs of arsenic poisoning are already present, gastric lavages or emetics should not be used. BAL should be given intramuscularly at 6–7 mg/kg of body weight three times a day until recovery. Fluids should be administered parenterally to rehydrate animals that have been vomiting or have had diarrhea. If uremia has developed, lactated Ringer's solution should be used; B-complex vitamins may be added to the Ringer's solution. After rehydration, 10% dextrose solution should be administered at 20 ml/kg of body weight; this should result in diuresis. The urinary bladder should be catheterized to determine the rate of urine flow. If flow increases considerably after the administration of 10% dextrose and the urine contains considerable sugar, the uremia may be controlled by administering lactated Ringer's solution and 5–10% dextrose alternately. If acidosis is present, 50% sodium lactate may be added to the lactated Ringer's solution at 2.5–5.0 ml/liter. Protein hydrolysates may be added to supply amino acids, but they must be given slowly to avoid inducing more vomiting. B-complex vitamins should be injected daily, and whole blood should be transfused if indicated by the occurrence of anemia or shock. There should be no effort to administer drugs or food orally during the period when the animal is vomiting. When emesis has stopped, kaolin–pectin preparations can be given orally to aid in controlling diarrhea. Antibiotics are indicated to prevent secondary infections, and meperidine should be given as needed to lessen abdominal pain. As improvement occurs, a high-protein low-residue diet should be fed, and other supportive therapy discontinued.[487]

Phenylarsonic Feed Additives

Organic arsenical formulations have been used as feed additives for disease control and improvement of weight gain in swine and poultry since the mid-1940's. These compounds are phenylarsonic acids—arsanilic acid, 3-nitro-4-hydroxyphenylarsonic acid, 4-nitrophenylarsonic acid, and 4-ureidophenylarsonic acid—and their salts. The most widely used compounds are arsanilic acid; its sodium salt, sodium arsanilate; and 3-nitro-4-hydroxyphenylarsonic acid.[51,587] The additives are considered to improve weight gain and feed efficiency and to aid in the prevention and control of some enteric diseases of swine and poultry.[76,114,268,558,559]

There is still considerable discussion regarding the mode of action of the organic arsenicals. However, it seems certain that the phenylarsonic compounds have an action different from that of inorganic and aliphatic organic arsenicals. The arsenic incorporated in the additives is in the pentavalent form, and it is likely that they have their primary action as pentavalent arsenicals, which may account for their characteristic rapid renal excretion.

There have been several theories as to the possible therapeutic and nutritional effects of phenylarsonic feed additives. First, it is known that some organisms cause a thickening of the intestinal wall; thus, the additives may inhibit these organisms by interfering with their enzyme systems, which would result in a thinner intestinal wall and better nutrient absorption. A second theory is that the additives, by interfering with the development of the bacterial cell wall or by inhibiting normal cellular production of proteins and nucleic acids, lower the harmful bacterial population. A third possibility is that these compounds have a sparing action on one or more of the nutrients required by growing animals.[51]

Some workers have suggested that both the toxicity and the efficacy of these compounds are due to their degradation and reduction to inorganic trivalent forms.[227,333,334,825] Eagle and Doak[227] reported that arsenoso compounds have direct activity, whereas arsonic acid compounds become active when they are converted to arsenoso compounds. Other research, however, clearly established that arsanilic acid and acetylarsanilic acid (4-acetylaminophenylarsonic acid) were excreted unchanged by chickens and that there is no evidence that these compounds are changed to any others or converted to inorganic arsenic.[183,555,613,614,616] Similar results were obtained in studies with 3-nitro-4-hydroxyphenylarsonic acid and 4-nitrophenylarsonic acid in chickens. Similar experiments by other workers with rats, rabbits, and swine indicated that the phenylarsonic acids for the most part are excreted unchanged by the kidneys, although some apparently undergo a limited amount of biotransformation.[556,557]

Because pentavalent arsenic compounds do not react readily with sulfhydryl groups and the phenylarsonic acids are apparently excreted unchanged, one must conclude that the mechanism of their action is something other than interaction with sulfhydryl-containing enzymes and proteins. The predominant lesions produced by these compounds in swine and poultry are peripheral nerve demyelination and gliosis, and it has been postulated that the phenylarsonic acids act to produce a vitamin B-complex deficiency, such as a deficiency of vitamin B_6 or B_1.[115] This postulation has not been studied experimentally.

When the phenylarsonic compounds are injected parenterally, they are mostly excreted in the urine within 24–48 h. When they are given orally, a considerable percentage is excreted in the feces. This indicates that they are poorly absorbed by the intestinal tract. The propor-

Biologic Effects of Arsenic on Plants and Animals

tion that is absorbed, however, apparently is excreted rapidly by the kidneys.[51,555-557,614]

Recommended Uses and Factors Affecting Toxicity

The registered uses of the phenylarsonic acid feed additives are listed in Table 5-3. Arsanilic acid and sodium arsanilate are recommended at 50–100 ppm (0.005–0.01%) in swine and poultry feeds for improving weight gain and feed efficiency and for other uses. They are recommended at 250–400 ppm (0.025–0.04%) in swine feed for 5–6 days for the control of dysentery. The margin of safety for arsanilic acid and its

TABLE 5-3 Arsenic Compounds Used as Feed Additives[a]

Compound	Concentration in Complete Feed, %	Species	Purpose
Arsanilic acid or sodium arsanilate	0.005–0.01	Chickens (broilers)	Increase growth rate and feed efficiency
		Growing turkeys	Improve pigmentation
		Laying hens	Improve egg production
		Swine	Increase growth rate and feed efficiency; prevent dysentery
	0.025–0.04	Chickens (up to 8 days)	Prevent coccidiosis
		Swine (5–6 days)	Control dysentery
3-Nitro-4-hydroxy-phenylarsonic acid	0.0025–0.005	Chickens and turkeys	Increase growth rate and feed efficiency
	0.0025–0.0075	Swine	Increase growth rate and feed efficiency
	0.02	Swine (5–6 days)	Control dysentery
4-Nitrophenyl-arsonic acid	0.01875	Growing turkeys and chickens	Prevent blackhead
4-Ureidophenyl-arsonic acid	0.0375	Growing turkeys	Prevent blackhead and increase growth rate

[a] Derived from the *Feed Additive Compendium*, 1975.[587]

salt is wide in normal animals.[269] However, the effective concentration and the chronic-toxicity concentration may impinge on one another under some conditions. The health of the exposed animals and management practices, especially those involving availability of water, are important contributing factors for adverse reactions to organic arsenical feed additives. Animals with diarrhea are usually dehydrated and thus are excreting very little urine. Because these arsenicals are excreted via the kidneys, their toxicity is greatly increased when they are given to animals with diarrhea. The morbidity is usually high, and the mortality very low. Experimentally, clinical signs appear after 3–10 days of exposure to high concentrations in the feed (e.g., 1,000 ppm) and within 3–6 weeks at lower concentrations (e.g., 250 ppm).[115]

The maximal safe dietary concentration of arsanilic acid for young turkeys (up to 28 days old) was reported to be between 300 and 400 ppm (0.03 and 0.04%).[12]

Roxarsone, 3-nitro-4-hydroxyphenylarsonic acid, is recommended at 25–50 ppm (0.0025–0.005%) for chickens and turkeys and at 25–75 ppm (0.0025–0.0075%) for swine for improving weight gain and feed efficiency. It is also recommended at 200 ppm (0.02%) for 5–6 days for the control of dysentery.[587] Swine may exhibit clinical signs after consuming 250 ppm in the feed for 3–10 days and have been chronically poisoned by a concentration of 100 ppm for 2 months.[112,114]

4-Nitrophenylarsonic acid has been recommended for chickens and turkeys at 188 ppm for prevention of blackhead. It has not been recommended for ducks or geese and has only limited use as a feed additive.

Carbarsone p-ureidophenylarsonic acid) is recommended for the prevention of blackhead in turkeys and increased growth rate at 375 ppm in the feed.

Arsanilic acid and sodium arsanilate are most commonly used as swine feed additives. Toxicoses may occur, however, with any of the phenylarsonics in any of the species. The circumstances usually associated with toxicoses related to the organic arsenicals used as feed additives include:

- Purposeful incorporation of excessive amounts in feed or water.[458]
- Mistaken feed formulation resulting in excessive amounts in feed.
- Prolonged and excessive administration in combination with other drugs.
- Treatment of animals with severe diarrhea and debilitation, which have increased susceptibility because of reduced renal excretion of the arsenical.

Biologic Effects of Arsenic on Plants and Animals

• Limiting of the water available to animals being exposed to therapeutic concentrations of organic arsenicals.[115,830]

Poisoning by organic arsenicals in swine is not uncommon and probably is second in frequency only to water-deprivation–sodium-ion-toxicosis syndrome.[458]

Signs and Lesions of Toxicosis

Acute clinical signs may appear after 3–5 days of exposure to high concentrations of phenylarsonic compounds in the feed. Signs include incoordination, inability to control body and limb movements, and ataxia. After a few days, swine and poultry may become paralyzed, but will continue to eat and drink (Figure 5–4). Arsanilic acid and sodium arsanilate may produce blindness, but this is rarely seen with 3-nitro-4-hydroxyphenylarsonic acid toxicosis. Erythema of the skin, especially in white animals, and sensitivity to sunlight may also be observed. The clinical signs are reversible up to a point. Removing the excess arsenical will result in recovery within a few days, unless the

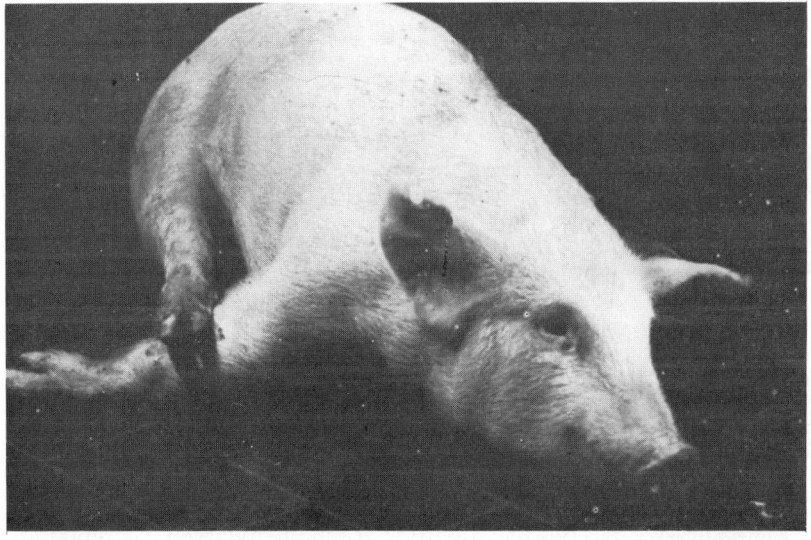

FIGURE 5-4 Pig with quadriplegia after 18 days of feeding arsanilic acid at 900 g/ton (992 g/tonne). Reprinted by courtesy of Marcel Dekker, Inc., from Ledet et al.[459 (p. 443)]

clinical signs have progressed to partial or complete paralysis resulting from irreversible peripheral nerve degeneration.[115,598]

Chronic poisoning occurs in swine and poultry when excessive but lower concentrations of phenylarsonic compounds are given in the feed or water for more than a few weeks. Animals will continue to eat and drink and remain alert while progressively developing blindness and partial paralysis of the extremities. The onset of signs is usually insidious and therefore not alarming to the herdsman. Goose-stepping, knuckling of the hock joints, and other manifestations of abnormal locomotion occur. Such animals usually have poor weight gain and feed efficiency.

Poultry usually become incoordinated and ataxic after consuming excessive concentrations of 3-nitro-4-hydroxyphenylarsonic acid, but more commonly exhibit ruffled feathers, anorexia, depression, coma, and death when exposed to excessive concentrations of arsanilic acid or sodium arsanilate.[112,114,539]

Postmortem findings in swine and poultry affected by organic arsenicals include no gross changes, except skin erythema in white pigs and muscle atrophy in chronic cases.[112,114,326] Harding et al.[326] reported abnormal distention of the urinary bladders in pigs poisoned by arsanilic acid.

Detectable histopathologic changes in swine are confined to the optic tracts, optic nerves, and peripheral nerves. Major lesions noted are necrosis of myelin-supporting cells, degeneration of myelin sheaths and axons, and gliosis of affected tracts (Figures 5–5 through 5–7). Damage is first seen after about 6–10 days of feeding on excessive arsenical and is characterized by fragmentation of the myelin into granules and globules and, several days later, by breaking up of the axons. There is an obvious increase in the severity of the lesions with the progression of the toxic syndrome. No microscopic changes are seen in the brain, cord, kidneys, liver, or other organ systems.[326,458,459]

Excretion and Recommended Withdrawal Time

In general, phenylarsonic compounds are rapidly excreted by the urinary system in domestic animals and poultry. Once they are absorbed from the gastrointestinal tract, 50–75% of the material is excreted within 24 h. Excretion of the remaining 25% is much slower and may take 8–10 days.[125,458,555–557] Although nervous tissue tends to accumulate relatively small amounts of the phenylarsonic compounds, their excretion rate from this tissue appears to be relatively low, less than 50% excretion 11 days after withdrawal.[458]

Biologic Effects of Arsenic on Plants and Animals 155

Ledet et al.[459] measured arsenic contents of various organs from swine after their consumption of arsanilic acid at 1,000 ppm in the diet (10 times the recommended concentration for continuous feeding for improving weight gain and feed efficiency) for 19 days. The results are presented in Table 5-4.

Evans and Bandemer[237] measured the arsenic content of eggs from hens fed diets containing arsanilic acid at 100 and 200 ppm for 10 weeks and found concentrations below the tolerance, established by the FDA, of 0.5 ppm.

Baron[51] reported on the accumulation and depletion of arsenic in tissues of chickens fed a ration containing 3-nitro-4-hydroxyphenyl-arsonic acid at 50 ppm (0.005%). Medication was started when the chickens were 4 weeks old, and the birds were killed at 1, 2, 3, 4, 5, 7, 9, 11, 14, 28, 56, and 70 days of medication and on day 1–14 after withdrawal of medication. Five birds of each sex from both the medicated and nonmedicated groups were killed on the days indicated. The arsenic concentrations found in kidneys, liver, muscle, and skin are presented in Table 5-5.

FDA regulations require that all labels of feeds containing any of the phenylarsonic compounds include a warning that such feed must be withdrawn from swine and poultry 5 days before slaughter. Elemental

TABLE 5-4 Arsenic in Swine Organs after Consumption of Arsanilic Acid[a]

Tissue	Elemental Arsenic (wet wt), ppm after withdrawal[b]				
	Control	0 Days	3 Days	6 Days	11 Days
Kidney	<0.02	8.33	2.90	2.24	1.90
Liver	<0.02	9.67	3.10	1.65	1.75
Muscle	[c]	0.92	0.29	0.29	0.31
Blood	<0.02	1.94	0.25	0.19	0.45
Rib	[c]	0.46	0.18	0.24	0.08
Peripheral nerve	<0.02	1.57	1.17	1.06	0.61
Spinal cord	<0.02	0.74	0.76	0.80	0.25
Brain stem	<0.02	1.04	0.90	0.91	0.62
Cerebellum	<0.02	1.23	1.58	1.10	0.85
Cerebrum	[c]	0.82	1.09	0.84	0.51

[a]Derived from Ledet et al.[459]
[b]Control, mean of three animals; 0 days, mean of three animals; 3, 6, and 11 days, mean of two animals.
[c]Negative to test.

TABLE 5-5 Arsenic in Chickens Fed Ration Containing 3-Nitro-4-Hydroxyphenylarsonic Acid at 50 ppm[a]

	Arsenic Concentration (wet wt), ppm							
	Medicated Chickens							
	On Medication				Off Medication			Nonmedicated Chickens
Tissue	Day 1	Day 7	Day 56	Day 70	Day 71	Day 75	Day 80	Day 84	
Kidney	0.93	0.76	0.52	0.64	0.22	0.10	0.09	0.08	0.05
Liver	1.31	2.43	1.26	1.26	0.69	0.43	0.32	0.19	0.08
Muscle	0.03	0.07	0.05	0.04	0.03	0.01	0.02	0.02	0.02
Skin	0.05	0.11	0.06	0.05	0.08	0.02	0.03	0.03	0.02

[a]Derived from Baron.[51]

arsenic tolerances of 2.0 ppm for uncooked swine liver and kidney tissues and 0.5 ppm for uncooked pork muscle and edible chicken and turkey tissue and eggs have been set.

Diagnosis of Toxicosis Produced by the Phenylarsonic Acids

Organic arsenical poisoning in swine and poultry can be diagnosed tentatively on the basis of the characteristic signs of wobbly, incoordinated gait and ataxia. Animals and birds that have paralysis of the extremities without central nervous system involvement, that undergo high morbidity with low mortality, that continue to eat and drink if food and water are made available (especially in the case of swine), and that show little or no gross change on postmortem examination should be suspected of having been exposed to excessive concentrations of phenylarsonic compounds.[51] (Figure 5-4 shows the appearance of a pig suffering from arsenic paralysis.)

Concentrations of arsenic in tissue are rarely diagnostic, because the organic arsenicals are excreted without being metabolized by the kidneys. If the animal has not been eating for 3–5 days, the arsenical will for the most part have been excreted from the body and will not be of diagnostic value. If liver and kidney specimens are obtained from animals that have been on feed containing excessive organic arsenical, an arsenic concentration of 3–10 ppm (wet-weight basis) would have diagnostic significance. Blood concentrations of 1–2 ppm would also be diagnostically significant. More important diagnostically is the concentration of organic arsenical in the feed.[112] Arsanilic acid and

3-nitro-4-hydroxyphenylarsonic acid concentrations of 250 and 100 ppm, respectively, should be viewed as significant if such other factors as diarrhea and limited water intake are evident in swine and poultry.

Microscopic examination of longitudinal sections of peripheral and cranial nerves is important in confirming a diagnosis of organic arsenical toxicity in swine and poultry. It should be kept in mind, however, that demyelination and gliosis will not be evident in the optic tract earlier than 10 days after the beginning of exposure, nor will these lesions be evident in sciatic and brachial nerves earlier than 2 weeks after the beginning of exposure[326,458] (see Figures 5-5–5-7).

AQUATIC ORGANISMS

Because arsenic compounds are poisonous to microorganisms and lower aquatic organisms, they have been used in wood preservatives and paints and in pesticides.

Arsenates have a limited use in power-plant cooling towers to control various fungi that attack and cause deterioration of structural wood. However, they are rarely used for this purpose, because of their relatively high toxicity; instead, a "preservative" (which may contain arsenate) is used. It has been suggested that some of the "preservative" may enter the aquatic environment.

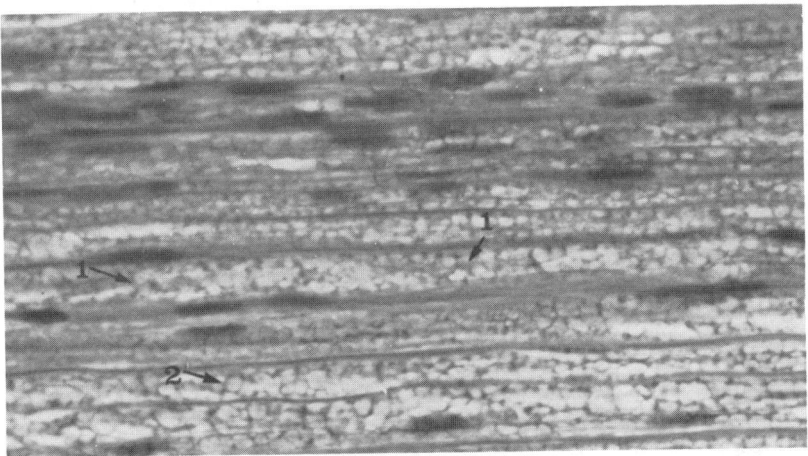

FIGURE 5-5 Sciatic nerve from control pig. An axon appears as a faint gray line between arrows 1. Note darkly stained neurokeratin network, arrow 2. Harris hematoxylin and eosin Y stain. Reprinted by courtesy of Marcel Dekker, Inc., from Ledet et al.[459 (p. 447)]

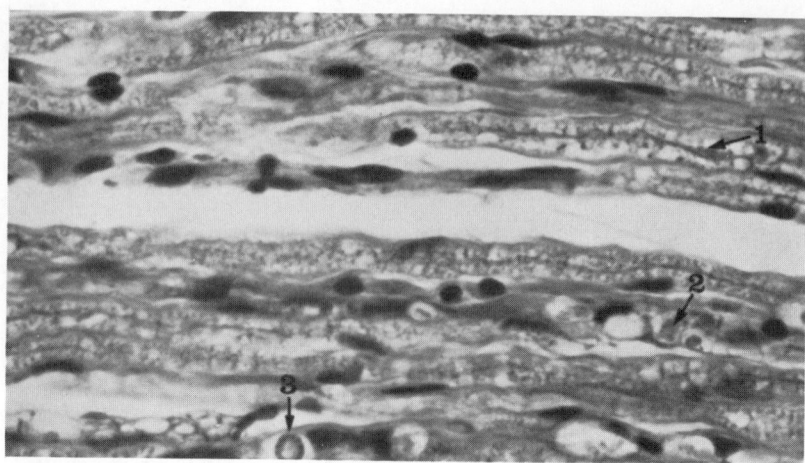

FIGURE 5-6 Sciatic nerve from pig fed arsanilic acid at 900 g/ton (992 g/tonne) for 16 days. Note contraction of myelin around intact axon, arrow 1; myelin fragment, arrow 2; and myelin ovoid, arrow 3. Harris hematoxylin and eosin Y stain. Reprinted by courtesy of Marcel Dekker, Inc., from Ledet et al. [459 (p. 447)]

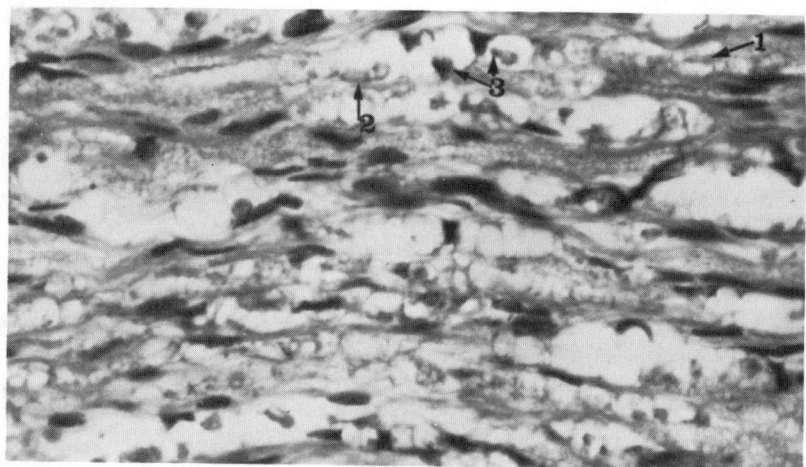

FIGURE 5-7 Sciatic nerve from pig fed arsanilic acid at 900 g/ton (992 g/tonne) for 27 days. Animal had developed quadriplegia. An estimated 60% of the nerve fibers were damaged. Note axon with myelin contracting around it, arrow 1; fragment of myelin, arrow 2; and myelin-containing fragment of axon, arrow 3. Fragmented axon is stained darker than myelin. Harris hematoxylin and eosin Y stain. Reprinted by courtesy of Marcel Dekker, Inc., from Ledet et al. [459 (p. 448)]

Arsenic has been found to be quite toxic to invertebrates and has therefore found application in the control of the shipworm *Bankia setacia* and other wood-borers. It tends to be accumulated by mollusks and may have chronic effects on them.

In addition to the acute toxicity of chemical compounds under controlled laboratory conditions, there is a need to examine pollutants for chronic toxicity. The long-term effects of exposure to sublethal concentrations may be as important as direct lethality, in that such exposure may limit development, growth, reproduction, metabolism, or other physiologic processes. For those who are charged with responsibility for managing the aquatic environment and its renewable resources, it may be important to know the sublethal concentrations of arsenic at which long-term chronic effects become manifest. In estuaries, for example, where migrating anadromous fish tend to linger in order to become acclimatized to changing salinity, the sublethal concentrations of a pollutant could have serious consequences. Although the fish may not be killed, the stress of sublethal concentrations of pollutants may have serious biochemical, physiologic, and behavioral implications. Adult fish migrating upstream may be unable to reach their spawning grounds or may be unable to reproduce for other reasons. Effects of long-term exposure to low concentrations of arsenic singly or in combination with other metals are generally unknown.

Pollutants are rarely found in the environment in isolation. Most laboratory bioassays are conducted on single chemicals under controlled conditions. This provides a simpler toxicologic experiment than do mixtures. It is known, however, that some substances can act synergistically or antagonistically. Arsenic renders selenium less toxic and has been experimentally added to feeds for cattle and poultry in areas high in selenium. The two elements appear to have an antagonistic effect on each other, causing a reduced toxicity. Copper and mercuric salts, however, are each more toxic when in the presence of the other.

Although considerable information has been published on the effects of arsenic on aquatic organisms, most of the research has concentrated on freshwater organisms;[173,348] very little is known about effects on marine organisms. Again, however, most of the data collected have been related to lethality, not sublethal physiologic stress.

In compiling data on the effects of arsenic on aquatic organisms, considerable use was made of two publications, *Water Quality Criteria*[531] and *Toxicity of Power Plant Chemicals to Aquatic Life*.[58] Although it was not possible to review all the original articles covered in those two documents, the information provided can be used to delineate the effects of arsenic on aquatic organisms, particularly fish and shellfish. Toxicity data on arsenic for fish and shellfish are compiled in Table 5-6. The toxicity data given for a particular compound can be highly variable, not only because of different responses by different aquatic organisms, but also because of such other factors as water quality. Among the characteristics of water that can influence the results of bioassays are temperature, pH, dissolved oxygen, conductivity, hardness, oxidation–reduction potential, dissolved chlorides, turbidity, and the presence of potentially toxic ions.

With respect to the lower forms of aquatic life, arsenic concentrations of 3–14 ppm have not harmed mayfly nymphs, and concentrations of 10–20 ppm have been harmless to dragonflies and damselflies.[692]

Surber and Meehan[774] carried out a comprehensive study of the toxicity of arsenic trioxide to many different fish food organisms, and their results indicated that those organisms could tolerate a concentration of 2.0 ppm.

According to Jones,[400] sodium arsenate is not highly toxic to fish. He found that sodium arsenate at 234 ppm, as arsenic, was lethal to minnows at 16–20 C.

Sodium arsenite has been used extensively as an herbicide for the control of mixed submerged aquatic vegetation in freshwater ponds and lakes. Commercial sodium arsenite contains various amounts of other arsenic compounds and impurities and is labeled in terms of equivalent arsenic trioxide. For the control of submerged vegetation in ponds and lakes, applications of 2–5 ppm as arsenic trioxide (1.5–3.8 ppm as arsenic) have been found effective.[455,772,773] These concentrations are generally considered to be safe for fish.

WILDLIFE

The association of arsenic with murder and suicide has made its agricultural and industrial uses particularly controversial. It has often been claimed, for example, that widespread kills of domestic animals, songbirds, and other wildlife were caused by extensive use of arsenicals as pesticides.

It must be borne in mind that the biochemical characteristics of this family of compounds vary considerably. Previous chapters have shown that the term "arsenicals" does not imply a homogeneous group of compounds, but rather a heterogeneous group that have highly individualistic properties and, in particular, greatly varying toxicity. Arsenic is a ubiquitous substance that is commonly found in animal tissues, even when pollution is not suspected. By and large, the organic forms of arsenic are less toxic than the inorganic forms, and the pentavalent compounds are usually less hazardous than trivalent.[475] Unfortunately, most published reports refer to total arsenic concentrations, and not to specific forms of arsenic.

Toxic oral doses of several arsenicals in some common wild species are listed in Table 5-7. Early work on this subject was concerned with the effects of the use of arsenicals in various insecticides. Chappellier and Raucourt[144] reported on extensive studies in France with domestic rabbits, wild rabbits (*Sylvilagus*), hares (*Lepus*), and the gray partridge (*Perdix perdix*) to evaluate the potential hazard of using lead arsenate, copper acetoarsenite, and calcium arsenate to control the potato beetle (*Doryphorus*). The arsenicals were incorporated into starch pellets and given orally to the experimental subjects. The authors noted that the wild hares and domestic rabbits succumbed to similar amounts of the arsenicals, but the former were able to tolerate doses for slightly longer periods—e.g., arsenic at 40 mg/kg as lead arsenate killed the domestic rabbit in about 24 h, compared with 60 h for the hare. These studies showed that the mammals were generally more susceptible to the arsenicals studied than the partridges, which in turn were significantly more sensitive than domestic fowl. Rabbits generally appeared to consider foliage treated with the three arsenicals repugnant and consumed other food if given the choice. The authors concluded that the practice of using these arsenicals to control the potato beetle did not pose a great threat to wildlife.

In a series of toxicity studies, Heath et al.[341] and Hill et al.[353] found that the mallard (*Anas platyrhynchos*) is even more tolerant to arsenicals than gallinaceans, such as quail and pheasants (Table 5-7). These observations are based on 8-day LC_{50} determinations; 2- to 3-week-old animals were fed arsenicals in the diet for 5 days and then given an arsenic-free diet for the remaining 3 days. The order of sensitivity among the several species of birds observed by these workers is bobwhite (*Colinus virginianus*) > Japanese quail (*Coturnix coturnix japonica*) > ring-necked pheasant (*Phasianus colchicus*) > mallard. Earlier reports[810] have shown the mallard to be tolerant to an arsenic dosage of 8 mg/day as sodium arsenite for a period that provided a total dose of 973 mg/kg.

Early work by Chorley and McChlery[149] and VanZyl[820] showed that arsenic-poisoned grasshoppers could be fed to domestic fowl without lethal effect and, in fact, were recommended as a supplement to poultry feed in Rhodesia. These studies were conducted with arsenic

TABLE 5-6 Toxicity of Various Arsenic Compounds to Freshwater and Marine Fish and Shellfish[a]

Compound	Test Organism	Habitat[b]	Test Conditions[c]	Concentration, ppm	Remarks	Reference
p-Sulfamylphenylarsonic acid	Rainbow trout (Salmo gairdneri)	A,F	SB,FW,LS	5.0	No effect, 24 h; 12.8 C	21
	Bluegill (Lepomis macrochirus)	F	SB,FW,LS	5.0	No effect, 24 h; 12.8 C	
p-Sulfophenylarsonic acid	Rainbow trout (Salmo gairdneri)	A,F	SB,FW,LS	5.0	No effect, 24 h; 12.8 C	
	Bluegill (Lepomis macrochirus)	F	SB,FW,LS	5.0	No effect, 24 h; 12.8 C	
Arsenic (form unspecified)	Bluegill (Lepomis macrochirus)	F	FW	15	Toxic	839
	Large-mouth bass (Micropterus salmoides)	F	FW	6.0	Survived 232 h	
				10.0	87% survival	
	Crappie (Pomoxis sp.)	F	FW	15	Toxic	
	Pike perch	—	FW	0.7–1.1	Tolerated, 48 days	538
				1.1–2.2	Lethal in 2 days	
	"Minnow"	—	FW	17.8	Toxic	118
	Carp (Cyprinus carpio)	F	FW	3.1	Toxic, 4–6 days	538
				2.2	Tolerated, 13 days	
	"Eel"	—	FW	3.1	Toxic, 3 days	
				2.2	Tolerated, 13 days	
	"Bleak"	—	FW	2.2	Toxic, 3 days	
				1.1–1.5	Tolerated, 11 days	
Arsenic (form unspecified)	"Fish"	—	FW	0.76	Tolerated	106
Arsenic trioxide	Sea lamprey (Petromyzon marinus), larvae	A	SB,FW,LS	5.0	No effect, 24 h; 12.8 C	21
	Rainbow trout (Salmo gairdneri)	A,F	SB,FW,LS	5.0	No effect, 24 h; 12.8 C	
	Bluegill (Lepomis machrochirus)	F	SB,FW,LS	5.0	No effect, 24 h; 12.8 C	
	Pink salmon (Oncorhynchus gorbuscha)	A	SB,SW,LS	9.5	Initial concentration, total kill in 7 days	361
				2.6–5.3	Indicated tolerance concentration, 10 days of exposure plus obser-	

Compound	Species				Effect	
Sodium arsenate	"Minnow" (*Phoxinus phoxinus*)	F	SB,FW,LS	250	Toxic, 16 h mean; loss of equilibrium	313
	"Minnow"	F	—	234	Lethal, 16–20 C	400
Sodium arsenite	Mud snail (*Nassarius obsoletus*)	S	SW,LS	2	Depressed oxygen consumption in 72 h	504
	"Minnow" (*Phoxinus phoxinus*)	F	SB,FW,LS	20	Toxic, 36 h mean; loss of equilibrium	313
	American oyster (*Crassostrea virginica*), eggs	S	SW,LS	7.5	48-h TLm; 26 C	124
	Spottail shiner (*Notropis hudsonius*)	F	SB,FW,LS	45	25-h TLm; sublethal effects	88
				29	48-h TLm; fin damage, diarrhea, scale damage, and hemorrhaging around fins	
				27	72-h TLm	
	Bluegill (*Lepomis macrochirus*)	F	FW,FS (pond)	4.0	Numbers reduced by 42%; monthly applications	455
	Golden shiner (*Notemigonus crysoleucas*)	F	FW,FS (pond)	4.0	No observed effect	230
	Fathead minnow (*Pimephales promelas*)	F	FW,FS (pond)	4.0	No observed effect	
	Large-mouth bass (*Micropterus salmoides*)	F	FW,FS (pond)	4.0	No observed effect	
	Bluegill (*Lepomis macrochirus*)	F	FW,FS (pond)	4.0	No observed effect	
	Channel catfish (*Ictalurus punctatus*)	F	SB,FW,LS	47.9	24-h TLm; 25 C	154
				25.9	48-, 72-, and 96-h TLm; 25 C	
	Rainbow trout (*Salmo gairdneri*)	A,F	FW	25.6	96-h TLm; 12 C	290
	Bluegill (*Lepomis macrochirus*)	F	FW	35.0	96-h TLm; 12 C	

TABLE 5-6 Continued

Compound	Test Organism	Habitat[b]	Test Conditions[c]	Concentration, ppm	Remarks	Reference
	Goldfish (*Carassius auratus*)	F	FW	34.0	96-h TLm; 12 C	189
	Rainbow trout (*Salmo gairdneri*)	A,F	—	60	48-h TLm; 12.8 C	189
	Bluegill (*Lepomis macrochirus*)	F	—	44	48-h TLm; 23.9 C	189
	Rainbow trout (*Salmo gairdneri*)	A,F	FW,LS	36.5	48-h TLm; 13 C	165
	Bluegill (*Lepomis macrochirus*)	F	FW,LS	44	48-h TLm; 24 C	165
	Bluegill (*Lepomis macrochirus*)	F	SB,FW,LS	0.5	48-h TLm	374
				0.7	24-h TLm	
	Chum salmon (*Oncorhynchus keta*)	A	SB,SW,LS	11.0	48-h TLm	8
	Channel catfish (*Ictalurus punctatus*)	F	FW	15	48- and 72-h TLM	154
				27.6	24-h TLm	
	Rainbow trout (*Salmo gairdneri*)	A,F	FW	20	Lethal or deleterious, 36 h	691
	"Minnow"	—	—	20	Lethal or deleterious, 36 h	
	Rainbow trout (*Salmo gairdneri*)	A,F	SB,FW,LS	5.0	No harmful effects, 24 h; 12.8C	21
	Bluegill (*Lepomis macrochirus*)	F	SB,FW,LS	5.0	No harmful effects, 24 h; 12.8C	
	Sea lamprey (*Petromyzon marinus*), larvae	A	SB,FW,LS	5.0	No harmful effects, 24 h; 12.8C	
	Pink salmon (*Oncorhynchus gorbuscha*)	A	SB,SW,LS	5.0	Initial concentration, 54% kill in 10 days	361
				2.5	Initial concentration, no kill in 10 days	

[a]Most of these data from *Toxicity of Power Plant Chemicals to Aquatic Life.*[58]
[b]A, anadromous; F, freshwater; S, seawater.
[c]SB static bioassay; FW, freshwater; SW, seawater; LS, laboratory study; FS, field study.

TABLE 5-7 Toxic Oral Doses of Some Arsenic Compounds in Wildlife

Compound	Animal	Toxic Dose[a] (as Arsenic)	Comment	Reference
Calcium arsenate	Wild rabbit	23.5 mg/kg	Dead at 3 days	144
	Hare	21.3 mg/kg	Lived	144
Copper acetoarsenite	Wild rabbit	10.5 mg/kg	Dead at 50 h	144
	Hare	10.5 mg/kg	Dead at 74 h	144
	Cowbird	99.8 ppm	50% mortality in 11 days	698
	Bobwhite quail	480 ppm	LC_{50}	341
	Japanese quail	1,204 ppm	LC_{50}	341
	Ring-necked pheasant	1,403 ppm	LC_{50}	341
	Mallard	>5,000 ppm	20% mortality at 5,000 ppm	341
Lead arsenate	Gray partridge	300 mg/kg	Approximate fatal dose	144
	Hare	40.4 mg/kg	Dead at 60 h	144
	Wild rabbit	40.4 mg/kg	Dead at 52 h	144
	Japanese quail	4,185 ppm	LC_{50}	353
	Ring-necked pheasant	4,989 ppm	LC_{50}	353
	Mallard	>5,000 ppm	No mortality	353
Sodium arsenite	White-tailed deer	923 mg	Yearling doe died in 12 h	93
	Mallard	1,000 ppm	50% mortality in 6 days	810
	Mallard	500 ppm	50% mortality in 32 days	810
	Mallard hen	323 mg/kg	LD_{50}	799

[a] mg/kg = dose per unit body weight; ppm = concentration of arsenic in the diet; mg = total dose.

trioxide-poisoned grasshoppers containing arsenic at up to 910 ppm as a dry meal. Lilly[470] fed grasshopper bait containing sodium arsenite or freshly poisoned grasshoppers to ring-necked pheasants without apparent ill effect. One bird consumed over 2,500 poisoned grasshoppers (approximately 8 mg of arsenic) in a 20-day period and, after a 7-day rest period, was sacrificed and analyzed for arsenic (Table 5-8). Little accumulation of arsenic was observed. The author noted that pheasants were reluctant to consume arsenic-containing baits, but readily consumed poisoned grasshoppers. The results indicate that there was little danger to this species from the grasshopper-poisoning activities. Helminen[342] also noted that spraying a potato field with an arsenical insecticide had little effect on pheasants penned on this field.

Several studies conducted by Whitehead[854] (Table 5-9) are questionable, although noteworthy because they are among the few that involved songbirds. Arsenic trioxide was used to poison western grasshoppers (*Melanophis bivittatus, M. femus-rubrum, M. bispinosus*), which were fed to bobwhite quail, mockingbirds (*Mimus polyglottos*), robins (*Turdus migratorious*), meadowlarks (*Sturnella magna*), redwing blackbirds (*Agelaius phoeniceus*), brown thrashers (*Toxostoma rufum*), dickcissels (*Spiza americana*), orchard orioles (*Icterus spurius*), scissortails (*Muscivora forficata*), and English sparrows (*Passer domesticus*). The author noted that, when quail consumed the maximal amount (25 g) of grasshoppers, less than 10% of a toxic dose was ingested; therefore, no detrimental effects were noted. Poisoned grasshoppers were force-fed to the various nestling birds in the wild. Many uncontrollable variables consequently also affected the outcome of these experiments. The results showed that fairly large numbers of poisoned grasshoppers (up to 134, containing a total of about 40 mg of arsenic) could be fed to nestling songbirds without any noticeable toxic effect. About 49% of all the birds fed poisoned grasshoppers in this experiment matured, compared with about 60% of those fed unpoisoned grasshoppers. Because there was great variability in these data, no significant detrimental effects were attributed to the arsenic consumption. Generally, the data indicated that songbirds experienced little danger from the ingestion of this pesticide in the form of poisoned grasshoppers.

Work undertaken at the Patuxent Wildlife Research Center[698] to evaluate the possible dangers of widespread use of copper acetoarsenite for mosquito control, particularly in southern marshes, indicated that there is little hazard when this compound is applied at the recommended rate of 0.75 lb/acre (0.84 kg/ha). Male cowbirds (*Molathrus ater*) were poisoned only when fed copper acetoarsenite at about

225 ppm (arsenic at 100 ppm) in the diet (Table 5-7) for 3 months; similar diets containing copper acetoarsenite at 25 and 75 ppm (arsenic at 11 and 33 ppm) appeared to have no effect on mortality. Arsenic residues (Table 5-8) were determined in birds that had died from consuming diets containing arsenic at 100 ppm (W. H. Stickle, personal communication). Whole-body concentration reached a peak of about 1.7 ppm (dry weight) in yearling male cowbirds after about 6 months of feeding arsenic at 11 ppm in the diet and thereafter appeared to level off. Birds given arsenic at 33 ppm reached a maximal whole-body concentration of about 6.6 ppm for the same period. Whole-body arsenic content continued to rise at this dose, reaching 8.6 ppm at 7 months. The latter concentration approaches toxicity.

The herbicidal properties of arsenic made its use as a tree-debarker an important factor in the northeastern U.S. wood pulp industry in the 1940's and 1950's. Cook[162] reported two cases in New York in which about 10 white-tailed deer (*Odocoileus virginianus*) consumed fatal amounts of sodium arsenite that was used to debark pulp trees. Field studies by Boyce and Verme[93] showed that 923–2,770 mg of arsenic (as sodium arsenite) was lethal to deer when licked from the bark of treated trees. No body weights were given, but, if we assume that one of the poisoned deer (a yearling doe) weighed about 27 kg, then we can calculate a minimal lethal dose of about 34 mg/kg. In a study to determine the palatability or acceptability of sodium arsenite, potassium arsenite, and ammonium arsenite to deer, the authors recorded the number of licks that the test deer made on trees coated with solutions of these compounds. They observed that sodium arsenite was as palatable as sodium chloride, whereas potassium arsenite was significantly less palatable, and ammonium arsenite was the least acceptable to the deer. The authors also report that wildlife kills from arsenic poisoning in Michigan's upper peninsula in 1952 amounted to five deer, four porcupines, and one rabbit on about 200 acres (81 ha) of commercially treated trees. In 1953 and 1954, apparently, only one wildlife mortality was found in over 5,000 acres, or 2,023 ha (which contained over 500 acres, or 202 ha, of treated trees), in lower Michigan. The practice of debarking trees with arsenicals for commercial use has been almost completely replaced by mechanical debarking equipment.

A well-documented report of a wildlife killoff attributable to arsenic was made by Swiggart *et al.*[776] They reported the poisoning of 23 white-tailed deer in Tennessee by the apparent misuse of arsenic acid as an herbicide to control Johnsongrass. The herbicide (USDA Reg. 295-6) was labeled for use in controlling crabgrass and Dallisgrass on

Bermuda-grass lawns and was applied to a 600-acre (243-ha) field in preparation for planting soybeans. A 5-gal mixture containing 0.5 gal of arsenic acid was applied per acre (0.05 m^3 of mixture containing 0.005 m^3 of arsenic acid per hectare). The dead deer were all found on the 600-acre field and appeared to have died on the same day. Apparently, the toxicity of this herbicide dissipated in a few days, inasmuch as no further mortalities were recorded. Autopsies showed that the deer died of massive hemorrhagic gastroenteritis. Analyses performed by the EPA Toxicology Laboratory showed that surface soil samples contained arsenic at up to 2.4 ppm, whereas water samples from the area averaged 0.42 ppm. Arsenic concentrations in the dead deer are shown in Table 5-8. It is interesting that the farmer and cropduster using the pesticide in this case were both taken to court by the Tennessee Health Department and sued for damages. In an apparently unprecedented decision, the defendants were made to pay for the poisoned deer—$109/head, the amount needed to transport new deer into the area (W. D. Turner, personal communication).

In March 1974, another deer kill involving at least two white-tailed deer was discovered in southwest Memphis and Shelby County, Tennessee, by R. C. Swiggart and W. D. Turner (personal communication). Although these deer were found in an area that had been treated with a cotton defoliant in the fall of 1973, the probable cause of death was determined to be the contamination of the water in a runoff ditch with MSMA. Several empty MSMA drums were found in the ditch, and mixing apparatus was nearby. Tissue analyses of these deer (Table 5-8) showed what are considered toxic concentrations of arsenic. This is in agreement with the studies of Dickinson,[176] who showed that the concentrations of arsenic in the livers of cattle fed toxic doses of MSMA were less than half those found in these dead deer. Analyses for chlorinated pesticides and other heavy metals were performed, but none were present in apparently toxic concentrations. As a point of perspective, these deer were found on land cultivated by the same farmer referred to by Swiggart et al.[776] Although both reports can be related to misuse of arsenicals, the Swiggart et al. report appears to refer to an instance in which wildlife died from consuming contaminated herbage. It is therefore in contrast with other reports cited here that indicated little hazard from the extensive use of some arsenic compounds. This is probably because of the varying toxicity of the numerous arsenicals, as well as the saturation effects of spraying huge acreages with arsenicals and leaving little untreated foliage for the local wildlife population to consume.

Little information is available on background or environmental concentrations of arsenic in various wild species. Bencko et al.,[64] however, stated that rabbits reproduced normally when exposed to air from a plant that discharged large amounts of arsenic for up to 12 months. They observed significant although apparently nontoxic accumulations of arsenic in the kidneys, hair, and nails of rabbits exposed for 9 and 12 months. Martin and Nickerson[524] monitored starlings (*Sturnus vulgaris*) from 50 sites in the United States during 1971; except for one sample in Michigan, all contained arsenic (whole body) at 0.04 ppm or less (Table 5-8). Similarly, Stickle (personal communication) found that trapped yearling male cowbirds not exposed to arsenic had brain, liver, kidney, muscle, and feather-skin concentrations of less than 0.78, less than 0.41, less than 1.48, less than 0.19, and 0.13 ppm, respectively.

Andren et al.[17] have monitored the ecosystem of the Walker Branch watershed in Tennessee for a number of trace elements, including arsenic. Unfortunately, arsenic was determined by spark-source mass spectrometry with a method that is only about 50% accurate. The quantitative validity of these data are therefore questionable, but the trends observed are worth noting. Such animals as earthworms (19 ppm) and cryptozoa (100 ppm), which are close to the soil surface and tree roots (11 ppm), contained high concentrations of arsenic. Similarly, tree-canopy insects also had high arsenic contents (10 ppm). Arsenic was the only element studied, however, that showed any decline in concentration with higher trophic levels. For example, fieldmice contained arsenic at 1 ppm of the whole body, but owls, which consume large quantities of mice, contained only 0.05 ppm (Table 5-8). It is noteworthy that the hawk sample contained 8 times as much arsenic as the owl, although one would expect that they consumed similar diets.

In 1969, a large dieoff of common auks—guillemots (*Uria allge*), razorbills (*Alca torda*), and puffins (*Fratercula arctica*)—was observed in the Irish Sea. Because the populations of these species of seabirds have been declining in recent years, an extensive study[360] of this dieoff was undertaken by the Natural Environment Research Council of Britain. These birds congregate in large groups in open water and spend most of the year at sea, except during March and April, when they gather at breeding grounds. It is significant that the killoff occurred in the late summer and early fall, when the birds are flightless because of molting. The dieoff period began in late July and ended in mid-October, when a total count of over 12,000 dead birds was recorded. Most of the dead and dying birds were washed ashore by storms, and nearly all the birds were severely emaciated. Although

TABLE 5-8 Tissue Arsenic Concentrations in Some Wildlife Species

Compound	Species	Tissue	Arsenic Concentration (wet wt), ppm	Comment	Reference
Copper acetoarsenite	Cowbird	Brain	6.1^a	Lethal	b
		Liver	40.6^a	Lethal	
		Kidney	22.8^a	Lethal	
		Muscle	19.0^a	Lethal	
		Skin	13.4^a	Lethal	
Sodium arsenite	Ring-neck pheasant	Cecum	0.42	No toxic effect	470
		Excreta	92.5	No toxic effect	
		Heart	0.37	No toxic effect	
		Gizzard	0.70	No toxic effect	
		Muscle	0.07	No toxic effect	
	White-tailed deer	Liver	40.0	Lethal	93
Arsenic acid	White-tailed deer	Liver	18.96	Found dead	776
		Kidney	17.78	Found dead	
		Rumen contents	22.50	Found dead	
MSMA	White-tailed deer	Liver	58.8	Found dead	c
		Kidney	63.0	Found dead	
		Rumen contents	332.0	Found dead	

Guillemots (murre)		Liver	7.1	Found dead	360
		Kidney	2.6	Found dead	
		Lung	0.62	Found dead	
		Liver	5.6	Shot	
		Kidney	0.3	Shot	
	Puffin	Liver	3.7	Shot	[d]
Unknown	Squirrel	Whole body	0.8[a]	Captured in wild	17
	Sparrow	Whole body	0.2[a]	Captured in wild	17
	Mouse	Whole body	1.0[a]	Captured in wild	17
	Hawk	Whole body	0.4[a]	Captured in wild	17
	Owl	Whole body	0.05[a]	Captured in wild	17
	Fox	Whole body	0.80[a]	Captured in wild	17
	Crow	Whole body	0.10[a]	Captured in wild	17
	Opossum	Whole body	0.20[a]	Captured in wild	17

[a] As dry weight.
[b] Personal communication, W. H. Stickle, USDI Fish and Wildlife Service, Patuxent Wildlife Research Center, Laurel, Maryland 20810.
[c] Personal communication, R. C. Swiggart and W. D. Turner, Tennessee Pesticide Study Project—EPA, Memphis and Shelby County Health Department, Memphis, Tennessee 38105.
[d] Personal communication, J. L. F. Parslow, Toxic Chemicals and Wildlife Section, Monks Wood Experiment Station, Abbots Ripton, Huntingdon PE 172LS, England.

TABLE 5-9 Results of Feeding Arsenic Trioxide-Poisoned Grasshoppers to Wild Birds[a]

Species	Arsenic Total Dose, mg	Comment
Bobwhite quail	141	No effect observed
Mockingbird (nestling)	27.2	Matured
Robin (nestling)	40	Matured
Meadowlark (nestling)	17.2	Matured
Redwing blackbird (nestling)	13.8	Matured
Brown thrasher (nestling)	5.7	Died
Dickcissel (nestling)	10	Matured
Orchard oriole (nestling)	10.9	Matured
Scissortail (nestling)	12.2	Matured
English sparrow (nestling)	10	Matured

[a]Derived from Whitehead.[854]

extensive pathologic, microbiologic, and chemical testing was conducted, no conclusive explanation for the deaths was determined. The arsenic content of livers from 36 guillemots ranged from less than 0.1 to 41 ppm (dry basis), with an average of 7.1 ppm. Of the 36 samples, only five contained arsenic at more than 10 ppm. Furthermore, apparently healthy birds shot in the same area were found to contain arsenic at 0.7–20 ppm (average, 5.6 ppm) in their livers. These data are similar to those obtained on the birds in the dieoff and do not indicate that arsenic was directly involved in this instance.

6

Biologic Effects of Arsenic on Man

TOXICITY

The medicinal use of arsenic, although practiced for hundreds of years, apparently reached a peak in the middle to late 1800's and was a major mainstay in the limited medical armamentarium of the time.[815] Fowler's solution, containing arsenic trioxide at 10 mg/ml (arsenic at about 7.6 mg/ml), was prescribed for symptomatic relief of many conditions, ranging from acute infections (although the germ theory of disease was not widely accepted until the time of Pasteur, 1822–1895, and Koch, 1843–1910) to epilepsy, asthma, and chronic, recurring skin eruptions, such as psoriasis and eczema. Thus, many patients received arsenic for periods of months and years. It was in such patients that the consequences of long-term administration of arsenic were first recognized to be palmar and plantar hyperkeratoses, characteristic pigmentary changes on the trunk, and a variety of cancerous and precancerous lesions on the hands, feet, and trunk. There was, in fact, some initial confusion: psoriasis was, for a while, mistakenly thought to be a precancerous condition.[331,852] Neubauer has provided an extensive review of these matters.[585]

The therapeutic usefulness of arsenic is apparently such that it has not been easily abandoned by the medical profession. Some justifications for its use were cited by Pillsbury et al. in 1956;[645] and a 1972 English text[860] stated that a possible use of Fowler's solution is "in elderly patients with bullous disease when steroids are contra-indicated." Fierz cited patient satisfaction in a large number of patients interviewed, including 55 of 64 with psoriasis.[253]

Although still used, especially in Europe,[253] Fowler's solution has not appeared in the *U.S. Pharmacopoeia* since 1950; arsenic trioxide is listed as a reagent in the eighteenth revision, published in 1970. However, both inorganic and organic arsenic preparations are still manufactured for medical and veterinary use in this country; and there is evidence that some goes to people who find it useful in "tonics" and for a wide variety of symptoms (more than 400 gal, or 1.5 m^3 of Fowler's solution were produced in 1974). In addition to the use of medicinal arsenic, there was, during the nineteenth and early twentieth centuries, widespread use of rat poisons and insecticides that contained arsenic and that left residua on fruits and vegetables.[128] The combination of these two major "reservoirs" appears to have resulted in a relatively high frequency of both deliberate and accidental arsenic poisonings, some of them grotesque, such as the mistaken use of powdered arsenic trioxide for talcum powder, which resulted in the deaths of 17 children.[362] Thus, physicians of the day were simultaneously using arsenic therapeutically and treating the consequences of excessive exposure from environmental sources. As DDT and organic pesticides fall into disfavor, increasing use of arsenicals as pesticides and herbicides may again increase the concentration of arsenic in the general environment. This, in turn, would require a renewed "index of suspicion" by modern physicians for the possibility of arsenic toxicity. Somewhat more recent, but overlapping with the earlier period, has been the involvement of physicians in recognition of and treatment for exposures to arsenic associated with the industrial revolution.

Reactions to Contact with Arsenic

Arsenic was at one time used in disreputable "cancer pastes" for its caustic properties. Causticity is a property of arsenic trioxide, and a greater or lesser degree of skin irritation, particularly in creases and where clothing binds, is the primary symptom in smelter workers or their families exposed to dusts with a high arsenic content.[79,382] A striking consequence of direct contact with the mucous membranes of the nose is perforation of the nasal septum, sometimes occurring after only a week or two of exposure.[79,222,648] Better working conditions, including improved opportunities for personal hygiene, have reduced the incidence of this problem.[382,842]

That topical exposure to arsenic results in local inflammation and vesiculation such as that seen with the war gas lewisite has been of interest to investigators, including those who developed dimercaprol (British antilewisite) at the time of World War II.[333] It is thought that the physical integrity of the epidermis depends on intact pyruvate metabolism and that the sulfhydryl-combining properties of arsenicals inhibit the sulfhydryl-containing enzymes related to this pathway.[334] This hypothesis has not been subjected to analysis by modern dermatologic biochemical techniques.

Besides acting as primary irritants, many arsenicals function as contact allergens, so that very low, noncaustic concentrations may result in either vesiculation or folliculitis in previously sensitized people. Holmqvist studied workers in a large copper-ore smelting facility over a 2-year period and concluded that most of their skin eruptions were based on this mechanism.[365] He noted that, on patch testing, 80% of arsenic workers reacted to concentrations of sodium arsenite, sodium arsenate, and arsenic pentoxide that caused reactions in only 35% of "other" and 30% of new employees. Holmqvist suggested that selection of nonsensitized workers or "hardening" of the skin of those who were allergic functioned to control the incidence of hypersensitivity reactions.[365] His extensive literature review and study of 71 patients did not suggest that any of the late cutaneous sequelae of arsenic ingestion are seen after chronic contact with the material, but no evidence (such as urinary arsenic content) was presented to indicate the extent to which these workers were absorbing arsenic through the skin and mucous membranes into the systemic circulation.

Evidence of systemic absorption of arsenic secondary to external exposure has been repeatedly recorded, usually in the form of increased urinary arsenic content correlated with the work week.[543,633,648,842] Little or no information is available to apply to questions of the quantity of arsenic, its physical and chemical form, and the duration of cutaneous or inhalation exposure required to result in significant systemic effects. It should be noted, however, that evidence of significant systemic concentrations of arsenic has been found in several studies of the incidence of lung cancer in populations exposed to arsenic dusts. The possibility that the effect, if any, of arsenic in this condition operates through a general body mechanism, rather than directly on lung tissue, should not be ignored.

Acute Arsenic Poisoning

Exposure to arsenic sufficient to cause severe acute systemic symptoms requiring prompt medical attention usually occurs through ingestion of contaminated food or drink. The signs and symptoms are somewhat variable in degree and timing and depend on the form and amount of arsenic, the age of the patient, and other unknown factors.[862] The major characteristics of acute arsenic poisoning are profound gastrointestinal damage and cardiac abnormalities.

According to Holland,[362 (p. 408)] symptoms may appear within 8 min if the poison is in solution, but may be delayed up to 10 h if it is solid and taken with a meal. The signs, which are variable, range from excruciating abdominal pain and forceful vomiting to cramps in the legs, restlessness, and spasms. "A feeble, frequent, and irregular pulse ushers in the other symptoms of collapse, the livid and anxious face, sunken eyes [dehydration?], cold and clammy skin [shock?]. . . . A small proportion of the cases are classed as 'nervous' or 'cerebral' because . . . the . . . conspicuous . . . phenomena are . . . prostration, stupor, convulsions, paralysis, collapse, and death in coma." Only a small fraction of patients will develop any kind of skin reaction secondary to acute arsenic poisoning. Presumably, the arsenic must be absorbed from the damaged gut and find its way to the skin. The usual reaction in these circumstances is an acute exfoliative erythroderma, probably reflecting the fact that arsenic is a capillary and epidermal poison.[333,362]

Subacute Arsenic Poisoning

Systemic exposure to amounts of arsenic sufficient to cause symptoms but inadequate to produce systemic collapse is of particular interest. The patient may go for weeks with gradually increasing or variable signs and symptoms related to several organ systems and giving the appearance of a progressive chronic disease state. If death occurs, it may appear to have been the consequence of the inexorable course of an obscure "natural" disease. This appearance has contributed to the popularity of arsenic as an agent of homicide. Skin manifestations of such victims are particularly important, in that they may offer critical clues in the unraveling of a mystery.

The method of arriving at a therapeutic dose of Fowler's solution was based on finding the patient's tolerance to increasing but nontoxic doses. As described by Holland,[362] the patient was given 5 drops (about 9 mg of arsenic trioxide, or 6.8 mg of arsenic) "well diluted, after meals [i.e., three times a day], increasing the dose one drop daily until the disease is under control or until the eyelids puff and the bowels move too freely. . . . The dose is then reduced to a safer quantity, and persisted in until the warning returns, when it is again reduced. . . . Occasionally persons are encountered [in whom] even the minimum dose will produce unpleasant effects," such as one case of erythroderma after 10 mg of arsenic trioxide (7.6 mg of arsenic) taken over a 2-day period.

Holland's descriptions of arsenic poisoning were based on personal observation and reports of suicides and criminal cases in which rat or fly poison, as well as Fowler's solution, had been used.[362] Occasionally, enthusiastic patients would overdo their use of medicinal arsenic, but this was uncommon, because of the associated discomfort. Holland described subacute poisoning as producing loss of appetite, fainting, nausea and some vomiting, dry throat, shooting pains, diarrhea, nervous weakness, tingling of the hands and feet, jaundice, and erythema. Longer exposure resulted in dry, falling hair; brittle, loose nails; eczema; darker skin; exfoliation; and a horny condition of the palms and soles.

In 1901, Reynolds reported on the clinical findings in over 500 patients that he had personally followed.[235] These patients had been drinking for many months 2–16 pints a day of beer contaminated with arsenic. The measured amount of arsenic in the beer was such that "a moderate drinker would only take a tithe of the quantity of arsenic which [would be prescribed for] an epileptic." Therefore, the possible additive role of alcohol to the observed symptoms merited consideration. Reynolds felt that the clinical manifestations were of four distinct "types" based on whether cardiac, skin, or neurologic symptoms predominated or were equally mixed, and he noted that these features and the sequence of their appearance were in accordance with several previously reported episodes of arsenic poisoning.[665]

First to appear were digestive symptoms, especially vomiting and diarrhea, to the extent that some patients gave up drinking beer, because it did not "agree with" them. Most, obviously, did not have so definitive a reason to stop their intake of the poison, and a few were said to have had a stimulation of the appetite.

Catarrhal symptons—conjunctivitis, rhinitis, laryngitis, and bronchitis—appeared in a few weeks, with various skin eruptions. The generalized mucous-membrane symptoms suggested a selective sensitivity of these organs. Hoarseness due to thickening of the vocal cords and hemoptysis were mentioned.

Insidious development of neurologic signs and symptoms began before the appearance of the classical skin lesions, but could be so vague as to go undiagnosed for many weeks. Involvement of the nervous system began with sensory changes, including paresthesias, hyperesthesias, and neuralgias. Marked muscle tenderness was found to be of major diagnostic value. Motor weakness of all degrees, including paralysis with muscle atrophy progressing from distal to proximal groups, was a frequent observation. Mental confusion, especially memory for time and place, was observed; but Reynolds felt that it was less frequent than in straightforward chronic alcoholism and so discounted any effect of arsenic on the cerebral cortex.

Left-side heart failure with severe peripheral edema was observed in one-fourth of the patients, and the 13 deaths in this series were all due to congestive heart failure. It is not clear whether this feature and the muscle tenderness described above were direct effects of arsenic on muscle fibers or secondary to its action on blood capillaries and nerve tissue supplying the affected tissue. Skin changes were present to some extent in all the patients, and a facial edema with an associated dusky red color was so typical that it provided a major clue to the diagnosis on first sight of the patient. The most outstanding problem was erythromelalgia: the patients complained of pain (possibly related to neuritis) combined with redness and swelling of the extremities, particularly the palms and soles. Excessive perspiration was regularly a feature of the painful, hot, red, swollen feet, and patients would not tolerate bedclothes or walking. Various short-lived generalized erythematous eruptions ranging from urticarial to measles-like were followed by slight thickening and darkening of the skin, especially in the folds.

Pigmentation was "generally not present in light-complexioned patients, or merely amounts to a darkening of pre-existing freckles. In darker people it is practically always present in greater or less degree [and] follows . . . the erythematous blush."[665] The distribution of the early stages of the pigmentation was noted to be around scars, the neck, the armpits, the nipples, and, generally more markedly, the trunk; and in some patients, it showed "well-marked lighter spots like 'rain-drops,'" leading to a punctiform or patchy appearance with the patches tending to run together to form a more or less continuous discoloration. A desquamation similar to that seen in scarlet fever might occur, with some lightening of the dark skin.

The familiar arsenical keratoses of the palms and soles were a late manifestation and took several forms: "it may be in a few isolated scaly masses, either thin or very heaped up in marked prominences, [or] the whole palm or sole is thickly covered with large white or dirty grey scales." Reynolds, who watched these processes evolve in his patients, noted that "in cases where there is no pigmentation keratosis may be present and forms a most valuable aid in the diagnosis of a case which might otherwise appear to be merely one of alcoholic paralysis. The process is very slow (many weeks) in its development."[665]

Reynolds also described the nail changes of subacute arsenic poisoning, observable some weeks after the intake of the poison was stopped, permitting normal nail to grow out and thus revealing the "transverse white ridge across the nail; proximal to this the nail is normal, but distal to it the nail is whiter, cracked, thin, and towards the tip almost papery and much flattened. In some cases there have been a series of parallel transverse ridges on the nails almost suggesting a series of week-end 'drinking bouts,'"[665] This feature of arsenic exposure, commonly given the appellation "Mees lines" on the basis of a 1919 description,[537] was also reported by Aldrich,[9] before Mees's report.

Viruses were not known in Reynolds's day, and his observation that 21 of his patients had herpes zoster led him to speculate that arsenic might play a role in the etiology of this condition. Modern recognition that herpes zoster is frequently seen in patients with depressed immunity suggests that the patients in Reynolds's series had had a suppression of their immune capacity. It is interesting to note that arsenic was used therapeutically for asthma, psoriasis, and eczema—conditions that also respond to therapy with a modern immunosuppressant, prednisone (see Harter and Novitch[330]).

Since Reynolds's time, reports of subacute arsenic intoxication have tended to confirm his observations, although none has provided such carefully detailed material on so large a group of affected people. Even acknowledging Reynolds's own misgivings about the contribution of alcohol to the neurologic manifestations and allegations that selenium, not arsenic, could have been at fault,[268] this article still stands as the definitive medical description of subacute poisoning with ingested arsenic.

The likelihood that selenium was also present in variable amounts in the contaminated beer deserves special attention, in view of the many interesting and unresolved questions about relationships between this element and arsenic. Tunnicliffe and Rosenheim[800] made the analyses on which they based their conclusion "that selenium compounds have played a definite rôle in the recent beer-poisoning epidemic." These authors went on to state, however, that this role was "subsidiary to that of arsenic." Willcox[863] evaluated the available tests for arsenic and concluded that "the poisoning could not have been due to selenium primarily and arsenic secondarily." Tunnicliffe's testimony before the

Royal Commission on Arsenical Poisoning[684] reaffirmed the secondary role of selenium in the epidemic, suggesting that cases of atypical wasting and unusually severe neurologic disease may have resulted from excessive selenium. Certainly, repeated testimony before the Commission by various chemists demonstrated repeatedly the presence of toxic amounts of arsenic in beer from several parts of the country.[31,60,428,477,631,683,685,686]

Mizuta *et al.* reported on 220 patients of all ages who had been poisoned by contaminated soy sauce, with an average estimated ingestion of roughly 3 mg of arsenic (probably as calcium arsenate) daily for 2–3 weeks. In this group, 85% had facial edema and anorexia; fewer than 10% were said to have exanthemata, desquamation, and pigmentation; and about 20% had peripheral neuropathy.[550] Except for headaches and fevers, the findings in these patients appear to be very similar to those reported by Reynolds, allowing for the more acute nature of the episode and the natural differences in emphasis between physicians separated by two generations and half the world.

The Japanese report offered additional information based on the availability of modern diagnostic techniques. Thus, although most patients' livers were enlarged, relatively few abnormalities were found in liver function tests; and the description of five liver biopsies was not particularly impressive. (Zachariae *et al.* found no differences between liver biopsies of 44 psoriatic patients with a history of arsenic therapy and 37 similar patients without such history.[888]) Conversely, there were no findings on clinical evaluation of the heart and no evidence of the congestive failure seen in Reynolds's somewhat more chronic patients; but electrocardiograms were abnormal in 16 of 20 patients, confirming the reports of Josephson *et al.*[403] and Nagai *et al.*[574]

It is of interest that the Japanese patients' symptoms tended to diminish after 5 or 6 days, despite continued intake of arsenic, and that neurologic symptoms became prominent as much as 2 weeks after arsenic ingestion was discontinued, at which time urinary arsenic content remained high. Hair was found to contain arsenic at 3.8–13.0 μg/g (ppm) near the root, compared with 0–1.5 μg/g near the end and 0.4–2.8 μg/g in control hair samples.

In the early 1960's, physicians in Antofagasta, Chile, noted dermatologic manifestations and some deaths, particularly among children, that were traced to a water supply containing arsenic at 0.8 ppm. This water supply had been in operation only since 1958. In 1971, Borgono and Greiber reported on a series of studies of the inhabitants of this city.[86] Of 21 children referred to Santiago for evaluation and treatment after 1962, 16 had recurrent bronchopneumonia during the first years of life, and all had bronchiectasis. All 21 had been referred because of abnormal skin color and hyperkeratosis. Peripheral vascular manifestations in these children included Raynaud's syndrome, ischemia of the tongue, hemiplegia with partial occlusion of the carotid artery, mesenteric arterial thrombosis, and myocardial ischemia. One autopsy showed hyperplasia of the arterial media.

In a survey of 27,088 schoolchildren, 12% were found to have the cutaneous changes of arsenism; one-fourth to one-third of these had suggestive systemic symptoms. Eleven percent had acrocyanosis. One hundred eighty inhabitants of Antofagasta were compared with 98 people who resided in a city (Iquique) having a normal water supply. Most of the people studied were less than 20 years old. Of the Antofagasta residents, 144 had abnormal skin pigmentation, compared with none in the 98 control subjects. In the 180, 30% and 22% had Raynaud's syndrome and acrocyanosis, respectively. Other findings are shown in Tables 6-1 and 6-2.

The vascular diseases and the repeated episodes of pneumonia with bronchiectasis observed in the children of this population are dramatic and deserve special attention. Clearly, exposure to significant amounts of arsenic from an earlier age may result in a clinical picture in growing children different from that seen in adults.

TABLE 6-1 Clinical Manifestations among 180 Antofagasta and 98 Iquique Inhabitants[a]

Manifestation	Incidence in Antofagasta, %	Incidence in Iquique, %
Bronchopulmonary disease history	14.9	5.3
Abnormal skin pigmentation	80.0	0.0
Hyperkeratosis	36.1	0.0
Chronic coryza	59.7	1.0
Lip herpes	12.7	0.0
Chronic cough	28.3	4.0
Cardiovascular manifestations:		
Raynaud's syndrome	30.0	0.0
Acrocyanosis	22.0	0.0
Angina pectoris	0.0	0.0
Hypertension	5.0	10.0
Chronic diarrhea	7.2	0.0
Abdominal pain	39.1	2.0

[a]Derived from Borgono and Greiber.[86]

TABLE 6-2 Clinical Manifestations among 180 Antofagasta Inhabitants according to Skin Pigmentation, 1969[a]

Manifestation	Incidence in Persons with Abnormal Skin Pigmentation (N = 144), %	Incidence in Persons with Normal Skin (N = 36), %
Bronchopulmonary disease history	15.9	6.2
Hyperkeratosis	43.7	3.1
Chronic cough	38.8	3.1
Lip herpes	14.5	3.1
Cardiovascular manifestations:		
Raynaud's syndrome	38.8	9.3
Acrocyanosis	24.3	12.5
Angina pectoris	4.1	0.0
Hypertension	6.2	0.0
Chronic diarrhea	40.9	0.0
Abdominal pain	39.1	28.1

[a]Derived from Borgono and Greiber.[86]

The Raynaud's phenomenon and acrocyanosis in this population are reminiscent of the report from Taiwan by Tseng et al. and suggest that chronic arsenism has effects on the vasculature (possibly the neural control of arteries) that are correlated with the more acute phenomena described by Reynolds and others as erythromelalgia and acrocyanosis.[798]

Tseng et al. surveyed a group of 40,421 (from a population "at risk" of 103,154) and found hyperpigmentation in 18.4%, keratotic lesions in 7.1%, and blackfoot disease—apparently secondary to arterial spasm in the legs—in 0.9%.[798] They also found an apparent tenfold increase in the incidence of skin cancer in patients over 59 years old. The latter figure is difficult to evaluate, because the usual incidence of these cancers in Taiwan was not given. All these phenomena were shown to increase with increasing arsenic concentration in the well water of the 37 villages studied. They also increased with age, but the earliest ages noted for specific findings were 3 years for the characteristic hyperpigmentation, 4 years for keratoses, and 24 years for skin cancer. The concentration of arsenic in the wells ranged from 0.017 to 1.097 ppm. No cases of melanosis, keratosis, or skin cancer were found in a group of 2,552 people living in an area where the wells contained almost no arsenic.

Feinglass reported on 13 persons exposed for 2.5 months to well water contaminated with buried insecticide.[244] Most patients were seen only once, and the most prominent feature was intermittent gastrointestinal symptoms related to water ingestion. Two of the 13 had nail changes, and five (of eight in whom it was measured) had increased arsenic content of the scalp hair. The author did not mention edema, exanthema, hyperpigmentation, or hyperkeratosis.

Heyman et al. studied 41 patients retrospectively in an effort to evaluate the response of arsenical neuropathy to BAL.[351] In the 21 patients for whom a history of skin lesions was mentioned, there was a prominence of branny desquamation 1-3 weeks after the exposure and a notable incidence of "herpetic lesions of the mouth."

There are many scattered case reports of subacute to chronic arsenic poisoning. Silver and Wainman provided a meticulous description of a patient who ingested approximately 8.8 mg of arsenic trioxide as Fowler's solution daily for a total period of 28 months, as a remedy for asthma.[733] Signs of arsenic poisoning, manifest as increased freckling and as darkening of the nipples, first appeared in association with gastrointestinal symptoms after 13 months; redness and puffiness about the eyes and hyperkeratoses developed at approximately 1.5 years. Neurologic symptoms in the form of paresthesias and weakness were the last to be noted, occurring after 2 years. When the arsenic intake was stopped, the pigmentation lightened, the hyperkeratoses remained, and the asthma became more difficult to control. This report is instructive, because the nature of episodes of accidental arsenic poisoning does not usually permit definitive analysis of the amount or duration of exposure necessary to produce reactions. However, many authors have suggested that there is substantial variation in individual susceptibility to any given symptom or sign. The increased likelihood that hyperpigmentation will occur in people whose skin is naturally darker supports this concept, as does the fact that relatively small fractions of the exposed population have any given feature.

Perry et al.[633] noted, however, that *all* of a group of chemical workers handling inorganic arsenic compounds had pigmentary changes and that one-third of them had "warts," although these were not well described. They reported that the cutaneous "changes were so evident that [the examiner] could readily tell whether the man . . . was a chemical worker."[633] All these handlers had increased urinary arsenic compatible in degree with the extent of exposure; this indicates systemic absorption of the arsenic from dust, probably through the lungs and skin.

Pinto and McGill studied urinary arsenic content in workers exposed to arsenic trioxide dust and related compounds.[648] The urinary arsenic in this group was about 8 times the normal value, but they were said not to have the pigmentary and keratotic changes seen in the group of Perry et al.[633] Neither paper described the average length of employment or the ethnic backgrounds of the workers, which might help to explain this discrepancy.

Chronic Arsenic Exposure

Neubauer has provided an exhaustive review of the literature up to 1947, covering all forms of arsenic exposure with analysis for many factors.[585] Fierz actually examined 262 patients who had received long courses of medicinal arsenic 6–26 years previously and found keratoses in 40% and typical skin cancer in 8%.[253] There was evidence of a dose relationship for both keratoses and skin cancer. Patients who had received more than 400 ml of Fowler's solution (4 g of arsenic trioxide) had an incidence of hyperkeratoses of greater than 50%, but as little as 60 ml (600 mg of arsenic trioxide) had resulted in keratotic changes in one patient. As little as 75 ml (750 mg of arsenic trioxide) had been consumed by one patient with skin cancer. The shortest time to cancerous change was 6 years, with an average of 14 years, compared with Neubauer's estimate of 18 years from review of the literature.[585] Fierz noted that 1,450 invitations for a free examination had been sent to patients who had been given the therapeutic arsenic.[253] Besides the 262 who came for examination, 100 patients provided written reports, and information was obtained about the deaths of 11. Five of the 11 deaths were due to systemic cancer, and three to lung cancer.

Sixteen of Fierz's 21 patients with cancer had typical keratoses,[253] and Arguello et al.[24] reported on a large group of patients seen for arsenical skin cancers in the Cordoba region in Argentina, which had a high arsenic content in the drinking water[73] and found keratoderma in "100% of our patients." Most patients also had associated hyperhidrosis and abnormalities of pigmentation, whereas those reported by Fierz did not.[253] Arguello et al. noted that the pigmentation appeared early and was variable among the patients.[24] It was described as small dark spots 1–10 mm in diameter, with a tendency to coalesce, and appearing predominantly on the trunk, that is, in the areas not exposed to the sun. These and other authors have noted that atrophy may be associated with telangiectasia and loss of color, or leukoderma, between the hyperpigmented areas (the "raindrop" appearance cited by Reynolds[665]).

The characteristics of the skin malignancies found in chronic arsenism have been reviewed by Yeh and Yeh et al. in their reports on the Taiwan cases.[886,887] A prominent, even necessary, clinical feature of arsenical skin cancer is its association with the characteristic keratoses or pigment irregularities on the trunk. Several authors have cited a similar association in exposed workers as evidence that arsenic may cause internal cancers, especially of the lung.[101,191,372,605,671,677,679] In addition, the skin lesions are characteristically multiple and predominantly on the areas of the body that are protected by clothing. Both these features are notable, inasmuch as "ordinary" skin cancers tend to be single and have been shown to have a body distribution directly correlated with the amount of sun exposure.[78,542] Arsenical lesions (both keratoses and cancers) also appear at an earlier average age than do solar (senile) keratoses and related carcinomas.

The histopathology of the multiple and varied lesions seen in arsenism has been the subject of considerable interest among dermatopathologists.[16,40,542,554,646,886,887] Lesions that clinically are keratoses may show proliferation of keratin of a verrucous nature, may exhibit precancerous derangement of the squamous portions of the epithelium equivalent to those seen in Bowen's disease and solar keratosis, or may even be frank squamous cell carcinomas. Lesions that are less keratotic and more erythematous may contain either squamous cell or basal cell carcinoma or a mixture of cell types. Most authors seem to agree that keratotic lesions appear to be able to progress to frank carcinoma, but observation of such an event is rare, and most cancers appear to arise independently of the keratoses.

The question of the association of Bowen's disease with arsenism has stimulated considerable controversy. Graham and Helwig analyzed 36 autopsies of patients with Bowen's disease in whom arsenic intake had been ruled out as much as possible.[303] It is striking that this group of patients differed from patients with arsenism in several respects: They lacked the typical keratoses and pigmentation; they had a tendency for the "typical Bowenoid" squamous cell carcinoma *in situ* to precede the other cutaneous malignancies by an average of 6 years; there was an incidence of approximately 80% of associated internal malignancies (some diagnosed only at autopsy); and they had suggestive evidence of a familial predisposition to the condition. Of more than 100 living patients with the diagnosis of Bowen's disease surveyed by the same authors, internal malignancy had been diagnosed in 23. These features seem sufficient to distinguish Bowen's disease from chronic arsenism, despite the confusion later introduced by Graham et al.[304] If

Graham and Helwig's cases are representative, the association of systemic cancers is much higher in Bowen's disease than has ever been suggested for chronic arsenism.

Late Effects of Exposure to Arsenic

One of the many unexplained puzzles about arsenic is that the characteristic skin cancers may appear years after exposure to the agent has ceased. Despite claims that arsenic could be demonstrated in the lesions,[304] there is a possibility that these findings are a result of artifacts,[209] and alternative explanations should be sought, especially because it is now known that the half-life of an epidermal cell is only a few weeks and any incorporated material can be presumed to be diluted in new cell generations. Interestingly, arsenic-induced pigment changes—which are irregular and associated with intermingled areas of atrophy, depigmentation, and telangiectasia—are reminiscent of those seen after chronic exposure to two well-known carcinogens: ultraviolet radiation and X rays. Cancers that are secondary to these agents also appear long after the relevant exposure. Conceivably, arsenic acts analogously in susceptible people, although it is clear that the carcinogenic "efficiency" of arsenic is far lower than that of X irradiation in causing skin cancers.

Braun reported on 16 patients who had been exposed to arsenic in their occupation as vintners many years before.[101] No known exposure to arsenic had occurred since. All had keratoses, nine had leukomelanoderma of the trunk, and seven had skin cancer or intraepidermal carcinoma *in situ*. Eight had lung cancer.

Roth also studied 27 vintners whose arsenic exposure had occurred 10–14 years earlier.[679] His population was selected by having come to autopsy. He found that 16 of the 27 had a total of 28 cancers, including five with skin cancer. There was hyperkeratosis of the palms and soles, "particularly in the patients with tumors." Melanosis was also present, but hard to evaluate in the postmortem state.

For a few months in 1955, a large number of babies in Japan received a formula made from powdered milk contaminated with arsenic.[525,596,597,702] The report by Hamimoto provides a fascinating view into the medical puzzle that the initial patients presented to their pediatricians.[325] The conscientious attention to both the solution of the mystery and the care of the patients is impressive. In the (translated) words of Hamimoto, the episode deserved "the reflection of all those concerned. This is necessary for the sake of the 62 young lives who disappeared."[325] The subacute symptoms of poisoning in these infants included the usual coughing, rhinorrhea, conjunctivitis, vomiting, diarrhea, and melanosis, but the striking presenting features were fever and abdominal swelling secondary to hepatomegaly. Abnormal laboratory findings included anemia, granulocytopenia, abnormal electrocardiograms, and increased density at epiphyseal ends of long bones similar to the familiar "lead line." Nagai et al. reported on a group of these children who were followed for more than 6 months.[574] Except for a measurable retardation in ulnar growth, they found that all other features of the syndrome had disappeared, including melanosis. Followup is continuing, and a report by the Japanese Pediatric Society in 1973[391] indicated that growth was still reduced and that there was a probable incidence of leukomelanoderma in the children (aged 17–20 at the time) of 15–30%. The children had a 15% incidence of keratosis.[885] Of greater concern, however, was the observation of increased incidences of mental retardation, epilepsy, and other findings that suggested brain damage in the arsenic-exposed children. Presumably, future studies in this population (more than 10,000 exposed infants) will help to resolve some of the standing questions regarding the latent effects of arsenic exposure.

Occupational Episodes of Toxicity

Sheep-Dip Factory Workers

The cancer experience between 1910 and 1943 in an English factory that manufactured a sodium arsenite sheep dip is described in the section on carcinogenesis. Clinical and environmental studies were done in 1945 and 1946,[633] including general air measurements, analysis of urine and hair for arsenic, and clinical examinations. High-exposure areas of the plant had arsenic concentrations ranging from about 250 to 700 $\mu g/m^3$. The relationship of urine and hair arsenic to the prevalence of pigmentation and warts is shown in Table 6-3.

Smelters

Holmqvist reported eczematous and follicular dermatitis in smelter workers, primarily on exposed skin.[365] Patch tests showed sensitivity to both trivalent and pentavalent arsenic. Birmingham et al. reported similar lesions that developed within a few months of the startup of a gold smelter that handled ores containing large amounts of arsenic sulfide.[79] Dermatitis developed in half the mill workers and in 32 of 40 students in a nearby elementary school.

TABLE 6-3 Arsenic Concentration and Prevalence of Pigmentation and Warts[a]

Workers	No. Persons	Arsenic Concentration, ppm		Prevalence, %	
		Urine	Hair	Pigmentation	Warts
Chemical workers	33	0.24	108	90	29
Maintenance workers and packers	32	0.10	78	38	3
Control[b]	56	0.09	13	18	4

[a]Derived from Perry et al.[633]
[b]Including two former chemical workers.

Vintners

Butzengeiger reported that, of 180 vinedressers and cellarmen with symptoms of chronic arsenic poisoning, about 23% had evidence of vascular disorders of the extremities.[122] Arsenical insecticides were used in the vineyards, and exposure occurred not only with spraying, but during work in the vineyards by inhalation of contaminated dusts and plant debris. Most of the workers consumed 1–2 liters of wine per day, and it was also believed to be contaminated with arsenic. All 15 workers with vascular disorders had hyperpigmentation, and all but two had palmar and plantar keratosis; six of the 15 had gangrene of the fingers and toes. The same association of vascular disorders, hyperpigmentation, and keratosis was observed in Taiwan.[886]

Urinary arsenic content averaged 0.324 mg/liter, and hair arsenic, 0.039 mg/100 g. Thus, the urine and hair had comparable concentrations, 0.3 and 0.4 ppm. Butzengeiger reported that the electrocardiograms of 36 of 192 vinegrowers with chronic arsenic intoxication were definitely abnormal, with no other evident cause.[121] The abnormalities included prolongation of the Q–T interval and a flattened T wave. In treated cases, these abnormalities diminished with the other evidence of toxicity. Similar findings were reported by Barry and Herndon[53] and Glazener et al.[293] Arsenic-induced myocarditis in these cases was similar to the evidence reported in the Japanese poisoning episodes described earlier.

Miscellaneous Considerations

Organic Arsenicals

Organic arsenicals occupy an exciting place in the history of scientific medicine, because they are the result of deliberate attempts to develop chemicals with increased therapeutic efficacy and reduced toxicity and are thus the first of a long line of synthetic chemotherapeutic agents.[333] Specifically, these agents were developed to exploit the antibacterial effects of inorganic arsenic while reducing its toxicity by attachment to an organic moiety. The goal was a cure for syphilis.

The major cutaneous side effects of the administration of organic arsenicals were rashes of various types, many of which were thought to be allergic. Although the actual incidence of such eruptions may have been quite small, considering the total number of doses given,[381] their nature was such as to cause considerable concern over and research into the problem.[771] Harvey stated that the ultimate basis of the action of the organic arsenicals is the inorganic arsenic moiety that results from degradation in the body.[333] It is interesting, however, that few, if any, patients receiving large doses of organic arsenic over long periods are reported to have developed the characteristic hyperkeratoses and irregular pigmentation associated with the use of Fowler's solution.[266,585]

Arsenic in Hair and Nails

The keratin of hair and nails is rich in disulfides, and it has been postulated that arsenic is incorporated into the growing portion of the hair root and the nail base.[721] The possibility raised by Lander and Hodge[449] that arsenic is excreted in the sweat in cases of acute poisoning must also be considered, although their methodology did not distinguish between eccrine and sebaceous gland secretions. It has been shown that arsenic in the environment reacts avidly with keratin and cannot be removed with repeated washings.[461] Thus, attempts to utilize growing hair or nails to determine exposure to ingested arsenic must be performed under circumstances that will guarantee an absence of external contamination.[219,721] Hair should be collected from control subjects simultaneously and analyzed in parallel. Even then, consideration must be given to the possibility of unsuspected contamination—e.g., from hair dyes and shampoos—if high arsenic concentrations are found. To avoid spuriously low concentrations, the timing of the hair collection must be such that the root portion has grown out from the hair canal (or the hair may be plucked out, roots and all). If the patient has been acutely ill, the exposure may have been sufficient to arrest hair growth temporarily and thus delay the contaminated hairs' arrival at the scalp surface still further.

Arsenic and the Immune Response

Several aspects of the medical side of the arsenic story suggest that arsenic has the capacity to function selectively as a suppressant of the immune response: the medical conditions for which arsenic was most popular were those for which steroid drugs are now the treatment of choice; the high incidence of herpes zoster and herpes simplex in cases of subacute arsenic poisoning is reminiscent of the same phenomenon in patients deliberately immunosuppressed to receive kidney transplants; the presentation of children in the Antofagasta episode with recurrent pulmonary infections is reminiscent of the story of children with congenital immunodeficiency syndromes; and the reputed capacity of arsenic to reduce the lymphocyte count in leukemia may reflect a selective sensitivity of this cell type to arsenic, which is again analogous to the effects of steroids.

Although the possible role of the immune response in protecting the body against cancer is not completely understood, that arsenicals may affect such a mechanism clearly warrants further study. Many of the techniques of modern immunology have become available only in the last 10 years and remain to be applied to the study of arsenic.

Arsenic as Therapy

Except for one brief positive report,[330] there is little published evidence that modern analysis has been applied to the question of whether arsenic may have a useful therapeutic role. As the limitations of some of our modern "miracle drugs" have become evident (e.g., growth retardation, osteoporosis, Cushingoid changes, and hypertension with steroids), serious consideration of reevaluation of this ancient remedy has become more important.

Uniqueness of Human Skin

Human epidermis has a number of distinguishing characteristics. Its relative hairlessness is associated with a squamous cell layer that is considerably thicker than the two or three cells of furred laboratory animals. In addition, there is a widespread proliferation of eccrine sweat glands not seen in any other animal, except a few primates.[553] In view of the propensity for arsenical keratoses to appear early and most prominently on the palms and soles, where these glands are heavily concentrated, it is conceivable that these structures are the mechanism through which arsenic exerts its effect; because they are uniquely prominent in human skin, a suitable laboratory model for arsenical changes could be unavailable.[553]

Other Dermatologic Conditions

Palmar keratoses may occur independently of exposure to arsenic, and several syndromes appear to be congenital. In the basal cell nevus syndrome, the palmar lesions are pitted (rather than protruding), tend to appear early in life, and are associated with such congenital abnormalities as jaw cysts and bifid ribs, as well as with multiple basal cell carcinomas that appear in adult life.[157]

A single report indicated that patients with internal malignancy may have an increased incidence of palmar keratoses. Dobson *et al.* examined 671 patients with diagnosed malignancies and 685 patients with other diseases.[208] Of the cancer patients, 32% had palmar keratoses, compared with 7% of the others. Patients with breast cancer were the most striking group, with a 39% incidence of keratoses. A standardized set of questions was used to ascertain a history of exposure to arsenic, and this revealed no difference between the tumor group and the control group (13% and 10%, respectively).

TERATOGENESIS

The teratogenic effects of arsenic compounds have been recognized only recently. However, potassium arsenate was one of the compounds used in the early studies in the 1950's that led to the chick embryo test for teratogenic agents.[668] Thus, Ridgway and Karnofsky found that injection of sodium arsenate into embryonate chicken eggs at 4 days in doses of 0.20 mg/egg caused no specific gross abnormalities in the resulting embryos 14 days later. Growth retardation (particularly of the legs), impaired feather growth, and abdominal swelling were noted.[668] This sort of response is commonly encountered in the chick embryo system and is generally regarded as nonspecific.

Even earlier, Franke *et al.* performed what might be called the first teratogenic study of an arsenic compound, when they tested the effect of sodium arsenite on the development of chick embryos.[264] Injection of sublethal concentrations of arsenic into the eggs produced ectopic conditions, but no monstrosities, such as produced by selenium.

More recent studies have shown that teratogenic effects result from the administration of sodium arsenate to hamsters, mice, and rats. In the hamster study,[250] sodium arsenate was administered intravenously as a single dose on specified days of gestation, and results were observed on the fifteenth day. It was found that the eighth day was critical; there was a high incidence of embryos with anencephaly and other defects, which occurred much less frequently if the arsenate was administered earlier or later than the eighth day of gestation. A more thorough study of the spectrum of treatment effects caused by the intravenous injection of sodium arsenate at 15, 17.5, or 20 mg/kg as a single dose on the eighth day of gestation has been reported.[251] Deionized water was administered to comparable hamsters as a control, and the data were collected on the fifteenth day of gestation. The incidences of dead, resorbed, and malformed embryos depended on dose. Thus, the fraction of the litter resorbed ranged from about 5 to 80%, and the incidence of malformations ranged from 20 to 90%. Up to 80% of the embryos had anencephaly; up to 65%, rib malformations; up to 30%, exencephaly; and approximately 20%, genitourinary malformations. Incidence of renal agenesis and cleft lip and palate were lower. Further analysis of the teratogenic consequences of sodium arsenate by Holmberg and Fern showed that sodium selenite injected at 2 mg/kg simultaneously with a teratogenic dose of sodium arsenate decreased the number of fetal resorptions and congenital malformations caused by the arsenical.[363] This observation is of interest, in light of the known metabolic antagonism between selenium and arsenic. The authors of the latter report stressed that the doses of arsenic and selenium used in their experiments exceeded the usual environmental contamination. However, they also pointed out that remarkable species variation can exist in the teratogenic response to any given teratogen (for example, thalidomide caused severe malformations in human embryos in relatively low therapeutic doses, whereas it took extremely high doses of the same compound to produce malformations in experimental animals). The paper concluded on a cautionary note, suggesting that all potential teratogens be carefully evaluated until individual species sensitivity to various teratogens is determined.

In mouse studies, Hood and Bishop administered a single dose (25 or 45 mg/kg) of sodium arsenate by intraperitoneal injection on a specified day from the sixth to the twelfth day of gestation and observed the results on the eigthteenth day.[367] The injections given on the ninth day were most teratogenic; 60% of 96 implantations were resorbed or dead, and 63% were grossly malformed. The defects included exencephaly, microagnathia, protruding tongue, agnathia, open eye, cleft lip, fused vertebrae, and forked ribs. Mice that received injections of distilled water served as controls. Although teratologic effects were seen at 45 mg/kg, 25 mg/kg was without effect. Sodium arsenite was more effective; preliminary data show that the extent of fetal anomalies caused by sodium arsenite at 10 mg/kg was comparable with that caused by sodium arsenate at 45 mg/kg. Hood and Pike reported that British antilewisite, when administered to mice at 50 mg/kg by intraperitoneal injection within 4 h of sodium arsenate at 40 mg/kg, prevented the arsenic-induced teratogenesis.[368]

Results similar to those reported for hamsters and mice were reported by Beaudoin for rats.[57] Each of a group of pregnant Wistar rats received an intraperitoneal injection of sodium arsenate during days 7–12 of gestation. The dosage of sodium arsenate varied; it was either 20, 30, 40, or 50 mg/kg of maternal body weight. The teratogenicity and lethality to embryos of arsenate depended on dosage and time; maximal effects were seen when the dosage was 30 mg/kg and the injection was given on day 8, 9, or 10. The most common malformations were eye defects, exencephaly, and renal and gonadal agenesis. Ribs and vertebrae were the skeletal elements most commonly affected.

It is of interest that potassium arsenate was fed to four pregnant ewes at 0.5 mg/kg during most of pregnancy without effect.[390]

MUTAGENESIS

As in the case of teratogenic effects of arsenic compounds, there have been only a few valuable mutagenesis studies. Most of the research has centered on chromosomal reactions to sodium arsenate. There are no data based on the host-mediated assay or the dominant-lethal technique.

One of the earliest observations that has meaning today was made by Levan in 1945.[462] Root meristem cultures of *Allium cepa* were treated for 4 h with an unspecified arsenic salt at 10 concentrations, from lethal to a no-effect. Chromosomal changes were observed, including spindle disturbances and metaphase arrests. Similar effects, with minor variations, were observed after treatment with salts of 24 other metals (mostly nitrates). The changes resembled those caused by colchicine, but they cannot be considered serious damage.

Petres and co-workers have reported chromosomal breakage in human leukocyte cultures after short-term *in vitro* exposure to sodium arsenate[637,638] and in cultures obtained after long-term exposure to arsenical compounds *in vivo*.[639]

The cytotoxic and mutagenic effects of sodium arsenate were tested *in vitro* on phytohemagglutinin-stimulated lymphocyte cultures in concentrations of 0.05–30 µg/ml of culture medium.[637,638] It was reported that 33% of metaphase plates were pulverized at 0.1 µg/ml and 80–100% at concentrations of 2 µg/ml or greater. The "mitosis index" and the "[^{3}H]thymidine labeling index" were decreased. Arsenate has also been found to increase the total frequency of exchange chromosomes in *Drosophila melanogaster* treated with selenocystine,[835] and several organic arsenicals have a harmful synergistic effect on the number of abnormalities in barley chromosomes caused by ethyl-methane sulfonate.[563] The overall significance of these chromosomal studies is difficult to assess, inasmuch as many unrelated compounds may cause similar effects. The fact that arsenic compounds have caused chromosomal damage in a number of biologic systems, however, should alert toxicologists to a possible role of arsenic in chemically induced mutagenesis.

The *in vivo* studies were made on 34 patients at the University of Freiburg skin clinic.[639] Thirteen of these patients had had intensive arsenic therapy, some more than 20 years before the experiment; most of these were psoriasis patients. The control group (21 patients) consisted of 14 psoriasis patients and 7 with eczema, none of whom had had arsenic treatment. Phytohemagglutinin-stimulated lymphocyte cultures were prepared from each patient for evaluation of chromosomal aberrations. The incidence of aberrations was remarkably greater in the cultures of patients who had been treated with arsenic. Expressed as the frequency per 1,000 mitoses, secondary constrictions were 49 in the arsenic group and 12 in the control, gaps were found in 51 in the arsenic group and 7 in the control, "other" lesions were 26 in the arsenic group and 1 in the control, and broken chromosomes were 65 per 1,000 mitoses in the arsenic group and 2 in the control. Aneuploidy was found at the expected frequency in the arsenic group. The extent of abnormalities attributed to treatment with arsenicals is impressive; it is important that this study be repeated.

Paton and Allison investigated the effect of sodium arsenate, sodium arsenite, and acetylarsan on chromosomes in cultures of human leukocytes and diploid fibroblasts.[620] Subtoxic doses of the arsenicals were added to leukocyte and fibroblast cultures at various times between 2 and 48 h before fixation. In leukocyte cultures treated with sodium arsenite at $0.29–1.8 \times 10^{-8} M$ for the last 48 h of the culture period, 60% of 148 metaphases examined were found to have chromatid breaks. No significant number of breaks were found in cultures treated with sodium arsenate at 0.58 $\times 10^{-8} M$, the highest nontoxic concentration. However, treatment with acetylarsan at 6.0 $\times$ $10^{-8} M$ resulted in 20% chromatid breaks in 50 metaphases examined. Sodium arsenite caused chromosomal damage in diploid fibroblasts to which sodium arsenite (0.29–5.8 $\times$ $10^{-8} M$) was added to the medium for the last 24 h of culture; chromatid breaks were found in 20% of 459 metaphases examined. These results supported the *in vitro* observations of Petres *et al.*[637,638]

CARCINOGENESIS

The purpose of this section is to review and evaluate the evidence of carcinogenic activity of arsenic compounds; the evidence is in four categories:

- Clinical reports of skin cancers associated with the medical use of arsenicals.
- Occupational studies of workers engaged in the manufacture of arsenic compounds, in smelting, or in the use of arsenicals.
- Population studies in areas of great exposure to environmental arsenic, primarily in water supplies.
- Experimental studies of arsenic carcinogenesis in laboratory animals.

Recent reviews of the literature on carcinogenicity studies in animals and man have been published by the International Agency for Research on Cancer[379] and by the National Institute for Occupational Safety and Health.[807]

Clinical Reports

The clinical association of skin cancer with the oral administration of arsenic compounds began with a report by Hutchinson in 1888.[377] He described six patients in whom skin cancer occurred and who had suffered for very long periods from diseases of the skin (five with psoriasis, one with pemphigus). In five of the cases, arsenic was known to have been used for a long time. Neubauer in 1947 summarized 143 published cases of medicinal arsenical epitheliomas in a review for the British Medical Research Council.[585]

A small, but undetermined, proportion of people treated with arsenicals developed cancers. Of the 143 patients, about 70% received arsenicals for skin disease; of these, half had psoriasis. Nearly all the 143 patients received arsenic in the inorganic trivalent form, the most common drug being potassium arsenite as Fowler's solution. A typical formula consists of 10 g of arsenic trioxide, 7.6 g of potassium bicarbonate, 30 ml of alcohol (or tincture of lavender), and distilled water to 1 liter.[642] Approximately 90% of the patients received Fowler's solution for more than 1 year, and 50% for more than 5 years. The total quantity of arsenic ingested was variable, averaging about 28 g.

Multiple horny keratoses, especially the punctate or warty form on the palms and soles, were commonly reported in patients who had received Fowler's solution. Keratoses occurred in about 90% of the cases of cancer ascribed to treatment with Fowler's solution; only in a few cases did the keratoses spare the hands and feet. Melanosis is a common sign of arsenic ingestion, and the hyperpigmentation is most marked at sites of normal pigmentation and at sites of pressure from clothing.

About half the skin cancers were squamous carcinomas arising in keratotic areas, with predilection for the hands (especially the palmar and lateral surfaces of the fingers and the borders of the palms), the heels, and the toes. About half were multiple superficial epitheliomas of the basal cell variety localized to the trunk and proximal parts of the extremities. Only a few of the 143 cases arose in psoriatic patches. There was a substantial frequency of mixed types of epitheliomas. Of the 143 patients, 70% had multiple lesions. Multiple lesions occurred even when squamous cancers arose in keratoses; there was an average of two lesions per case.

The elapsed time from the beginning of administration of the arsenical drug to the beginning of the epitheliomatous growth was variable, but averaged 18 years, regardless of the type of lesion. In cases with keratosis, the latent period to the onset of keratosis was about half the latent period to the onset of the epithelioma—i.e., about 9 years. In spite of the long induction period, arsenic-related skin cancers started when the patients were relatively young, one-third when they were 40 or younger, and 70% when they were 50 or younger.

Of the 143 patients, 13 had or developed miscellaneous cancers at other sites, but such cases were not reported systematically; the reports commonly presented one or a few case histories. For example, Regelson *et al.* reported a case of hemangioendothelial sarcoma of the liver in a 49-year-old man who had taken Fowler's solution intermittently for 17 years to control psoriasis.[663]

Occupational Exposure

There have been numerous reports of arsenic-induced occupational cancer, such as those of the excess lung-cancer mortality among Southern Rhodesian miners of gold-bearing ores containing large amounts of arsenic[605] and of the occurrence of lung and liver cancer and clinical arsenism among German vineyard workers exposed to arsenic-containing insecticides.[101,678,679] The association of cancer with a high degree of arsenic exposure has often been based on the existence of palmar or plantar keratoses.[753] However, because of the increased concentration of arsenic in the lesions of Bowen's disease, arsenic has been considered as a possible cause of the disease and accompanying visceral tumors,[304] without overt prior exposure to arsenicals (see also discussion under "Chronic Arsenic Exposure").

A number of relatively quantitative studies of cancer attributable to occupational exposure to arsenicals will be discussed in some detail.

A death-record examination was made of a British plant that manufactured sodium arsenite sheep dip.[352,633] The factory was in a small country town within a specific birth and death registration subdistrict. In this and adjacent subdistricts, death certificates of 75 factory workers and 1,216 men (not factory workers) in three other occupational groups were obtained for the period 1910–1943. Of the 75 deaths among factory workers, 22 (29%) were due to cancer; of the other 1,216 deaths, 157 (13%) were due to cancer. The proportion of deaths due to cancer was even higher among men who actually worked with the manufacture and packaging of the arsenic-containing material: 16 of the 31 deaths of men so classified were due to cancer. The number of deaths due to cancer according to site for the two groups is shown in Table 6-4, in which those deaths are expressed as a fraction of cancer deaths and as a fraction of total deaths. The absolute numbers of deaths and the fractions of cancer deaths are from the author's paper; the fractions of total deaths were calculated for this report. The data suggest a relative excess in the factory workers of cancers of the respiratory system and skin, whether calculated on the basis of cancer deaths or of total deaths; the corresponding deficits in cancers of the digestive organs and peritoneum disappear when calculated on the basis of total deaths.

Although Hill and Faning stated that the numbers of cancer deaths are small, they concluded that "there is a suggestion in the figures that the factory workers have been especially affected in the lung and skin."[352] Hence, there was an investigation of the environmental conditions at the factory and the clinical condition of the workers in

TABLE 6-4 Deaths Due to Cancer, by Site[a]

Site	No. Cancer Deaths		Fraction of Cancer deaths,[b] %		Fraction of Total Deaths,[b] %	
	Factory Workers	Other 3 Occupational Groups	Factory Workers	Other 3 Occupational Groups	Factory Workers	Other 3 Occupational Groups
Buccal cavity and pharynx	2	10	9.1	6.4	2.7	0.8
Digestive organs and peritoneum	5	91	22.7	58.0	6.7	7.5
Respiratory organs	7	25	31.8	15.9	9.3	2.1
Genitourinary organs	2	13	9.1	8.3	2.7	1.1
Skin	3	2	13.6	1.3	4.0	0.2
Other or unspecified	3	16	13.6	10.2	4.0	1.3
Total	22	157	99.9	100.1	29.4	13.0

[a] Derived from Hill and Faning.[352]
[b] There were 75 deaths among the factory workers and 1,216 deaths in the other three occupational groups (see text).

question, compared with employees in other branches of the factory who were not exposed to arsenic.[633] The median air arsenic content for the chemical workers at the various operations ranged from 254 to 696 $\mu g/m^3$. As an upper limit, this was stated to represent the inhalation of about 1 g of arsenic per year. This amount of arsenic is roughly equivalent to the amount received by patients getting arsenic medication for skin diseases.

The excretion of arsenic in the urine of 127 current employees was determined; the scatter of these values was very wide. Some exposed workers excreted from 1 to nearly 2 mg/day, whereas many excreted less than 100 μg/day. A few of the persons in the control group had very high excretion rates, for which the authors found no explanation. It is important to note that 20 of 31 factory workers had been exposed to airborne sodium arsenite for more than 20 years, and five of them for 40–50 years. Furthermore, the median age of the 31 exposed workers was 52 years, and the average age was 50. None of these men's lungs had pathologic signs attributable to their exposure to sodium arsenite (radiographs were made, and vital capacity and exercise capacity were measured).

The mortality experience of 8,047 white male smelter workers exposed to arsenic trioxide during 1938–1963 was compared by Lee and

Biologic Effects of Arsenic on Man

Fraumeni with that of the white male population in the same state.[460] There was a threefold excess total mortality from respiratory cancer in smelter workers, and this reached an eightfold excess for employees working more than 15 years and heavily exposed to arsenic. When respiratory cancer deaths were grouped according to degree of arsenic exposure, the observed mortality was significantly higher than expected in all three groups: approximately 6.7, 4.8, and 2.4 times the expected mortality in the heavy-, medium-, and light-exposure groups, respectively. In addition to arsenic trioxide dust, smelter workers were concurrently exposed to sulfur dioxide. Exposure to silica and ferromanganese and lead dusts occurred in parts of the refineries where arsenic concentrations were low. Therefore, a similar classification was made for relative sulfur dioxide exposure. Respiratory-cancer mortality was directly related to sulfur dioxide exposure, with observed deaths ranging from 6.0 down to 2.6 times the expected in heavy-, medium-, and light-exposure groups. Most work areas having heavy arsenic exposure were also medium-sulfur dioxide areas, and all jobs with heavy sulfur dioxide exposure were medium-arsenic areas. It was observed that workers with the heaviest exposure to arsenic and moderate or heaviest exposure to sulfur dioxide were most likely to die of respiratory cancer.

A study by Pinto and Bennett[647] involved a smelting plant in the state of Washington that produced arsenic trioxide as a by-product. The plant had an average employment of 904 during the years 1946–1960. During that period, a total of 229 deaths were reported among active plant employees and pensioners. Thirty-eight of the dead were classified as exposed to arsenic. Of the 38, six died of cancer, including three cases of cancer of the respiratory tract. The total cancer experience of the arsenic-exposed workers was not higher than that of the unexposed, although there was twice as much respiratory cancer in both exposed and unexposed smelter workers as expected from male mortality experience in Washington. Mortality among workers at the same plant was restudied by Milham and Strong, who published their survey in 1974.[543] They criticized the methods of the Pinto and Bennett study. The records of workers from the same plant revealed 40 deaths from lung cancer, which was significantly higher than the 18 expected on the basis of rates in the general U.S. population.

Snegireff and Lombard[747] made a statistical study of cancer mortality in a metallurgic plant (A) in which arsenic was handled and in a control plant (Z) in which "working conditions approximate those of Plant A except that no arsenic is handled." From 1922 to 1949, there were 146 deaths among the employees of Plant A who handled large quantities of arsenic trioxide. Of these deaths, 18 were due to cancer, including seven cases of cancer of the respiratory system. In the control plant, 12 of 109 deaths between 1941 and 1949 were due to cancer, including six due to lung cancer. The authors stated that total cancer mortality in the two plants was not significantly different from the figures for the state as a whole, and they concluded that handling of arsenic trioxide in the industry studied does not produce a significant change in cancer mortality of the plant employees. However, as pointed out in the National Institute for Occupational Safety and Health (NIOSH) publication, *Occupational Exposure to Inorganic Arsenic, New Criteria—1975*,[807] there are a number of deficiencies in the report. Specifically, reanalyses of the data have revealed that actually there was a large excess (approximately fivefold) of lung-cancer deaths relative to mortality from all causes among workers in both plants. Thus, the data demonstrated evidence of a carcinogen for the respiratory system among the workers of both the plant in which arsenic trioxide was handled and the control plant.

Findings of increased risk of lung cancer among copper-smelter workers are not limited to the United States. A retrospective study by Kuratsune *et al.* in Japan revealed that, of 19 males who died of lung cancer in a particular town, 11 had been employed as smelter workers in a local copper refinery, and in all cases the disease had become manifest after the men had stopped working at the refinery.[443] The authors' conclusion was that prolonged exposure to arsenic, and possibly also other compounds, seemed to be associated with cancer of the lungs. Additional groups exposed to inorganic arsenic—such as gold miners in Rhodesia,[606] hard-rock miners in the United States,[833] and nickel refinery workers[672]—have shown an increased mortality from lung cancer, but evaluation of the role of arsenic is difficult, because of the presence of other suspected carcinogens in the working atmosphere.

A study at the Dow Chemical Company examined the incidence of respiratory cancer among 173 decedents who were exposed primarily to lead arsenate and calcium arsenate and 1,809 decedents who worked in the same plant and were not exposed to those compounds.[609] Data were presented on the relationship between cumulative arsenic exposure and the ratio of observed to expected deaths from lung cancer. The average exposure of each worker was calculated on the basis of records of job assignments and data on the arsenic content of the air in various parts of the plant. Deaths from respiratory malignancy were 7 times greater than expected for total inhaled quantities of 29.8 g and 2–4 times greater for 0.13–6.56 g. There was no association between the extent of exposure and the time from beginning of exposure to death; most of the respiratory cancers occurred 20–40 years after initial exposure, regardless of total exposure.

The ratio of observed to expected deaths was even higher (3.85 : 1) in another category—malignant neoplasms of the lymphatic and hematopoietic tissues except leukemia—than it was in malignant neoplasms of the respiratory system (3.45 : 1). Six lymphomas were reported, with the following diagnoses on the death certificates: four cases of Hodgkin's disease, one of lymphoblastoma, and one of reticulum cell sarcoma.

By contrast with the Dow Chemical Company workers, orchard workers who sprayed lead arsenate showed no evidence of increased cancer.[584] A mortality study involving a cohort of 1,231 workers in Wenatchee, Washington, who had participated in a 1938 morbidity survey of the effects of exposure to lead arsenate insecticide spray was conducted in 1968–1969. Air concentrations of arsenic during spraying averaged 0.14 mg/m^3. The population was grouped according to exposure in three categories and compared in terms of standardized mortality ratios with the mortality experience of the state of Washington. There was no evidence of increased mortality from cancer, heart disease, or vascular lesions.

In 1974, the mortality experience of retired employees of an Allied Chemical Company pesticide plant in Baltimore was analyzed (Baetjer et al.;[43] A. M. Baetjer, personal communication). The employees had been exposed to a number of industrial chemicals, including arsenicals; there were no data on the extent of exposure to the various chemicals. Incidence of death among the retirees was 3.5 times that among the general Baltimore population. The excess mortality was concentrated in cancer-caused deaths (14 times the expected), particularly respiratory cancer and lymphatic cancer. The noncancer deaths were at the expected rates. These calculations were based on a total of 22 deaths in men from all causes during the period 1960–1972.

Several human studies not generally available were reviewed in the NIOSH document on occupational exposure to inorganic arsenic,[807] including unpublished reports to Kennecott Copper Corporation in 1971 and 1974; unpublished papers presented at the conference on occupational carcinogenesis in New York City on March 24–27, 1975; and an evaluation by NIOSH of the study by Nelson et al.[584] In the last examples, independent sources of information investigated by NIOSH contradicted, rather than confirmed, the report by Nelson et al. The conclusion drawn was that the report apparently did not accurately depict the cancer experience of persons exposed to lead arsenate spray in the Wenatchee Valley.[807]

Population Studies

High incidences of skin cancer have been reported in several population groups exposed to high concentrations of arsenic in drinking water, including people in the district of Reichenstein in Silesia,[288] Cordoba Province in Argentina,[73] and Taiwan.[798]

A study by Tseng et al.[798] was done on the southwest coast of Taiwan, where there were artesian wells with high concentrations of arsenic that were used for more than 45 years. The arsenic concentrations in the well water of the surveyed villages ranged from 0.05 ppm to over 1.0 ppm, with a median of approximately 0.5 ppm. The chemical form of arsenic in the Taiwanese artesian-well water is also unknown; however, the reported occurrence of methane gas in the water could preclude the existence of arsenic in the pentavalent form (K. J. Irgolic, personal communication). The total population of the area was approximately 100,000, and the survey encompassed the 40,421 inhabitants of 37 villages. The overall prevalence rates for skin cancer, hyperpigmentation, and keratosis were 10.6/1,000, 183.5/1,000, and 71.0/1,000, respectively. The male : female ratios were 2.9 : 1 for skin cancer and 1.1:1 for hyperpigmentation and keratosis. Generally speaking, the prevalence of each of the three conditions increased steadily with age, although there was a decline for cancer and hyperpigmentation in women above 69. The prevalence rate for each condition varied directly with the arsenic content of the well water. The systematic effects of age and arsenic content of well water on the prevalence of skin cancer are shown in Figure 6-1. "Blackfoot disease" (a local term for a vascular disorder of the extremities), particularly of the feet, had an overall prevalence rate of 8.9/1,000. A dose-response relationship between this disease and the amount of arsenic in the well water was similar to that observed for skin cancer.

The existence of arsenical waters in an eastern area of the province of Cordoba, Argentina, has been known for many decades and is associated with the occurrence of hyperpigmentation, keratosis, and skin cancer. A study made in 1949–1959 indicated a higher proportion of deaths from cancer in the arsenical region than in the rest of the province—23.8% versus 15.3%.[73] The excess was due mainly to cancer of the respiratory and digestive tracts in both men and women. The excess cancer was unrelated to socioeconomic differences.

Experimental Animal Studies

This section presents examples of tests of oral, topical, and parenteral administration of arsenicals to rats, mice, and fish. A number of

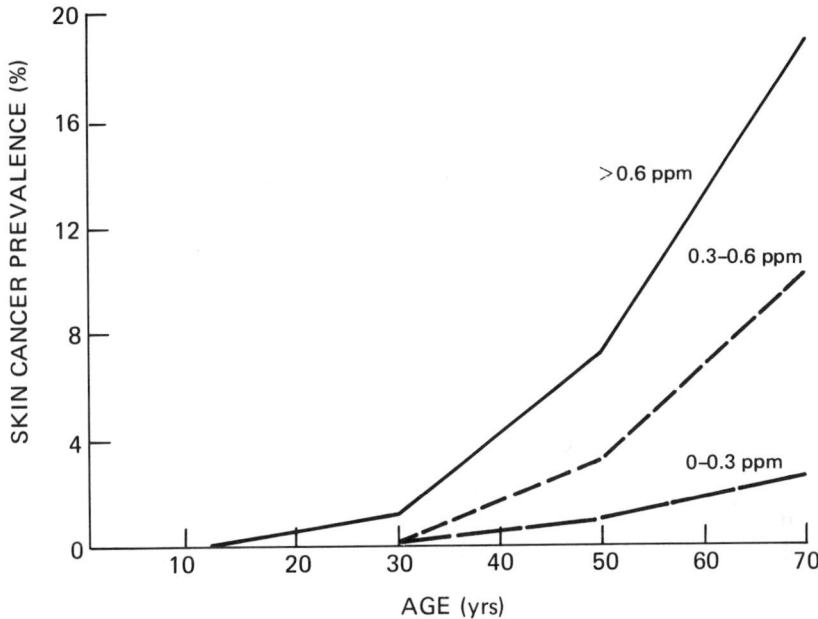

FIGURE 6-1 Prevalence of skin cancer with respect to age and arsenic concentration in well water for both sexes.[798]

laboratory animal studies designed to test arsenic compounds for carcinogenicity are not included here, for such reasons as inadequate numbers of test animals, too short a test period, too low an exposure, and poor survival. To our knowledge, no adequate animal studies have been omitted that would add substantially to the examples that follow.

In general, animal studies have not shown carcinogenicity for arsenic compounds, even when administered at near the maximally tolerated dosage for long periods. Two notable exceptions are described first, and then several of the negative studies.

In 1962, Halver reported the occurrence of hepatomas in trout fed a synthetic diet containing carbarsone at 480 mg/100 g of diet (the data were reviewed by Kraybill and Shimkin;[439] the original report is not readily available). Of 50 trout exposed to carbarsone, five developed hepatomas. There were no hepatomas in a large control group fed the synthetic diet without carbarsone. However, aflatoxin contamination of the diet may have been a confounding variable.

More recently, Osswald and Goerttler[607] reported that subcutaneous injections of sodium arsenate in pregnant Swiss mice caused a considerable increase in the incidence of leukemia in both the mothers and their offspring. A 0.005% aqueous sodium arsenate solution was injected daily during pregnancy for a total of 20 injections, each containing arsenic at 0.5 mg/kg. Some groups of offspring from the arsenic-treated females were given an additional 20 subcutaneous injections of arsenic (0.5 mg/kg) at weekly intervals. Leukemia occurred in 11 of 24 mothers (46%), 7 of 34 male offspring (21%), 6 of 37 female offspring (16%), and, in the offspring given the additional 20 injections, 17 of 41 males (41%) and 24 of 50 females (48%). Leukemia developed in only 3 of 35 male (9%) and in none of 20 female offspring of untreated control mice. Furthermore, 11 of 19 mice (58%) developed lymphoma after 20 weekly intravenous injections of 0.5 mg each of arsenic as sodium arsenate.

Long-term studies of effects of arsanilic acid on chickens, pigs, and rats were reported by Frost et al.[273] No adverse effects were seen in the chickens and pigs after 4 years of feeding, nor in pigs fed 0.01% arsanilic acid for three generations. Male and female weanling rats from the F_2 generation of a six-generation breeding study in which 0.01% and 0.05% arsanilic acid was fed were held on the 0.01% arsanilic acid diet or on the control diet for 116 weeks. The overall tumor incidence was the same in all groups and resembled the historical incidence of tumors in the colony, 35–45%. The significance of these data lies in the fact that transplacental exposure to a carcinogen followed by lifetime exposure to the same carcinogen is often the most sensitive technique for detecting carcinogenicity of a substance,[793] but this test was negative.

Boutwell[91] used female mice (Rockland and a specially bred strain highly susceptible to skin tumors) in a test for cocarcinogenicity of potassium arsenite. It was tested as an initiator, both orally by stomach tube (a total of 2.4 mg in 5 days) and locally (a total of 1.2 mg in eight applications during 5 days). This initiating treatment was followed by topical application of croton oil twice a week for 18 weeks. He also tested potassium arsenite as a promoter by daily applications (a total of 2.3 mg/week) after a single 75-μg dose of dimethylbenzanthracene (DMBA). The prolonged skin applications of potassium arsenite were hyperkeratotic and ulcerogenic. Other experiments were done to determine whether arsenic would increase the yield of skin cancers caused by a suboptimal regimen of DMBA plus croton oil given either at the time of DMBA initiation or during the 24-week period of croton oil promotion. Under the latter condition, the mice were fed potassium arsenite at 169 mg/kg of food. This dietary concentration of 169 ppm (as potassium arsenite) is very high, compared with the 0.5 ppm usually found in the human diet. In no case was there an effect of arsenite on skin carcinogenesis in these experiments. Many tumors developed in the positive control mice, beginning as early as 6 weeks after treatment began.

Baroni, van Esch, and Saffiotti[52] carried out a similar study with male and female Swiss mice, testing the oral effects of potassium arsenite (100 ppm in drinking water) as an initiator with croton oil promotion and as a promoter with DMBA and urethane initiation. Local skin applications of sodium arsenate were tested as a promoter after initiation with DMBA or urethane. The arsenicals had no effect on tumorigenesis; and only a very slight degree of keratosis was observed.

Milner[546] used three strains of mice that differed in susceptibility to the induction of skin tumors by the application to the skin of methylcholanthrene-impregnated paraffin disks for 2–3 weeks. The treated site was transplanted syngeneically and observed for 8 weeks for tumor formation. Arsenic trioxide (100 ppm in drinking water) was administered either during methylcholanthrene exposure, to animals with transplanted skin, or both. Arsenic exposure produced a small increase in the yield of papillomas in the low-susceptibility strain, a small decrease in the high-susceptibility strain, and no effect in the intermediate-susceptibility strain.

Byron et al.[123] fed either sodium arsenite or sodium arsenate to Osborne–Mendel rats in a 2-year study at dietary concentrations of 15–250 ppm for arsenite and 30–400 ppm for arsenate. No carcinogenic activity of either material was found. These investigators also did a 2-year arsenic feeding experiment on dogs, with negative results; however, this was an inadequate observation period for studying carcinogenic responses in dogs.

Hueper and Payne[373] incorporated arsenic trioxide in the drinking water (either plain or with 12% ethanol) of groups of rats and mice. The initial concentration of 4 mg/liter was increased by 2 mg/liter each month to a maximum of 34 mg/liter at 15 months. Thus, the daily intake of arsenic trioxide ranged from 0.1 to 0.8 mg/rat. The administration of arsenic trioxide was continued until 24 months. Neither the rats nor the mice developed any cancers in suspected target organs—skin, lung, and liver.

Kanisawa and Schroeder[406] and Schroeder et al.[711] found no carcinogenic effects on mice exposed from weaning to senescence to potassium arsenite at 5 ppm in drinking water[406] or on rats on the same regimen.[711]

Kroes et al.[440] studied the carcinogenicity of lead arsenate and sodium arsenate with SPF–Wistar-derived male and female rats. In addition, some groups were intubated with a subcarcinogenic dose of diethylnitrosamine to investigate a possible synergistic action leading to lung tumors. Food intake and body weights were recorded, and complete gross and microscopic examinations were made on all animals. Lead arsenate that was incorporated in the diet at 1,850 ppm was toxic and caused increased mortality; an adenoma of the renal cortex and a bile duct carcinoma were found in this group, but no significance can be attached to one or two tumors in any group. No cancer was associated with the feeding of lead arsenate at 463 ppm or sodium arsenate at 416 ppm. No synergism with the nitrosamines was observed. There was a high spontaneous-tumor incidence in this experiment. The test diets were fed to female rats from the time of parturition until the young were weaned, and these young were the test animals. Surviving rats were killed after 29 months of feeding.

As Fraumeni has pointed out, it is largely because laboratory studies have not succeeded in producing tumors in animals that arsenic has not been accepted universally as a carcinogen.[267]

Evaluation

Skin Cancer

There is evidence from clinical observations and occupational and population studies that inorganic arsenic is a skin carcinogen in man. There is a characteristic sequence of skin effects of chronic exposure to arsenic that involves hyperpigmentation initially, then hyperkeratosis (keratosis), and finally skin cancer.[887] This sequence has been observed under a variety of circumstances involving chronic exposure: potassium arsenite (Fowler's solution) was used medicinally,[585] vineyard workers used sprays and/or dusting powders containing arsenic compounds and drank arsenic-contaminated wine,[101,679] chemical workers manufactured sodium arsenite for use as a sheep dip,[633] and residents of a southwest area of Taiwan had as their only source of drinking water for over 45 years artesian wells contaminated by arsenic from geologic deposits.[798] The similarity of responses under these diverse circumstances is important, because studies in human populations always involve variables that cannot be controlled as in laboratory experiments; hence, the credibility of information derived from human studies depends on the demonstration of comparable effects under different conditions. This requirement has been amply met with arsenic as a cause of skin cancer.

The earliest skin effect of chronic arsenic exposure, hyperpigmentation (melanosis), occurs in a dappled pattern predominantly in unexposed areas. After the onset of melanosis, the skin begins to atrophy in a patchy way in hyperpigmented areas, with the formation of keratoses that are the pathognomonic lesions of chronic arsenic exposure.[887] Only a small proportion of the keratoses evolve into skin cancer, and this takes place only after very many years. The sequence is illustrated by the Taiwan data—the prevalence of melanosis, keratosis, and skin cancer reached 10% in the male population roughly at ages of 18, 30, and 60 years, respectively.[798] Chronic exposure to inorganic arsenic thus causes a slowly progressive form of patchy skin damage involving the epidermis and adnexal structures, as well as the underlying dermis, with the precancerous keratoses and cancers forming in the areas of chronic atrophy. The chronic damage and tumorigenesis resulting from arsenic are similar to the effects of ionizing and ultraviolet radiation on the skin.

Arsenical skin cancer is readily distinguished from skin cancer induced by sunlight, in that it occurs predominantly on surfaces that are shielded from sunlight and multiple lesions are much more common; for example, in 428 of the 429 cases of skin cancer studied in Taiwan, there was more than one cancer.[887]

Substantial doses of inorganic arsenic are required to produce an appreciable incidence of skin cancer. The average intake of persons treated with Fowler's solution who developed skin cancer was around 20–30 g. The prevalence of skin cancer in Taiwanese men exposed to drinking water containing arsenic at 0.3–0.6 ppm was about 15% at age 60 and over. The normal incidence is 2–3%. On the basis of a 2-liter/day water intake for the period over which the artesian wells were used (45 years), the total arsenic intake must have been about 15 g, which is roughly in the same domain as that in clinical cases of the use of Fowler's solution. Thus, the Taiwanese data that demonstrated the requirement for large doses of arsenic to obtain even a modest yield of skin cancer are consistent with the relatively low frequency of skin cancer in patients treated with Fowler's solution. The low potency of inorganic arsenic may explain why no skin effects have been reported in people treated for syphilis with organic arsenicals, inasmuch as the total doses amounted to only a few grams. However, it is also possible that the metabolism of the organic arsenicals is sufficiently different to preclude the occurrence of skin cancer and other forms of arsenical damage even at higher doses.

The relative frequency of melanosis, keratosis, and skin cancer was roughly similar in the Taiwanese population and the chemical workers who manufactured sheep dip. On direct examination, the latter showed a 90% prevalence of melanosis and a 30% prevalence of keratosis, for a ratio of melanosis to keratosis of 3 : 1. At comparable ages, the Taiwanese showed a ratio of about 4 : 1. Two of the nine keratosis patients in the sheep-dip factory had already been treated for skin cancer, and the proportionality between keratosis and skin cancer was about the same in Taiwan. As in the Taiwan experience, the sheep-dip chemical workers had been exposed to large doses of inorganic arsenic (up to 1 g/year), but much of this was by inhalation.

It is possible that the trivalent and pentavalent forms of inorganic arsenic produce the same effects on skin. This is of interest, particularly in view of the different metabolic patterns of trivalent and pentavalent inorganic arsenic—the former by interaction with sulfhydryl groups and the latter by substituting for phosphate. The clinical use of Fowler's solution and the manufacture of sodium arsenite as a sheep dip both involved exposure to trivalent inorganic arsenic. The two categories of people developed similar skin responses. The Rhodesian gold miners, in whom the incidence of typical arsenical keratoses was very high, were exposed to arsenopyrite, in which the arsenic becomes trivalent on weathering; the reactions of arsenopyrite in the body are unknown (K. J. Irgolic, personal communication). The chemical form of arsenic in the Taiwanese artesian-well water is also unknown; however, the reported occurrence of methane gas in the water could preclude the existence of arsenic in the pentavalent form (K. J. Irgolic, personal communication).

Lung Cancer

Of the published reports on mortality from respiratory cancer in copper smelters, the most impressive is that of Lee and Fraumeni.[412] The study involved a population of 8,047 white male smelter workers who were followed for 26 years; for each employee, information was available on time, place, and duration of employment, maximal arsenic and sulfur dioxide exposures (descriptive, rather than numerical), and cause of death. The life-table method was used to evaluate age-specific mortality rates for the various causes of death, and the rates were compared with those of the states in which the smelters were. The number of deaths available for analysis was very substantial—1,877. The study demonstrated a systematic gradient for respiratory cancer according to the magnitude and duration of exposure to both arsenic and sulfur dioxide. These agents, however, were inseparably linked, because of the nature of the smelter operations. The amount of excess cancer was impressive, with an eightfold increase in the workers who had the heaviest arsenic exposure for the longest duration, i.e., more than 15 years. The latent period—the interval between first employment and death from respiratory cancer—was extraordinarily long and was inversely related to the magnitude of exposure: 34, 39, and 41 years for the categories of heavy, medium, and light arsenic exposure. There were deficiencies in the study, some of which were unavoidable. For example, no indication was given of whether the study population was representative of the total worker population; the exposure rankings were based on the maximal arsenic concentrations, rather than weighted averages derived from work histories. No quantitative data were available on exposure. No attempt was made to validate the stated causes of death. No smoking histories were obtained. However, none of these deficiencies could be seriously regarded as invalidating the conclusions of the study.

The Kuratsune report dealt with a smaller study that compared lung-cancer mortality rates calculated from the 22 deaths that occurred in a 30-year period in a smelter town with the lung-cancer experience in the same period in a neighboring city and in Japan as a whole.[443] The standardized mortality rate for males in the smelter towns was 4 times higher than that for the rest of the country, but equal to that for women. This fourfold excess is comparable with the 3.3-fold excess observed in the Lee–Fraumeni study. Although many of the men in the town worked in the refinery, a much higher proportion of the lung-cancer cases, compared with controls, occurred in men who were heavily exposed to arsenic as smelter operators. As in the case of the Lee–Fraumeni study, the latent period from first exposure to the diagnosis of lung cancer was very long, ranging from 26 to 48 years. The duration of employment was also very long, with a median of about 30 years, although two cases occurred in people who worked for only 2–3 years.

Two lung-cancer studies of the American Smelting and Refining Company smelter have produced conflicting results. The 1963 Pinto and Bennett report examined the proportional mortality from lung cancer in a total of 229 deaths in the period 1946–1960.[647] This study dealt only with pensioners and workers who died during their employment and did not include people who had left the plant. The reported data showed that the 18 lung-cancer deaths in the plant population as a whole indicated a rate that was higher than the rate in the state of Washington. However, the excess lung cancer for the plant as a whole was due to the high occurrence in controls, i.e., in workers who were considered *not* to have arsenic exposure. Milham and Strong, by contrast, found, in the years 1950–1971, that there were records of 39 deaths due to respiratory cancer in Pierce County (the smelter locale) in people who were stated to have worked at the smelter.[543] Applica-

TABLE 6-5[a] Observed Deaths and Standardized Mortality Ratios (SMR) at Ages 65 and Over for the Period January 1, 1949, through December 31, 1973, among 530 Men Retiring from the Tacoma Smelter, by Cause of Death and Arsenic Exposure Index at Retirement[b]

Cause of Death[d]	Arsenic Exposure Index[c]											
	Total		Under 3,000		3,000–5,999		6,000–8,999		9,000–11,999		12,000+	
	Obs	SMR	Obs	SMR	Obs	SMR	Obs	SMR	Obs	SMR	Obs	SMR
All causes	324	111.1[e]	87	98.1	124	110.3	70	129.2[e]	24	117.7	17	130.0
Cancer (140–205)	69	146.6[e]	15	107.9	28	156.0[e]	14	151.6	7	218.7	5	217.2
Digestive (150–159)	20	120.3	6	121.2	9	140.4	2	62.7	3	264.7	0	0.0
Respiratory (160–164)	32	300.3[e]	5	165.6	11	279.4[e]	7	306.9[e]	4	568.5[e]	5	810.5[e]
Lymphatic (200–203, 205)	2	94.9	1	166.1	1	126.1	0	0.0	0	0.0	0	0.0
Other cancer	15	84.8	3	56.3	7	102.8	5	150.4	0	0.0	0	0.0
Stroke (330–334)	44	114.7	18	150.3	12	80.0	7	104.5	6	218.4	1	64.7
Heart disease (400–443)	144	107.7	33	81.4	63	122.4	36	144.2[e]	5	53.6	5	83.2
Coronary (420)	118	105.9	25	74.9	52	122.2	31	145.1[e]	4	51.7	5	95.5
Other heart	26	116.6	8	111.5	11	123.2	5	138.4	1	62.9	0	0.0
Respiratory disease (480–493, 500–502)	10	91.6	4	116.8	3	70.9	1	52.4	2	250.8	0	0.0
All other causes	57	91.2	17	89.2	18	74.8	12	104.1	4	91.3	6	212.4

[a]Pinto, S. S., V. Henderson, and P. Enterline. "Mortality experience of arsenic exposed workers." Unpublished data.
[b]Expected deaths were estimated on the basis of Washington State experience, 1949–1970. Includes four men with unknown exposures.
[c]Arsenic exposure index derived from A. Baetjer, A. M. Levin, and A. Lilienfeld, "Analysis of mortality experience of Allied Chemical plant," unpublished data.
[d]*Manual of the International Statistical Classification of Diseases, Injuries, and Causes of Death.*[880]
[e]Statistically significant ($p < 0.05$).

tion of U.S. mortality rates to the published figures for the smelter population at risk yielded an expected number of 18 respiratory-cancer deaths, compared with the 39 deaths observed.

Pinto et al. (S. S. Pinto, V. Henderson, and P. Enterline, "Mortality experience of arsenic exposed workers," unpublished data) recently resolved the discrepancy between the Pinto and Bennett[647] and Milham and Strong[543] papers in a study of the same smelter that reevaluated the exposure categories used in the Pinto and Bennett paper[647] (which were apparently in error) and also included a longer observation period and therefore more deaths. The data, in Table 6-5, include a total of 32 respiratory-cancer cases and show a progressive increase in standardized mortality ratio with increasing arsenic exposure. The arsenic-exposure index was calculated as a weighted average based on urinary arsenic concentration and duration of employment. It is of interest that the eightfold excess in respiratory cancer for workers with the highest exposures and the threefold excess for all the smelter workers reported by Pinto et al. (see Table 6-5) were very close to the figures reported by Lee and Fraumeni[460] and Kuratsune.[443]

The studies described here indicated that excess respiratory cancer occurs in copper-smelter workers as a function of the magnitude and duration of exposure to arsenic, with latent periods of three to four decades from the time of initial exposure. However, the studies do not permit a resolution of the issue of whether concomitant exposure to sulfur dioxide and other smelter dusts is necessary for the carcinogenic response. Evidence from studies involving entirely different circumstances of exposure—including workers in three pesticide manufacturing plants,[352,609]* vintners who applied pesticides,[101,679] and Rhodesian gold miners[606]—suggests that sulfur dioxide and other unspecified smelter dusts are not essential cofactors for the respiratory carcinogenicity of arsenic. All the nonsmelter studies had obvious limitations, but the lung-cancer excess in each study was relatively large and, taken as a group, they provide significant evidence that arsenic is a lung carcinogen.

The Hill–Faning study of 75 deaths in a sheep-dip factory used the indirect method of proportional mortality to evaluate the small group of 22 deaths from cancer; seven of them were cancers of the respiratory tract, compared with an expected 2.4 deaths.[352] The Dow arsenic workers[609] were evaluated in two ways: by an analysis of death records of those who died from lung cancer (28, or 16.2%, of 173 chemical-

*Also, A. Baetjer, M. Levin, and A. Lilienfeld, "Analysis of mortality experience of Allied Chemical plant," unpublished data.

worker deaths, compared with 104, or 5.7%, of 1,809 control-case deaths), and then, as a retrospective cohort study, a comparison of the mortality from respiratory cancer (obtained from the records used in the first approach) among 603 persons identified as having worked in the arsenic plant from 1940 to 1973 with the mortality among the corresponding U.S. white male population. The two approaches gave essentially the same results—a threefold to fourfold excess. However, the puzzling aspect of the data is that almost 60% of the respiratory-cancer deaths were in people who had worked with arsenic for less than a year, three decades earlier. Most of the arsenic workers were unskilled short-term employees, of whom a large proportion left the company after a brief period of employment. The followup study, however, dealt only with the people who remained in the company. A confirmation of the excess lung cancer in a followup of short-term arsenic workers who left the company would be very useful. Nevertheless, there were about a dozen cases in people who worked longer than a year and who were in the highest dose categories, where the excess risk was maximal—fourfold to sixfold. It is possible that the apparent twofold excess in lung cancer in the lower exposure categories, including those who worked with arsenic for less than a year, would not be ascribable to arsenic, because there was no change in cancer risk over a very wide range of total doses (0.04–1.56 g). Furthermore, these low dose categories consisted predominantly of short-term unskilled workers who as a group might have had higher exposures to other hazardous chemicals than the controls.

The Allied Chemical Company pesticide manufacturing operations produced a range of products, including some arsenical compounds. A preliminary study of the proportional mortality among retired employees showed a sevenfold excess of lung cancer that accounted for about 40% of all deaths (A. M. Baetjer, personal communication). Both the Dow and Allied studies also showed a few excess deaths from lymphoma and Hodgkin's disease. The results of a more detailed study of the Allied Chemical Company that is now in progress will be very useful.

Arsenic sprays and dusts were widely used in Germany between 1925 and 1942, at which time they were banned.[101,679] Vineyard workers also drank wine containing arsenic. Hundreds of workers developed acute and chronic arsenic poisoning. In the 1950's, vineyard workers with lung cancer began to appear in hospitals serving the vineyard regions. An association between arsenic and lung cancer is further suggested by the high proportion of vineyard workers with lung cancer who had the characteristic hyperpigmentation and keratoses associated with chronic arsenic exposure.

The same high degree of association of skin arsenism and lung cancer occurred in Rhodesian gold miners who were heavily exposed to arsenopyrite dust.[606] In the period 1957–1963, the occurrence of 37 cases of lung cancer in gold miners represented an incidence of 206/100,000, compared with 34/100,000 for adult males in the Gwanda region of Rhodesia. This represents a sixfold difference in lung cancer in miners.

The probability of death from lung cancer in persons with keratosis shown in Table 6-6 ranges from 32 to 56%, which is roughly 5–10 times higher than might be expected.

The data suggest that there is a very high risk of lung cancer when the exposure to inorganic arsenic dust is high enough to cause keratoses.

Liver Cancer

The only evidence that arsenic is a liver carcinogen comes from German vintners. Thirteen of the 27 persons whose autopsies were reported by Roth[679] had cirrhosis, and three had angiosarcoma, a rare form of liver cancer associated with exposure to a vinyl chemical and Thorotrast. Only two cases of angiosarcoma have been reported in people treated with Fowler's solution.[663] There is no evidence of either cirrhosis or liver damage in any of the other studies on arsenic. It is possible that the combined effect of a high alcohol intake and arsenic is

TABLE 6-6 Frequency of Lung Cancer in Persons with Keratoses Who Had Heavy Exposure to Arsenical Dusts

Subjects	(a) No. Cases of Keratosis	(b) No. Cases of Lung Cancer	b/a, %	Reference
Rhodesian gold miners	40	13	32	606
Vintners (Braun)	16	9	56	101
Vintners (Roth)	30	10	33	679
Sheep-dip workers[a]	12	5	42	633
Total	98	37	38	

[a] Assumes that 41 chemical workers who died in 1910–1943 had the same skin changes as chemical workers examined in 1946.

responsible for the unusual forms of cirrhosis and liver cancer observed in vintners. It should also be pointed out that the chemical form of arsenic in wine is unknown.

Experimentally Induced Cancer

The fact that there is no established method for producing cancer by treatment with any form of arsenic in an animal model system is an enigma. One must conclude either that arsenic is not a carcinogen or that particular circumstances not yet achieved are essential to demonstrate a role for arsenic in experimental carcinogenesis. A conclusion that carcinogenesis by arsenic is restricted to humans (or cows, horses, and deer[420]) is highly suspect. Therefore, much effort should be spent in attempting to find conditions in which the presence or absence of arsenic determines the appearance or nonappearance of cancer in an animal model. Some questions need to be explored (their answers may account for the variable incidence of human cancer associated with arsenic exposure):

• Potassium arsenite, arsenic trioxide, and possibly other compounds of arsenic appear to have an unusual propensity to alter epithelial morphology (at least in humans), often acting as irritants and causing hyperplasia, as well as hyperkeratosis. Thus, appropriate forms of arsenic should be tested with known lung carcinogens for synergistic action. Possibilities include the ferric oxide–benzopyrene model in the hamster developed by Saffiotti *et al.*[699] and the sulfur dioxide–benzopyrene inhalation model of Kuschner and Laskin.[444] Controls designed to test exposure to arsenicals alone should be included; properly controlled long-term inhalation studies have not been done.

Although both Barone *et al.*[52] and Boutwell[91] based their tests in mouse skin on a possible cocarcinogenic role for arsenic and found none, additional experiments of this nature are reasonable.

Moreover, because morphologic changes in epithelial tissue are ascribed to arsenic, and because vitamin A and some retinoids control normal epithelial morphology,[754] it is appropriate to design experiments in which vitamin A deficiency is induced in animals as a test system for arsenical carcinogenicity (and cocarcinogenicity). In experimental animals, vitamin A deficiency increases susceptibility to chemical carcinogenesis, and high dietary concentrations of retinoids have remarkable ability to prevent chemical carcinogenesis in epithelial tissues,[754] including skin, breast, and lung.

Again, because arsenicals alter epithelial morphology, the possibility that the function of mucus-secreting cells or of the ciliated cells of the lung is interfered with by respirable particles bearing arsenic[580] should be investigated. Interference with mucus secretion or ciliary action would facilitate the action of a carcinogen, such as tobacco smoke, entering the lungs.

- Because compounds of arsenic and the heavy metals that may be associated with them are enzyme poisons, it is possible that chronic exposure to abnormal amounts of these substances partially poisons enzymes that inactivate carcinogens. Model systems might be devised to test this possibility.
- The interaction of arsenic with some essential nutrients, such as sodium selenite and potassium iodide, is known. This should be considered in designing animal models.

Peoples[626] has shown that potassium arsenite and sodium arsenate are detoxified via methylation pathways. Biologic changes attributable to arsenic might be accentuated in animals fed diets that are low in labile methyl groups.

- The administration of some carcinogens to pregnant females may result in an unusually high incidence or early development of cancer in the offspring. Because one such test, by Osswald and Goerttler,[607] resulted in an unusual incidence of leukemia in mice, it is especially urgent to design appropriate transplacental tests. Repetition of such a test is essential. The credibility of the Osswald and Goerttler study is limited by their failure to give the vehicle solution to the controls.
- Because of the failure of repeated tests in lower animals to show carcinogenicity due to arsenicals, consideration should be given to the use of nonhuman primates as test animals.

These are only a few examples of approaches to the problem of ascertaining whether an animal model may be devised to account for the association of human cancer with exposure to arsenic.

7

Summary and Conclusions

CHEMISTRY

The compound of arsenic produced in largest quantity is arsenic trioxide. It is a by-product of the copper-smelting industry. Arsenic exhibits oxidation states of III and V and forms a great variety of inorganic and organic compounds. In addition to arsenic trioxide, some widely encountered inorganic compounds are arsenic pentoxide, arsenous acid, arsenic acid, tetraarsenic tetrasulfide (realgar), arsenic trisulfide (orpiment), and arsenic pentasulfide. Some of the more common organic compounds are methanearsonic acid, cacodylic acid, methyldihydroxyarsine, dimethylhydroxyarsine, trimethylarsine, and trimethylarsine oxide. Some aromatic arsenic derivatives with veterinary and medicinal uses are arsanilic acid, 3-nitro-4-hydroxyphenylarsonic acid, 4-nitrophenylarsonic acid, and 3-nitro-4-ureidophenylarsonic acid.

Cationic species of As(III) are probably not present in aqueous solution. Arsenous acid likely exists as $As(OH)_3$. The fact that the hydroxides of iron(II), iron(III), chromium(III), and aluminum strongly adsorb or form insoluble precipitates with arsenites and arsenates is important in the control of arsenic pollution. The ability of various molds and bacteria to convert arsenic compounds to various methyl-

Summary and Conclusions

ated arsines is well known. Because the methylated arsines are sparingly soluble in water, volatile, and sensitive to air, they are returned to the environment as methanearsonates, cacodylates, and trimethylarsine oxide. Arsenic–sulfur bonds are less subject to hydrolysis than arsenic–oxygen bonds, and the formation of arsenic–sulfur bonds with sulfur-containing biologic molecules is considered to be of great importance.

DISTRIBUTION

Arsenic is ubiquitous in the environment and is found in all living organisms. Natural sources include a variety of sulfur-containing minerals, of which arsenopyrite is the most common. The amounts of arsenic in soil and water depend largely on the geologic inputs from mineral weathering processes, whereas the amounts in indigenous plants and animals reflect species differences. Some species of marine plants, such as algae and seaweed, and marine organisms, such as crustaceans and some fish, often contain naturally high concentrations of arsenic.

Man-made sources of arsenic are generally by-products of the smelting of nonferrous metal ores, primarily copper and to a lesser degree lead, zinc, and gold. In the United States, the sole producer and refiner of arsenic trioxide is the copper smelter of the American Smelting and Refining Company in Tacoma, Washington. Major imports of arsenic come from Sweden, the world's leading producer.

The largest use of arsenic is in the production of agricultural pesticides, in the categories of herbicides, insecticides, desiccants, wood preservatives, and feed additives. Arsenic trioxide was the raw material for the older inorganic pesticides, including lead arsenate, calcium arsenate, and sodium arsenite. The newer major organic arsenical pesticides include three herbicides, monosodium and disodium methanearsonate and cacodylic acid, and four feed additives that are substituted phenylarsonic acids. Arsenic has several minor uses, primarily as an additive in metallurgic applications, in glass production, as a catalyst in several manufacturing processes, and in medicine. Arsenical drugs are still used in treating tropical diseases, such as African sleeping sickness and amebic dysentery, and are used in veterinary medicine to treat parasitic diseases, such as heartworm (filariasis) in dogs and blackhead in turkeys and chickens.

The major arsenic residues resulting from use of agricultural pesticides and fertilizers are found in soils and to a lesser degree in plants and animals living on contaminated soils. The highest pesticide residues occur primarily in orchard soils that received large applications of lead arsenate. Large accumulations of arsenic also occur in soils around smelters. Two important closely related effects measurable in plants are arsenic residues and phytotoxicity. Some soils that received massive applications of arsenate are currently incapable of supporting plant growth.

Arsenic in air has three major sources: smelting of metals, burning of coal, and use of arsenical pesticides. Two known acute incidents of arsenic pollution from smelters have occurred in the United States. The most serious air-pollution problem, however, is associated with manufacturing processes and occupational hazards to workers. Some arsenic in water results from industrial discharges. Several endemic poisonings of water supplies have been reported.

Safe disposal of arsenic wastes still constitutes a major administrative and technologic problem. The major sources of arsenical wastes are residues in empty pesticide containers; surplus pesticides stored by government agencies, manufacturers, state and municipal facilities, and users; and soil contaminated by extensive use of arsenical pesticides. Recommended procedures for management of arsenical wastes are recycling and reuse (preferred), long-term storage, recovery of other metals and long-term storage of arsenic trioxide, and disposal in landfill sites.

Several arsenic cycles have been proposed to interrelate the source, emission, movement, distribution, and sinks of various forms in the environment. Arsenic is continuously cycling in the environment, owing to oxidation, reduction, and methylation reactions. Man's activities can alter the distribution of arsenic in finite geographic areas or in selected components of the environment, but man has little control over the natural processes.

METABOLISM

Arsenic compounds must be in a mobile form in the soil solution in order to be absorbed by plants. Except for locations around smelters or where the natural arsenic content is high, the arsenic taken up is distributed throughout the plant body in less than toxic amounts.

In nature, arsenic absorption by plants from the air is negligible. Although smelter fumes and dusts may deposit on plant leaves, there is no evidence that arsenic from this source is taken into plants.

Translocation of arsenicals in plants is demonstrated by the fact that arsenical solutions applied to foliage of some weeds results in the killing of root tissue. Metabolic experiments with radiolabeled organic arsenic compounds have indicated that these compounds or metabolites thereof form complexes with some plant constituents.

Bacteria and fungi can metabolize inorganic arsenic salts to form methylated derivatives. Algae can biosynthesize complex organic arsenicals that are associated with the lipid fraction of these microorganisms. Mollusks and crustaceans can contain rather high concentrations of arsenic, but there appears to be no relationship between their arsenic content and the collection date or geographic location; this suggests that industrial pollution is not a factor. Fish also can contain arsenic, which apparently is derived from their diet. The arsenic that occurs naturally in seafood is metabolized quite differently from inorganic arsenic. The form of arsenic in shrimp, for example, is not retained by the human body and is rapidly excreted.

The rat has a unique arsenic metabolism that renders it unsuitable for metabolic studies with arsenic compounds. This rodent stores arsenic in the hemoglobin of its red cells, which release the arsenic only when they break down. The resulting very slow excretion led to the belief that arsenic is a cumulative poison. Trivalent sodium arsenite seems to be almost entirely oxidized to pentavalent sodium arsenate *in vivo*. Evidence of the opposite process—i.e., the *in vivo* reduction of arsenate to arsenite—is much less clear.

Arsenic in normal urine of man, dog, and cow is principally in the methylated form. When the dog and cow are fed large doses of trivalent or pentavalent inorganic arsenic, about half the arsenic appears in the urine as methylated derivatives. This methylation process is true detoxification, inasmuch as methanearsonates and cacodylates are only one two-hundredth as toxic as sodium arsenite.

EFFECTS ON ANIMALS AND PLANTS

A number of different factors can influence the toxicity of arsenicals, including chemical form, physical form, mode of administration, species, and criterion of toxicity. Several reports have suggested that arsenic can exert biologic effects at concentrations below those generally considered "safe," but the physiologic significance of such findings is not known.

The trivalent forms of arsenic apparently exert their toxic effect chiefly by reacting with the sulfhydryl groups of vital cellular enzymes. Pyruvate dehydrogenase seems to be a particularly vulnerable site in metabolism, because it contains the dithiol lipoic acid that is especially reactive with trivalent arsenicals. The biochemical basis of the toxic action of pentavalent arsenic compounds is known with less certainty, but such arsenicals may well compete with phosphate in phosphorylation reactions to form unstable arsenyl esters that spontaneously hydrolyze and thereby short-circuit energy-yielding bioenergetic processes.

The use of phenylarsonic animal feed additives as recommended is beneficial and does not constitute a human or animal health hazard. Animal losses and excessive arsenical residues in poultry and pork tissues occur only when the arsenicals are fed at excessive dosages for long periods. The mechanism of action of phenylarsonic animal feed additives remains obscure, and these compounds are for the most part absorbed and excreted without metabolic change.

Toxicoses caused by the phenylarsonates are manifested by an entirely different syndrome from those caused by the inorganic and aliphatic organic arsenicals. The latter produce the typical signs and lesions usually associated with arsenic poisoning, whereas the former are less toxic and produce demyelination and gliosis of peripheral and cranial nerves.

Poisoning of forage-eating livestock by inorganic and aliphatic organic arsenical compounds, especially those used as herbicides and defoliants, has been reported. Most cases result from accidental or careless contamination of forage that becomes accessible to livestock.

The large-scale use of arsenicals in the United States has caused some scientists to suspect that the use of these compounds may have a deleterious effect on wildlife. However, there is little evidence to confirm such suspicions in the scientific literature. Wildlife kills that have been attributed to arsenic compounds were all associated with misuse of the compounds in question. But several laboratory studies have shown that wild species are generally more sensitive to arsenic poisoning than many domestic species; therefore, some ecologic vigilance is appropriate.

Most data on the effects of arsenicals on aquatic organisms, particularly on freshwater organisms, were collected in short-term, direct-lethality studies. Practically nothing is known about the sublethal long-term effects of arsenic, singly or in combination with other pollutants, on aquatic organisms.

Although early workers were not able to demonstrate any adaptation in animals to toxic concentrations of inorganic arsenic, some recent work has suggested that there may be a rather limited adaptive response to inorganic arsenicals under some conditions.

Summary and Conclusions

Abnormal physiologic responses have been noted in animals exposed to arsenic trioxide aerosols at concentrations considerably below currently accepted air-quality standards. Unfortunately, these experiments were carried out with the rat, which has a unique ability to accumulate arsenic and is therefore a poor animal model for studying arsenic metabolism. It is difficult to draw valid conclusions about the public-health or environmental implications of these investigations.

High concentrations of arsenicals have been shown to decrease the ability of mice to resist viral infection, presumably by inhibiting interferon formation or action. However, low concentrations of arsenicals appear to enhance the antiviral activity of interferon.

Arsenic is known to protect partially against the effects of selenium poisoning over a wide variety of conditions. Arsenic decreases the toxicity of selenium by enhancing its biliary excretion, thus clearing it from the liver, the primary target organ in selenosis.

Preliminary results have suggested a role for arsenic as a nutritionally essential trace element. Improved methods in trace-element research—such as the use of ultrapure water, highly refined diets, and plastic animal housing—apparently have enabled nutritionists to uncover a function for arsenic in normal metabolism.

The biologic effects of arsenic compounds on microorganisms appear to be mediated very much by the same mechanisms as in mammals. However, some microorganisms have a substantial ability to adapt to toxic concentrations of arsenicals. This adaptation seems in most cases to be due to decreased permeability of the microorganism to arsenic.

Arsenicals clearly can be toxic to plants, but the biochemical basis of such toxicity is less understood than that of the toxicity of arsenicals to animals. As in animals, arsenates are generally less toxic to plants than arsenites. One of the first symptoms of plant injury by sodium arsenite is wilting caused by loss of turgor, whereas the symptoms due to arsenate do not involve rapid loss of turgor, at least through the early expression of toxicity.

The phytotoxicity of organic arsenical herbicides is characterized by a relatively slow kill; the first symptoms are usually chlorosis, cessation of growth, and gradual browning followed by dehydration and death. Several variables can influence the response, including stage of growth, senescence, moisture availability, temperature, light intensity, and insect or mechanical wounding of foliage before treatment.

Arsenic can interact with several plant nutrients in either soils or nutrient solutions. Phosphate can increase or decrease the toxicity of arsenicals, depending on the experimental conditions. The toxicity in some species grown on arsenic-contaminated soils could be reduced by foliar or soil application of zinc or iron.

EFFECTS ON MAN

The past medicinal use of inorganic arsenic preparations has provided the basis for reasonably clear definition of the consequences of chronic systemic arsenic exposure—specifically, characteristic hyperkeratosis and, less frequently, irregularities in pigmentation, especially on the trunk. Association of these features with other, less common disorders, such as arterial insufficiency and cancer, in exposed populations must be regarded as supportive evidence of a causal function of arsenic. It should also be noted that many studies of populations "at risk" have failed to evaluate cutaneous changes adequately. Proper examination of the skin of people subjected to chronic low-dose arsenic exposure has the potential for providing valuable information related to the dose and duration of exposure necessary to cause changes in given populations. In a word, these benign skin lesions may be regarded as sensitive indexes of exposure to an agent that has potentially serious consequences.

The present generation of physicians has not used arsenic and has little direct knowledge of its toxic manifestations. Thus, the "index of suspicion" of the average practitioner may be relatively ineffective in diagnosing isolated cases of arsenic toxicity.

There is also considerable reason to believe that, judiciously used, arsenic may have therapeutic value. The time may be ripe to rediscover an old remedy with modern analytic techniques.

Several occupational and nonoccupational episodes of arsenic toxicity have occurred. Two of the best characterized and yet least known nonoccupational episodes occurred in Japan in 1955. One involved tainted powdered milk; the other, contaminated soy sauce. In the former, 12,131 cases of infant poisoning were recorded, with 130 deaths. Evidence of severe damage to health, including retarded growth and brain dysfunction, was found in a followup study 15 years later.

Experimental teratogenic effects of arsenic compounds have been reported, but none of the studies has been sufficiently exhaustive to allow accurate assessment of the human hazard. For example, the doses that were administered to achieve effects far exceeded likely environmental exposure, and accurate no-effect doses were generally not determined.

Summary and Conclusions

There is some evidence that arsenicals can be mutagenic in humans: An increased incidence of chromosomal aberrations was observed in phytohemagglutinin-stimulated lymphocyte cultures prepared from psoriasis patients who had been previously treated with arsenic.

There is strong epidemiologic evidence that inorganic arsenic is a skin and lung carcinogen in man. Skin cancer has occurred in association with exposure to inorganic arsenic compounds in a variety of populations, including patients treated with Fowler's solution, Taiwanese exposed to arsenic in artesian-well water, workers engaged in the manufacture of pesticides, and vintners using arsenic as a pesticide. The Taiwan data demonstrated a gradient of incidence with degree of exposure and age. All these populations had a pathognomonic sequence of skin changes leading to cancer.

Lung cancer has been observed to be associated with inhalation exposure to arsenic in copper smelters, workers in pesticide-manufacturing plants, Moselle vintners, and Rhodesian gold miners. Two of the three smelter studies showed a gradient in the incidence of lung cancer with the degree of arsenic exposure; one of these studies also suggested that sulfur dioxide may be a carcinogenic cofactor for the lung.

Although hemangioendothelioma has been reported occasionally in people who have been exposed to arsenic, the case for arsenic as a liver carcinogen is not clear.

The absence of a useful animal model is a serious handicap to the study of arsenic as a skin carcinogen and is probably due to metabolic differences between humans and the animals tested so far. The failure to induce skin cancer in test animals is perhaps not surprising, inasmuch as neither melanosis nor keratosis has been duplicated in animals and these effects appear to be inseparably linked to the tumorigenic action of arsenic in the skin of man. The carcinogenicity of arsenic for the lung in animals has not yet been evaluated by inhalation studies.

MEASUREMENT

The preparation of material for the determination of arsenic requires the usual care to ensure that the portion of the sample submitted for analysis truly represents the whole. Special hazards related to arsenic compounds are the possible loss of arsenous oxide by volatilization and the rapid adsorption of some arsenic compounds from solution onto the walls of storage vessels.

If total arsenic is to be measured in plant or animal tissue or in coal, the sample is first wet-ashed with some combination of nitric, perchloric, and sulfuric acids. Arsenic originally present in the sample at very low concentrations must often be preconcentrated before it can be measured. If the sample is a solution, the arsenic can be coprecipitated on metallic hydroxides or precipitated with organic reagents. It can also be isolated from its original matrix by liquid–liquid extraction or by volatilization as a trihalide or as arsine.

Until recently, total arsenic was usually determined colorimetrically, by either the molybdenum blue method or the silver diethyldithiocarbamate method. Arsenic is now usually determined by atomic absorption, with the sample solution introduced into a flame as an aerosol or deposited as a droplet inside a tube or on a metallic strip, which is then strongly heated. Greater sensitivity has been achieved with atomic absorption, however, by converting the arsenic to arsine and introducing this gas into a heated tube. Equal sensitivity can be achieved by introducing the arsine into an arc in helium and measuring the resulting spectral emission. Low detection limits for arsenic can also be reached by neutron-activation analysis (often without chemical treatment). Electrochemical methods, such as differential pulse polarography, can achieve comparable sensitivity in the presence of natural pollutants (e.g., sludge).

CONCLUSIONS

Environmental contamination with and human exposure to arsenic compounds have resulted from incidents of air pollution from smelters, the improper use of arsenical pesticides, and episodes of tainted food and drink. The degree of arsenic air pollution due to smelter operations and pesticide use should decrease if currently proposed occupational and environmental standards are promulgated. The technical and economic feasibility of the changes in engineering controls or work practices needed to achieve compliance with such standards, however, has yet to be determined.

Although the total amount of arsenic injected into the atmosphere in the United States as a result of coal-burning is very large, the sources of such air pollution are widely dispersed, and arsenic exposure due to fossil-fuel combustion does not seem to constitute a health hazard. This contrasts with the situation in some other countries (e.g., Czechoslovakia), where the arsenic content of coal is high and high ambient-air concentrations of arsenic result. Although petroleum gen-

Summary and Conclusions

erally contains only small quantities of arsenic, oil from shale can contain significant amounts; therefore, if use of this fossil fuel becomes common, removal of arsenic from the oil or more careful environmental monitoring of arsenic is indicated.

The food supply normally contains small amounts of arsenic, but these are not considered harmful. Some seafood has appreciable natural concentrations of arsenic, but in such a form that it is rapidly and completely excreted by humans after ingestion. Arsenic residues in foodstuffs due to arsenical pesticide or feed-additive use do not seem to warrant concern. There have been isolated epidemics of food poisoning due to arsenic as a result of manufacturing accidents, but they are rare.

Water supplies generally contain negligible quantities of arsenic, although some cases of endemically poisoned waters have been reported. Industrial effluents have been shown to contain arsenic, but the self-purifying tendency of rivers and streams and improved quality of wastewater discharges should help to minimize this problem.

The use of arsenical pesticides in food crops declined greatly after introduction of the chlorinated hydrocarbon and organophosphorus chemicals. However, as more and more restrictions are placed on the use of the latter two families of compounds, the use of arsenical pesticides may once again assume importance. If this occurs, more careful monitoring of arsenic in the environment and food supply would be imperative.

Our greatest area of ignorance about arsenicals in the environment has to do with the ecologic cycling of arsenic compounds. Little or no quantitative information is available regarding the fate of arsenicals in the ecosphere, so it is not possible to state with certainty whether arsenic is building up in any sector of the ecosystem. For example, organic arsenicals are widely used as herbicides and desiccants, but we do not know whether such use will eventually render the soil phytotoxic, as has happened in some orchards in which lead arsenate was heavily applied. More research is needed to investigate such problems.

Suitable methods for arsenic determination are available for environmental analysis. However, sample-handling may present difficulties because of losses of arsenic compounds via sublimation, especially during air monitoring, and analytic personnel should be alerted to this possible procedural pitfall.

Individual arsenic compounds can be determined only after isolation by an appropriate method, such as volatilization, paper chromatography, gas chromatography, or electrophoresis. When the nature of the compound is known, the quantity present can be measured by measuring the amount of arsenic present.

The continued concern about the association between inorganic arsenic and cancer has raised questions regarding the implications of widespread dispersion of inorganic arsenicals in the environment. Clearly, the ecologic uncertainties about arsenic compounds deserve more effort and attention.

8

Recommendations

Review of the scientific literature by the Subcommittee on Arsenic identified several subjects on which additional information is needed. If the following recommendations for research are successfully carried out, the new knowledge thereby generated should allow a more accurate assessment of the environmental impact of arsenic compounds.

1. *Further epidemiologic and laboratory experimental research should be conducted on the question of the possible carcinogenicity of arsenic compounds.* The possible carcinogenicity of arsenic remains controversial, and it is urged that more studies be done to settle this issue. A group of experts should be convened to address this question specifically and to recommend and oversee studies in man and experimental animals designed to resolve the enigma. Experts in the following subjects should be on the working group: pathology of cancer; epidemiology; statistics; chemistry, biochemistry, and metabolism of arsenic; and experimental design (especially as the last relates to the many possible confounding factors that may modify carcinogenesis). Numerous opportunities exist for additional epidemiologic work, and followup studies should be performed on populations that have been inadvertently exposed to arsenic. The problem of experimental arsenic cancer in laboratory animals also requires more effort, and a series of

studies designed as rationally as possible should be carried out, to determine whether arsenic can be demonstrated to be a carcinogen under experimentally controlled conditions. In such studies, careful attention should be given to various experimental characteristics, such as the species of animal, the dosage of arsenical administered, the nature of arsenical tested, the duration of arsenical exposure, and the route of exposure to the arsenical. Possible cocarcinogenic effects of arsenic compounds with other chemicals should also be considered.

2. *More research is required to clarify the effects of long-term low-dose exposures to arsenic on man, domestic animals, wildlife, and aquatic organisms.* Recent studies using sensitive indicators of biochemical toxicity, such as alterations in enzyme activity, or physiologic criteria of poisoning, such as impaired reproductive performance, have suggested subtle changes in association with exposures of arsenic that were previously thought to be innocuous. How pertinent such results are to environmental problems is not certain, but at least the preliminary experiments should be confirmed or refuted and an attempt made to put such experiments into perspective.

3. *Additional studies on the possible teratogenic and mutagenic effects of arsenicals need to be carried out.* All experimental teratology studies that have been carried out with arsenic compounds have used doses far in excess of those likely ever to be encountered as a result of environmental contamination. Research with more realistic doses should be encouraged, to evaluate whether arsenic in the environment actually constitutes a teratogenic risk. Experiments carried out with humans previously treated medically with arsenicals revealed chromosomal abnormalities, which suggest a mutagenic potential for some arsenic compounds. Again, however, the doses of arsenic given to patients in the past were higher than any reasonable degree of environmental arsenic exposure that one would expect. Nevertheless, the positive results argue strongly for further work along these lines.

4. *Much more effort is required regarding the inhalation toxicology of arsenic.* The physiologic significance of some of the experiments in this field is open to debate, but the observation that biologic changes occur under some conditions apparently is not. Alterations in metabolic or biochemical characteristics are observed in association with exposures that seem very low. This work needs to be repeated, and any possible physiologic relevance of these data needs to be pointed out.

5. *Possible metabolic interrelationships of arsenic with other pollutants should be explored.* Metabolic antagonisms between arsenic and some minerals suggest that arsenic may have antagonistic or synergis-

tic effects with other pollutants. This illustrates the fact that environmental standards for pollutants cannot be set in isolation, but should take into account possible interactions among pollutants.

6. *The use of the rat as an experimental animal in studies of arsenic metabolism should be strongly discouraged.* The rat has a unique arsenic metabolism that is totally unlike that of man or other mammals. Therefore, research conducted with rats is difficult to apply to man; such research has led to many misinterpretations. One such misconception is the idea that arsenic is retained in the body to the same extent as heavy metals, such as lead, mercury, and cadmium.

7. *More information about the chemical nature of arsenic in soil, water, foodstuffs, and plant and animal tissues is desirable.* The behavior of arsenic in the food chain cannot be fully understood without increased knowledge of the various chemical forms of arsenic. The data are very incomplete, although it is clear that the naturally occurring arsenic in foods is metabolized quite differently from inorganic arsenicals. The recent attempts to characterize the arsenolipids in marine oils show what can be accomplished in this direction, but more effort is warranted. The forms of arsenic in foods have unknown toxicity and environmental behavior. Further examination of their identity, toxicity, and fate in the environment is needed, so that their significance to both man and his environment can be assessed.

8. *Better analytic techniques and sample-handling procedures for arsenic compounds need to be developed.* Most current analytic techniques for arsenic give values only for the total amount of arsenic in the sample and do not characterize the various chemical forms of arsenic present. Because the toxicity and ecologic behavior of arsenic depend strictly on its chemical forms, means to identify these forms are needed. Recent evidence has also suggested that the equilibrium vapor pressure of some arsenic compounds (e.g., arsenic trioxide) is great enough for appreciable losses to occur as a result of sublimation when dust particles are collected on high-volume air samplers. Sublimation losses may also occur during sample storage or drying. Surveillance personnel need to be alerted to these possible problems of analysis, and alternative procedures may have to be worked out. Once acceptable methods for the determination of arsenic compounds are established, routine monitoring of arsenic in environmental samples should be undertaken.

9. *An economic assessment should be made of the possible effects that not using arsenical pesticides would have on food and fiber production.* The organic arsenical pesticides play an important role in protecting crops and livestock from damaging pests. Current use is

estimated at 15,000–20,000 tons (13,500–18,000 tonnes) a year. Loss of these pesticides or major price adjustments due to low availability of starting materials (arsenic trioxide) could have a major economic impact on American agriculture. It is urgent to assess the domestic and foreign consequences of the loss of these compounds.

10. *Guidelines on the disposal of arsenical wastes should be developed.* Arsenic is an unavoidable by-product of smelting operations. It must be used, stored, or disposed of safely. For pesticides, the safe disposal of containers is important. Slag from smelting operations, as well as the arsenic trioxide that is collected, must be used or disposed of in an acceptable manner. Perpetual storage should most likely be avoided.

11. *Additional work is needed to elucidate the biochemical mechanisms responsible for arsenic poisoning.* Although the toxic effects of trivalent arsenicals are accounted for reasonably well on the basis of their reactivity with sulfhydryl groups, the mechanism of action of pentavalent arsenicals, both organic and inorganic, is much less understood. Careful metabolic studies should be carried out to determine whether pentavalent arsenicals are reduced to trivalent arsenicals *in vivo* and, if so, to what extent.

12. *Experiments should be carried out to establish whether animals can adapt to the toxic effects of arsenic.* It seems to be well documented that microbial systems can adapt to toxic concentrations of arsenic, although the precise molecular mechanism of this effect is unknown. Recent results that indicated that mammals also can adapt to arsenic to a limited extent should be followed up, and additional work along these lines should be encouraged.

13. *The possible effect of arsenicals in decreasing the ability to resist infection needs to be investigated further.* The mechanism of this effect of arsenic, inhibition of interferon formation or action, is of both theoretical and practical interest. If this work can be verified, the implications for public health could be considerable.

14. *Arsenic should be studied as a possible nutritionally essential trace element.* The occasional favorable effects of arsenic in animal metabolism suggest that it may play a physiologic role at very low concentrations. Such a role has recently been shown in experiments using modern techniques in trace-element research, but these studies need to be verified and expanded.

15. *The mechanism of action of arsenical "growth-promoting" agents should be studied.* Although many theories have been advanced in an attempt to explain the growth-promoting effect of organic penta-

Recommendations

valent arsenicals, none of these hypotheses seems totally satisfactory. If these compounds are to be continued in use, a better understanding of their mode of action might allow the design of equally active yet less toxic compounds.

16. *Studies on environmental characteristics that can affect the redistribution of arsenic within the ecosystem should be undertaken.* Environmental conditions can seriously affect the toxicity of arsenical residues in soils. Dissipation of applied arsenicals is subject to changes in rate and is a function of the environment and the arsenical. Information is needed on how these dissipation rates can be changed to prevent the buildup of toxic residues.

17. *An estimate of annual arsenic use in agriculture is needed.* The exact annual production, distribution, imports, exports, and inventories of arsenical pesticides are unknown. Furthermore, it is impossible with current estimates to predict market trends as influenced by shortages in petroleum-based feedstocks, development of new pesticides, or any other economic change. Consequently, the short- or long-term environmental impact of continued arsenic use on agricultural production cannot be determined.

Appendix A:

Arsenic Content of Plants and Plant Products

Plant or Product	Treatment[a]	Arsenic Concentration, ppm (dry wt) Treated	Nontreated	References
Cereals:	S	14.6	—	248
Wheat	—	—	0.007–0.3	50,96,129,399, 726,769,828, 864
	SP	trace–0.0[b]	—	357
	6S	0.09–0.30	0.09–0.16	20
	7S	0.06–0.50	0.09–0.16	20
Wheat flour	—	—	0.01–0.09	44,49,410,769
Corn, grain	—	—	<0.01–0.4	96,129,388,389, 401,828,864
	1	0.04–0.07	<0.01–0.05	146
	6S	<0.05–0.8	0.05–0.07	20
	7S	<0.05–0.19	<0.05–0.10	20
Corn, stalk and leaves	—	—	0.04[b]	388,389
	3	0.09–17.1	0.6–2.5	874
	6S	1.82–3.75	1.83–1.90	20
	7S	0.25–4.36	0.10–1.94	20
	1S	2.76	0.71	401
Corn, seedling	3S	1.8–252	3.0	878
Corn, pop	—	—	0.1	129
Barley	—	—	<0.1–0.55	129,389,399,726, 864
	S	4	—	84
	SP	0.0–0.9[b]	—	357
Barley, straw	SP	14.3[b]	—	357
Rye	—	—	<0.1	726
Oat	—	—	<0.1–2.28	312,389,399,726
	1S	0.74–1.03	0.09–0.13	147
	SP	0.1[b]	—	357
Straw	1S	2.07	0.28	147
Millet	—	—	<0.1	726
Rice, grain	—	—	<0.07–3.53	49,96,389,410, 726,767
Rice	S	0.5–5.0	0.4	662
Rice, whole plant	2	0.9–9.4	0.8–5.0	236
Bread	—	—	0.016–0.03	516
Whole wheat	—	—	0.008–0.02	516
Ginger	—	—	0.05–0.07	519
Vegetables:				
Soybean	—	—	0.08	410
	6S	0.05–1.31	0.05–1.22	20
	7S	0.06–2.03	0.05–1.22	20
Soybean, fodder	6S	0.09–2.44	0.07–2.12	20
	7S	0.48–3.08	0.07–2.12	20

Appendix A: Arsenic Content of Plants

Plant or Product	Treatment[a]	Arsenic Concentration, ppm (dry wt)		References
		Treated	Nontreated	
Soybean, oil	—	—	0.09	96
Soy sauce	—	100[c]	—	550
Beans, green	—	—	0.1[b]–0.4	49,129,389
	1S	trace–0.22	0.01–0.08	146,147,387,532
	SP	trace[b]	—	357
	3S	1.2–28.5	trace	156
	4S	trace–26.6	trace	156,387
Beans, pod	1S	0.79	0.27	387
Beans, leaves	1S	1.92	0.21	387
Beans	—	—	0.05–0.40	532,864
	N	4.50	0.07	503
Bean, vines	1S	1.82	0.18	401
Bean, roots	1S	5.78	0.29	401
Bean, kidney	—	—	0.33	407
Bean, lima	—	—	0.4	129
Bean, yellow eye, leaf	1S	0.25–3.00	0.08–1.14	147
Bean, black wax, leaf	1S	4.58	1.57	147
Bean, black wax	1S	0.25	0.08	147
Pea	—	—	<0.01–0.49	389,401,532,726, 828
	1S	0.04–0.48	0.01–0.40	401,509
Peas, pod	1S	0.88	0.05	401,509
Peas, vine	1S	2.04–5.70	0.12–2.82	401,509
Peas, root	1S	1.20	22.70	401
Peas, sweet	SP	trace–0.1[b]	—	357
	—	—	0.3	129
Peanut	—	—	0.01–0.30	96,828,864
Carrot	—	—	0.03–0.80	96,129,145,389, 532,726,864
	1S	trace–0.27	<0.01–0.08	146,147,532
	SP	0.0–2.9[b]	—	357
Carrot, tops	1S	0.57	0.00–0.57	96,401
Carrot, roots	1S	0.18	0.32	401
Potato	—	—	0.0076–1.25	96,129,389,408, 724,828,864
	1S	0.06–0.11	0.01–0.05	146,147
	SP	0.0–0.1[b]	—	357
	5S	≤1.0	0.2	730,731
	4S	trace–0.6	trace–0.1	387,569,758
Potato, peelings	4S	0.2–83.0	0.4–2.4	758
Potato, sweet	—	—	0.00	96
Onion	—	—	0.015–1.54	129,389,407,532, 828,864
	1S	0.16–0.36	0.08–0.36	147,401
	SP	trace–3.2[b]	—	357

Plant or Product	Treatment[a]	Arsenic Concentration, ppm (dry wt)		References
		Treated	Nontreated	
Onion, tops	1S	8.85	3.19	401
Turnip	—	—	0.036–0.83	146,389,864
	1S	0.10	<0.01	146
Turnip, greens	—	—	0.03	96
Rutabaga	—	—	0.80	864
Parsnips	—	—	0.20	129,864
Beets, tops	1S	0.08–1.46	0.07–3.48	147,401,532
Beets, roots	SP	0.0–0.4[b]	0.1–1.3	129,401,407,532, 724,864
	1S	0.08–1.28	0.34	401,416,532
Beets	1S	20.2	1.27	401
Radish	—	—	0.01–2.02	96,129,357,389, 407,532,864
	SP	trace	—	357
	1S	0.02–0.22	—	532
Tomato	—	—	0.01–2.95	96,129,407,724, 864
	1S	trace–0.09	0.08–0.09	147,401,532
	4S	0.68–39.5	<0.2	156,284
	3N	3.75–145.28	trace	156
	4N	trace–18.1	trace	156
Tomato, stem and leaves	4S	334	<0.2	284
	1S	11.4	6.75	401
Tomato, root	4S	1,707	<0.2	284
	1S	1.93–12.83	0.26–0.49	401
Eggplant	—	—	0.18–0.77	407,724
	1S	trace–19.68	0–6.14	532
Eggplant, roots	1S	9.84	0.98	401
Cucumber	—	—	0.02–2.4	96,407,532,724, 840
	1S	0.2	—	840
Pickle, sweet	—	—	0.14	129
Lettuce	—	—	0.01–3.78	49,96,389,401, 532,828
	SP	0.0–2.1[b]	—	357
	1S	0.08–0.32	0.12	401,532
Lettuce, roots	1S	10.98	0.47	401
Parsley	—	—	0.1–8.0	129,261,281,864
Watercress	—	—	1.84–2.10	389,407
Spinach	—	—	0.04–2.25	96,389,407
Kale	—	—	0.11–0.22	456
	1S	0.98	0.01–0.99	96,401
Kale, roots	1S	17.49	0.39	401
Swiss chard	1S	0.04–0.27	<0.91–0.08	146,147
Kohlrabi	SP	trace–0.1[b]	—	357

Appendix A: Arsenic Content of Plants

Plant or Product	Treatment[a]	Arsenic Concentration, ppm (dry wt) Treated	Nontreated	References
Cabbage	—	—	0.0–2.01	96,129,357,389, 407,724,864
Chicory	—	—	0.62	49
	—	—	0.1[b]	389
Lentil	—	—	0.70	49
	—	—	0.1[b]	389
Celery	—	—	0.2–0.75	129,145,389
Celery, whole plant	—	—	2.32	389
Celery, stalks	—	—	0.60	864
Celery, root	—	—	1.00	145
Salsify	—	—	0.11[b]	389
Asparagus	—	—	0.1	389
Mushroom, canned	—	—	0.45–0.79	389,516
Broccoli	1S	trace	—	532
Cauliflower	—	—	0.86	389
Endive	—	—	0.21	828
Pepper	1S	trace–0.47	0.39	401,532
	—	—	0.00	96
Pepper, roots	1S	6.89	1.57	401
Squash	—	—	0.023–0.034	532

Fruits:

Plant or Product	Treatment[a]	Treated	Nontreated	References
Apple	—	—	0.04–1.72	129,339,724,755, 792,828,864
	SP	trace–0.1[b]	—	357
	I	0.33–14.2	0.03–1.91	80,389,670
Apple, skin	I	5.0	0.07–1.35	595,755,780
Apple, butter	—	—	0.43–2.41	129
Apple, juice–cider	—	—	0.065–0.165	755
	I	0.18–0.47	—	
Orange	—	—	0.11[b]–0.35	49,389,544
Orange, juice	I	0.08	0.008–0.12	384,544
Pear	—	—	0.17[b]–0.39	339,389
	I	4.0	—	82
Pear, skin	—	—	0.40–0.60	780
Peach	—	—	0.07–1.5	96,160,828
Peach, leaves	S	1.38–2.39	—	55
Apricot	—	—	0.15–1.5	160
Lemon	—	—	0.50	49
Lemon, leaves	3N	11.0	0.35	468
Lemon, roots	3N	1,200	—	468
Pineapple	—	—	0.08[b]	389
Banana	—	—	0.06[b]	389
Pumpkin	—	—	0.09[b]	389
Blueberry	2S	<1.4–4.3	—	54

Plant or Product	Treatment[a]	Arsenic Concentration, ppm (dry wt)		References
		Treated	Nontreated	
Blueberry, leaves	2S	6.74–14.97	0.78	14
Blueberry, stems	2S	7.6–13.3	0.27	14
Blueberry, roots	2S	93.7–164.2	2.40	14
Grapes	—	—	0.75–1.20	780
	6S	0.24–0.28	0.05	195
	1S	0.6–3.8	—	
Grape, leaves	—	—	2.3	349
Grape, juice	—	—	None detected	349
Grapefruit, leaves	—	—	2.0–3.0	682
Mandarin	—	—	0.85	389

Beverages:
Wine	—	—	0.005–0.15	95,516
	1S	0.0–4.0	—	285
	2S	0.4–1.0	0.01–0.02	240
	2	2.76	<0.1	636
	1	0.02–0.18	—	826
Wine, white	—	—	0.06–0.56	158
Wine, red	—	—	0.03–1.38	158
Wine, fruit	—	—	0.06–0.11	192
Wine, port	—	—	0.02–0.07	279
Lemonade	—	—	0.000–0.005	516
Whiskey	—	—	0.02–0.07	95
Beer	—	—	0.01–2.0	95,516,522,831
Ale	—	—	<0.02	522
Malt	—	—	0.26–0.35	522
Hops, sundried	—	—	0.08–0.15	160
Hops, sulfured	—	0.15–19.5[c]	—	160,471,760
	—	—	0.03–0.82	471,760
Coffee, bean	1	0.5–1.5	—	630
Liquid fruit products	—	—	0.09–0.21	192

Trees:
Pine, short leaf	—	—	0.1–0.2	17
Fir, Douglas, needles	—	—	4.0–8,000	201
Fir, Douglas, twigs (ash)	—	—	<100	838
Fir, Douglas, twigs	AM	>1,000	—	838
Cypress, Italian	—	—	1.4	547
Fir (*Abies alba*)	—	—	0.11	547
Pine (*Pinus laricius*)	—	—	0.13	547
Chestnut (*Castanea vesca*)	—	—	0.05–0.11	389,547
Pine, Scotch	—	—	<0.05	547
Beech, European	—	—	<0.05	547
Spruce, white	—	—	1.0–2.4	674
Spruce, black	SP	1.0–96	—	457

Appendix A: Arsenic Content of Plants

Plant or Product	Treatment[a]	Arsenic Concentration, ppm (dry wt) Treated	Nontreated	References
Oak, chestnut	—	—	0.05–0.40	17
Oak, chestnut, acorns	—	—	0.1	17
Oak, chestnut, roots	—	—	11.0	17
Hickory	—	—	0.10–0.40	17
Poplar, tulip	—	—	0.08–0.40	17
Walnuts	—	—	0.07	49
Walnut, black	—	—	0.13[b]	389
Hazelnuts	—	—	0.78	49
Date	—	—	0.12[b]	389
Filbert	—	—	0.11	389
Peach, leaves	S	2.0	—	472
Almond	—	—	0.3	389
Hemlock, foliage	—	2.0–4.8	0.2–0.4	734

Forage Crops:

Plant or Product	Treatment[a]	Treated	Nontreated	References
Grass	—	—	0.1–0.7	37
	1S	0.5–2.0	0.50–0.94	129,147
	S	0.5–75.5	0.5	248,864
	SP	2.5–12.0[b]	—	357
	4	938–1,462	—	581
	1,5	15,000–60,000	—	111
Clover	—	—	<0.10–0.17	562
	1S	1.32	0.46	147
	S	12.0	—	864
Clover, red	—	—	0.37	129,389
	4S	0.09–0.84	0.11–0.39	728
Clover, white	1S	6.24	3.64	401
Hay	1S	1.26	0.52	147
Alfalfa	—	—	0.05–3.38	389,562
	SP	0.4–5.7[b]	—	357
	S	14.0–860	—	129,816
	1S	3.37	1.97	401
Alfalfa, roots	1S	0.78	3.15	401
Sudan-grass	—	—	0.70	503
	3N	9.6–384.8	trace	156
	4N	3.1–68.4	trace	156
	4S	0.38–33.4	—	156
Vetch	1S	1.92	1.22	401
Vetch, roots	1S	15.82	7.15	401
Sunflower	—	—	<1.0–2.0	129
Sunflower leaf	SP	3.3[b]	—	357

Marine Algae, Seaweed:

Plant or Product	Treatment[a]	Treated	Nontreated	References
Macrocystis pyrifera	—	—	4.0–60.0	299,864,866
Chondrus crispus	—	—	3.8–18.0	143,398,456

Plant or Product	Treatment[a]	Arsenic Concentration, ppm (dry wt)		References
		Treated	Nontreated	
Laminaria digitata lamina	—	—	107–109	495
Laminaria digitata	—	—	47.0–93.8	398,456
Laminaria digitata, oil	—	—	221.0	491
Laminaria digitata, fatty acid	—	—	36.0	491
Laminaria saccharina	—	—	45.0[b]–52.5	398,456
Laminaria saccharina, oil	—	—	155	491
Laminaria saccharina, fatty acid	—	—	7.5–52.5	398,456,491
Halidrys siliquosa	—	—	26.0–30.0	398,456
Fucus nodosus	—	—	45.0	398
Entarompha compressa	—	—	11.2	398
Ahnfeltia plicata	—	—	39.0	456
Fucus vesiculosus	—	—	24–65	398,495
Fucus vesiculosus, oil	—	—	35.0	491
Fucus vesiculosus, fatty acid	—	—	5.1	491
Fucus serratus	—	—	28–67.5	398,495
Fucus serratus, oil	—	—	27.0	491
Fucus serratus, fatty acid	—	—	6.1	491
Piocamium coccineum	—	—	7.5	398
Ulva latissima	—	—	6.0	398
Gigartina mammillosa	—	—	4.5–17.2	398,495
Laminaria hyperborea, oil	—	—	197	491
Laminaria hyperborea, fatty acid	—	—	16	491
Ascophyllum nodosum, oil	—	—	7.8–49.0	491
Ascophyllum nodosum, fatty acid	—	—	5.2–21.0	491
Fucus spiralis	—	—	15–34	495
Fucus spiralis, oil	—	—	5.7	491
Fucus spiralis, fatty acid	—	—	5.0	491
Pelvetia canaliculata	—	—	15–22	495
Pelvetia canaliculata, oil	—	—	10.8	491
Pelvetia canadiculata, fatty acid	—	—	7.3	491
Algae:				
Algae	—	—	0.5–12.0	129,519,864
Algae, *Odegodeum*	7	4.5–71.4	—	383
Sceletonema costatum, oil	—	—	1.3	497

Appendix A: Arsenic Content of Plants

Plant or Product	Treatment[a]	Arsenic Concentration, ppm (dry wt) Treated	Nontreated	References
Chlorella ovalis, oil	—	—	0.7	497
Chlorella pyrenoidosa, oil	—	—	0.5	497
Phaedactylum tricornutum, oil	—	—	3.6–4.8	497
Oscillatoria rubescens, oil	—	—	0.4–0.5	497
Pterygophera californica	—	—	12.0	864
Agarum fimbuetum	—	—	4.0	864
Rhodemia pertusa	—	—	1.0	864
Casteria castata	—	—	1.0	864
Moss:				
Hylocomium splendens	SP	<4–99	<4	457
Pleurozium schreberi	SP	<1–10	2–3	457
Aquatic Plants, New Zealand:				
Ceratophyllum demursum	GTA	20–1,060	1.4	448,660,661
Lagarosiphon major	GTA	29–1,450	—	448,660,661
Elodea canadensis	GTA	307–700	3.0	448,661
Potamogeton sp.	GTA	45–436	<6.0	448,661
Lemna sp.	GTA	30	2.5	448,661
Nitella hookeri A. Braun	GTA	182	13.0	448,661
Enteromorpha nana	GTA	14–40	—	448,660,661
Compsopogon hookeri	GTA	550	—	660,661
Typha orientalis Presl	GTA	8	—	448,661
Egeria densa	GTA	266–310	—	
Atriplex confertifolia	—	—	3.2	339
Myriophyllum propinquum	GTA	456	—	448
Miscellaneous:				
Baking powder	—	—	1.0	44
Cottonseed	6	0.05–0.08	0.05	46
Cottonseed products	5	0.68	—	96
	—	—	0.58	447
Cotton leaves	6	0.13–41.4	0.055	861
Sugar	—	—	0.15	49
Glucose	—	—	0.2	516
Honey	—	—	0.14	129
	1	0.9	—	226
Pectin	—	—	1.0–3.55	102,129
Organic food color	—	—	3.0	102

Plant or Product	Treatment[a]	Arsenic Concentration, ppm (dry wt)		References
		Treated	Nontreated	
Gelatin	—	—	1.0	102
Polyphosphates	—	—	<0.3–3.0	102,640
Chocolate	—	—	0.07–1.53	49,516
Jam	—	—	0.00–0.1	516
Jam and marmalades	—	—	0.04–0.08	192
Tobacco	—	—	trace–42.8	129,318,476,573, 737,738,889
Johnsongrass	—	—	0.65	447
Sugar cane	—	—	2.0	624
Mustard, paste	—	—	0.28	864
Rhubarb	—	—	<0.1	864
Astragalus bisulcatus	—	—	2.0	864
Russian thistle	—	—	<1.0	864
Turpentine weed	—	—	≤1.0–2.0	864
Wild aster	—	—	2.0	864
Ironweed	—	—	1.0	864
Ragweed	—	—	1.0	864
Tulipa sp.	—	—	2.0	864
Scarlet mallow	—	—	1.0	864
Oreocarya sp.	—	—	<1.0	864
Stanleya pinnata	—	—	<1.0	864
Cocklebur	—	—	<1.0	864
Spurge	—	—	<1.0	864
Aplopappus fremontii	—	—	1.0	864
Astragalus pectinatus	—	—	<1.0	864
Lambsquarters, common	—	—	1.0	864
Mustard, common	S	<1.0	1.0	864
Clintonia borealis	SP	<2–52	<2–4	457
Sorrel	—	—	0.005	
Dandelion	S	7.0	—	864
Wild leek	S	8.0	—	864
Buckhorn plantain	S	16.0	—	864
Sourgrass	S	18.0	—	864
Daisy	S	12.0	—	864
Milkweed, tops	S	1.0	—	864
Sour dock, tops	S	1.0	—	864
Burdock, leaves	S	<1.0	—	864
False indigo	S	<1.0	—	864

[a]1 = lead arsenate; 2 = calcium arsenate; 3 = sodium arsenate; 4 = sodium arsenite; 5 = arsenic trioxide; 6 = MAA; 7 = cacodylic acid; AM = arsenic mineralization; GTA = geothermal area; N = nutrient solution; S = soil; SP = smelter pollution.
[b]Wet weight.
[c]Contaminated.

Appendix B:

Arsenic Content of Animals

Animal	Exposure[a]	Arsenic concentration, ppm (fresh wt) Exposed	Normal	References
Human:				
Hair	—	—	0.3–1.75	95,145
Distal	—	—	0.79	287
Proximal	—	—	0.03[b]–1.92	95,287,409,526, 742,818
	1	0.4–816	<3.0	122,219,543,651
	2	3.58	0.997	61
Brain	—	—	0.001[b]–0.14	287,409,742
	3	1.0–1.4	—	310
	4	1.9	—	533
Teeth	—	—	0.003–0.635	742,821
Esophagus	4	168	—	533
Thyroid	—	—	0.06–0.13	75,287
	—	—	0.001–0.314[b]	742
	—	—	0.003–0.332[b]	742
	2	0.002–0.093	—	437
Lung	—	—	0.08–0.17	287,409
	3	2.3–2.6	—	310
	4	20.0	—	533
	—	—	0.006–0.514[b]	742
Female	—	—	0.006–0.038	552
Heart	4	64.0	—	533
	—	—	0.002–0.078[b]	742
	—	—	0.001–0.016	287,409,850
Liver	—	—	0.09–0.30	95,287,409
	3	4.4–6.9	—	310
	4	12.8–143	—	533
	—	—	0.005–0.246[b]	742
Kidney	—	—	0.07–0.14	287,409
	3	0.4–1.3	—	310
Left	4	15.8–92	—	533
Right	4	81	—	533
	—	—	0.002–0.363[b]	742
Pancreas	—	—	0.07	287
	4	94	—	533
	—	—	0.005–0.410[b]	742
Bladder	—	—	0.06	287
Gallbladder	4	41	—	533
Stomach	—	—	0.04	287
	3	0.1–0.3	—	310
Walls	4	5–246	—	533
Contents	4	5–8,836	—	533
	—	—	0.003–0.104[b]	742

Appendix B: Arsenic Content of Animals

Animal	Exposure[a]	Arsenic concentration, ppm (fresh wt) Exposed	Normal	References
Intestine	—	—	0.07	287
Small	4	132	—	533
Large	4	259	—	533
Spleen	—	—	0.08–0.13	75,287,409
	3	0.5–2.2	—	310
	4	12.8	—	533
	—	—	0.001–0.132[b]	742
Bone	—	—	0.16–0.50	287,409
Calvarium	—	—	59–61 (in ash)	592
Rib	—	—	20–27 (in ash)	592
Nail	—	—	1.70	287
	5	7.1–17.8	0.04–0.11	380
	—	—	0.02–2.90[b]	742
	4	20–130	—	819
Blood	6	0.82–3.0	—	213
	—	—	0.01–0.59	287,317,526
	4	5.0	—	533
	—	—	0.001–0.920[b]	742
	7	0.03–0.27	0.01–0.13	832
Women, venous	—	—	0.06–1.44	317,830
Menstrual	—	—	0.18	830
Serum	—	—	0.000–0.0028	194,526
Skin	—	—	0.009–0.59[b]	742
Spinal cord	4	20.6	—	533
Urine	1	0.04–0.9	0.01–0.22	122,392,543,617
	—	—	0.000–0.11	287,526
	4	27.2	—	533
Uterus	—	—	0.010–0.188[b]	742
Membrane	—	—	45.6	317
Aorta	—	—	0.003–0.570[b]	742
Adrenal	—	—	0.002–0.293[b]	742
Breast	—	—	0.030–0.221[b]	742
Muscle, pectoral	—	—	0.012–0.431[b]	742
Ovary	—	—	0.013–0.260[b]	742
Prostate	—	—	0.010–0.090[b]	742
Domesticated Animals:				
Beef	—	—	0.008	50
Calf muscle	—	—	0.52	641
Calf liver	—	—	0.15	
Liver	—	—	0.063	604
Milk	—	—	0.0005–0.07	50,411,516
	7	<0.05–0.27	—	248,521

Animal	Exposure[a]	Arsenic concentration, ppm (fresh wt) Exposed	Normal	References
Milk, dried	—	—	<0.5	782
Milk, sterilized	—	—	0.03–0.04	516
Milk, condensed	—	—	0.01–0.014	516
Butter	—	—	0.07	49
Veal	—	—	0.005–0.010	50
Pork				
Muscle	—	—	0.22–0.32	49,641
	7	0.29–0.92	<0.02	459
Salami	—	—	0.14–0.20	49,129
Chicken	7	0.2–1.2	—	168
Meat	7	0.01–0.4	0.02	51,168
Kidney	7	0.08–1.2	0.05	51,168
	—	—	0.02	286
Liver	—	—	≤2.2	168
	—	—	0.02	286
	7	0.19–2.43	0.08	51
Bone, marrow	—	—	0.0–0.4	168
Eggs	7	0.40	—	238
Yolk	—	—	0.005	50
Rabbit, muscle	7	1.0–2.0	—	725
Liver	7	3.0	—	725
Kidney	7	3.0	—	725
Heart	7	trace	—	725
Lungs	7	trace	—	725
Meat, canned	—	—	0.01–0.18	641
	—	—	0.20–4.13[b]	726
Fat	—	—	0.13–0.54[b]	726
Wild Animals:				
Squirrel	—	—	0.8[b]	17
Sparrow	—	—	0.2[b]	17
Mice	—	—	1.0[b]	17
Hawk	—	—	0.4[b]	17
Owl	—	—	0.05[b]	17
Fox	—	—	0.8[b]	17
Crow	—	—	0.1[b]	17
Opossum	—	—	0.2[b]	17
Starling	—	—	0.01–0.21	524
Bee, dead	4	3.22–12.0	—	226,502
	4	20.8–31.2	—	479
Pollen	2	1–120	—	775
	4	7.75–30	—	226,228
Larvae, dead	4	4.95–13	—	226,228
Pupae	4	10	—	228

Appendix B: Arsenic Content of Animals

Animal	Exposure[a]	Arsenic concentration, ppm (fresh wt) Exposed	Normal	References
Honey	4	16–22	—	228
	4	1–2	—	479
Aquatic Organisms:				
Shrimp	—	—	1.27–41.6	129,143,171,501
English potted	—	—	8.2–18.8	143
Edible portion	—	—	0.95–31.2	172
Canned	—	—	0.08	203
Pandalus borealis, oil	—	—	10.1	491
Pandalus borealis, fatty acid	—	—	4.8	491
	—	—	13.0–42.0[b]	496,502
Palamon serratus, cooked	—	—	1.0–2.7	167
Parapeneus longirostris	—	—	1.7–38.2	167
Crab	—	—	27.0–52.5	143
Dressed	—	—	18.8–62.6	143
Canned	—	—	0.71	203
Muscle	—	—	6.1	369
	7	≤7.95	—	790,791
Carcinus maenas, cooked	—	—	2.5–7.0	167
Cancer pagurus, cooked	—	—	2.1–33.4	167
Clam, minced	—	—	0.85	129
	—	—	1.42–2.56	129,853
Canned	—	—	0.36	203
Pecten maximus	—	—	11.6	492
N-liquor	—	—	18.0	492
Oil	—	—	4.8	491
Fatty acid	—	—	1.9	491
Prawns	—	—	34.1	129
Dublin Bay	—	—	27.0–130.5	143
American tinned	—	—	10.5–30.0	143
Japanese tinned	—	—	15.0–63.8	143
Oyster	—	—	0.3–3.7	129,176,356,506, 853
English	—	—	2.2–7.5	143
Portuguese	—	—	24.8–52.5	143
American tinned	—	—	0.4–0.8	143
Canned	—	—	0.22	203
Smoked	—	—	1.00	203
Ostrea edulis	—	—	2.6–8.2[b]	456,492
Ostrea edulis, N-liquor	—	—	9.8	492
Gryphea angulata	—	—	1.2–3.6	167

Animal	Exposure[a]	Exposed	Normal	References
Lobster				
(*Homarus vulgarus*)	—	—	2.27–54.5	129,143,167,202
Canned	—	—	0.94	203
Fillet	—	—	5.3	492
Fillet, N-liquor	—	—	14.0	492
Cooked	—	—	10.8–17.2	167
Muscle	—	—	0.022	50
Whole	—	—	0.453	50
Norwegian, cooked (*Nephrops norvegicus*)	—	—	7.2–19.4	167
Scallop	—	—	27.0–63.8	129,143
Mussel	—	—	2.58–89.2	129,143,202,496
Mytilus edulis	—	—	0.08–8.0	167,202,299,492, 501,502
	—	—	9.5–15.0[b]	456
Whole	—	—	0.0[b]	496
N-liquor	—	—	9.7	492
Oil	—	—	18.0	491
Fatty acid	—	—	22.0	491
Mytilus edulis, whole	7	0.04–3.73	0.01	202,703
Mytilus magellonicus	—	—	10.5–26.1[b]	567
Cockle				
Cardium edule	—	—	5.1–8.4	456
	—	—	12.8–30.0	129,143
	—	—	1.3–2.4	167
Tapes decussatus	—	—	3.7–6.6	167
Whelk	—	—	9.0–30.0	143
French edible snail	—	—	0.4	143
Buccinum undatum	—	—	11.0[b]	456
Periwinkle				
Littorina littorea	—	—	12[b]	456
	—	—	14.0–19.0[b]	456
Littorina littorea, oil	—	—	84.0	491
Littorina littorea, fatty acid	—	—	32.0	491
Cooked	—	—	3.6–6.3	167
Crawfish				
Palinurus vulgaris, cooked	—	—	12.0–54.6	167
Palinurus vulgaris	—	—	15.0–33.8	143
Astacus pallipes	—	—	0.8–1.5	143
Squid				
Omnastrephes sagittatus	—	—	6.5	492

Appendix B: Arsenic Content of Animals

Animal	Exposure[a]	Arsenic concentration, ppm (fresh wt) Exposed	Normal	References
N-liquor	—	—	17.0	492
Loligo vulgaris, raw	—	—	0.8–7.5	167
Loligo vulgaris, cooked	—	—	0.4–3.3	167
Fatty acid	—	—	0.7	491
Starfish (*Asterias rubens*)	—	—	10[b]	456
Starfish, oil	—	—	9.1	491
Starfish, fatty acid	—	—	7.5	491
Cuttlefish				
Sepia officinalis, gills	—	—	198[b]	456
Sepia officinalis, mantle	—	—	73[b]	456
Sepia officinalis, raw	—	—	6.2–11.5	167
Sepia officinalis, cooked	—	—	0.8–6.8	167
Anchovy	—	—	7.1–10.7	499
Octopus				
Octopus bimoculatus, tentacles	—	—	0.12	299
Octopus vulgaris, raw	—	—	2.6–40.3	167
Octopus vulgaris, cooked	—	—	3.0–31.0	167
Cod (*Gadus morrhua*)	—	—	3.69–24.3[b]	129,496
Fillet	—	—	2.2	492
Fillet, N-liquor	—	—	13.0	492
Muscle	—	—	0.4–0.8	696
Liver	—	—	0.7–3.2	696
Liver, oil	—	—	1.4–10.0	129,364,491,502, 696
Black marlin				
Muscle	—	—	0.1–1.65	505
Liver	—	—	0.1–2.75	505
Tuna	—	—	0.71–4.6	129,604
Tunny (*Thunnus thynnus*)	—	—	9.6[b]	496
Haddock (*Melanogrammus aeglefinus*)	—	—	5.54–10.8[b]	129,496
Mullet, red	—	—	1.54	49
Dogfish	—	—	0.53	49
Plaice	—	—	4.5–7.5	143
Fillet, oil (*Pleuronectes platessa*)	—	—	6.1	491
Fillet, fatty acid	—	—	5.2	491

Animal	Exposure[a]	Arsenic concentration, ppm (fresh wt)		References
		Exposed	Normal	
Sole (*Solea solea*)	—	—	5.2	143
Dab	—	—	2.2–3.0	143
Caviar, Russian	—	—	3.8	143
Pike (*Esox lucius*)	—	—	0.8	143
Pike	7	0.0	0.0–0.11	790,791
Perch (*Perca fluviatilis*)	—	—	0.6	143
Tench	—	—	0.4	143
Bream	—	—	0.4	143
Roach	—	—	0.4	143
	7	≤0.09	—	790,791
Trout, viscera	2	5.3	—	231
muscle	2	2.4	—	231
	—	—	0.069–0.149	653
Whitefish, viscera	2	3.6	—	231
muscle	2	2.7	—	231
Sucker, spotted, whole	—	—	0.062–0.253	233,653
Sucker, white	—	—	0.11	644
Shiner, golden	—	—	0.55–1.95	233
Bass, black, liver, oil	—	—	7.37–77.31	233
Bass, black, largemouth (*Micropterus salmoides*)	7	0.07–0.93	0.01–1.86	233,653,857
Bass, white	—	—	0.28–0.48	233,644
Carp	—	—	0.055–0.51	233,644,653
	7	≤0.19	—	790,791
Catfish	—	—	0.07–0.298	644,653
Herring, fillet (*Clupea harengus*)	—	—	3.8	492
N-liquor	—	—	6.4–24.0	492,500
Meal	—	—	2.7–6.9[b]	490,496
Oil	—	—	3.1–20.2	491,494,499,696
Muscle	—	—	2.0	696
Mackerel (*Scomber scomber*)	—	—	0.027–9.2[b]	496
Meal	—	—	2.7–3.8	490
Fillet, N-liquor	—	—	3.2–17.0	492,500
Fillet	—	—	2.2[b]–3.5	456,492
Fillet, oil	—	—	8.2	491
Fillet, fatty acid	—	—	4.1	491
Liver, oil	—	—	13.0	491
Liver, fatty acid	—	—	6.2	491
Oil	—	—	4.3–15.0	494,499
Capelin, meal	—	—	2.6–19.1	490,496

Appendix B: Arsenic Content of Animals

Animal	Exposure[a]	Arsenic concentration, ppm (fresh wt) Exposed	Normal	References
Capelin, N-liquor	—	—	10.3	500
Oil (*Mallotus villosus*)	—	—	5.2–23.2	491,494,499
Fatty acid	—	—	6.3	491
Pout, Norway, meal	—	—	3.9	490
Pout, Norway, oil	—	—	11.8	499
Whale (*Balaenoptera physalus*)	—	—	0.4	492
N-liquor	—	—	0.9	492
Coalfish (*Pollachius virens*)	—	—	7.2[b]	496
North Atlantic Finfish				
Catfish (*Bagre marinus*)	—	—	<1.0	867
Eel (*Anguilla rostrata*)	—	—	<1.0[b]	867
Flounder (*Paralichthys lethostigma*)	—	—	<1.0[b]	867
Decapterus punctatus	—	—	1.8[b]	867
Eel (*Conger* sp.)	—	—	<1.0[b]	867
Anchovy (*Anchova mitchelli*)	—	—	2.1[b]	867
Mullet (*Mugil cephalus*)	—	—	<1.0[b]	867
Hygophum hygomi	—	—	<1.0[b]	867
Ceratoscopelus warmingil	—	—	<1.0[b]	867
Notoscopelus caudispinous	—	—	<1.0[b]	867
Lobianchia dofleini	—	—	<1.0[b]	867
Lepidophanes indicus	—	—	<1.0[b]	867
Diaphus mollis	—	—	<1.0[b]	867
Lampanyctus pusillus	—	—	1.0[b]	867
Ophichthus ocellatus	—	—	1.0[b]	867
Ophichthus gomesi	—	—	1.0[b]	867
Morone saxatilis	—	—	1.8[b]	867
Sea trout (*Cynoscion nebulosus*)	—	—	2.5[b]	867
Euthynnus alletteratus	—	—	1.1[b]	867
Scomberomorus maculatus	—	—	1.8[b]	867
Centropristes striatus	—	—	6.4[b]	867
Coastal Organisms, England				
Halichondria panicea	—	—	2.8[b]	456
Tealia felina	—	—	72.0[b]	456

Animal	Exposure[a]	Arsenic concentration, ppm (fresh wt)		References
		Exposed	Normal	
Nereis diversicolor	—	—	5.2[b]	456
Palaemon elegans	—	—	16.0[b]	456
Patella vulgata	—	—	11–24[b]	456
Crepidula fornicata	—	—	8.1–13.0[b]	456
Nucella lapillus	—	—	16.0–38.0[b]	456
Styela clava	—	—	4.8[b]	456
Botryllus schlosseri	—	—	6.6[b]	456
Anguilla anguilla, muscle	—	—	1.7[b]	456
Marone labrax, muscle	—	—	7.1[b]	456
Platichthys flesus, muscle	—	—	8.7[b]	456
Shellfish, Portugal				
Rock shell (*Murex trunculus*) cooked	—	—	14.6–26.4	167
Donax trunculus	—	—	1.8–3.7	167
Solen marginatus, cooked	—	—	1.9–4.2 1.4–2.7	167 167
Aristeus antennatus	—	—	4.4–19.6	167
Aolliceps cornucopia, cooked	—	—	1.2–8.6	167
Miscellaneous				
Bluegills (*Lepomis macrochirus*)	— 7	— 0.09–11.60	0.52 —	233 290
Gar, long-nosed	—	—	0.35–0.40	233
Shad, gizzard	—	—	0.13–1.47	233,644
Small-mouthed buffalo	—	—	0.05–2.75	233
Brook silversides	—	—	0.30–1.26	233
Drum, freshwater	—	—	0.09	644
Salmon, coho	—	—	0.09	644
Minnows	—	—	0.14–1.95	233
Pickerel	—	—	0.13–0.73	233
Black bullhead	—	—	0.22	233
Horned dace	—	—	0.42–0.65	233
Gambusia	7	0.07–11.20	—	383
Insects	—	—	10[b]	17
Cryptozoa	—	—	100[b]	17
Earthworms	—	—	19[b]	17
Snail	7	0.61–68.3	—	383
Snail, garden	—	—	0.3	143
Crustacea, planktonic	—	—	3.2–5.5	233

Appendix B: Arsenic Content of Animals

Animal	Exposure[a]	Arsenic concentration, ppm (fresh wt)		References
		Exposed	Normal	
Sea star (*Pisoster ochraceus*)	—	—	1.26[b]	299
Fish, muscle	—	—	3.06–6.8	369
Daphnia magna	7	3.9–254	—	383

[a] 1 = industrial; 2 = pollution; 3 = AsH_3; 4 = poisoned; 5 = arsenic polyneuritis; 6 = aerosol treatment; 7 = fed arsenic.
[b] Dry weight.

Appendix C:

Determining Traces of Arsenic in Natural Materials

This discussion is intended primarily for the consumer of analytic information, i.e., for the physician, biologist, or ecologist who collects and selects samples and wishes to obtain the most useful information from them. The principal paths by which arsenic can be accidentally added to or lost from the system are mentioned, and the advantages and disadvantages of the more commonly used analytic techniques are pointed out, so that the investigator can choose among the available services and critically evaluate the results. The general approach is that followed in the recent review by Talmi and Feldman,[778] although new material has been added and some of the less accessible techniques omitted.

COLLECTION, SUBDIVISION, AND STORAGE OF SAMPLES

The sample collected should be large enough to represent the material studied. Because a single mean value is desired for the concentration of each arsenical species of interest, the sample must be homogenized and a subsample of suitable size for analysis must be taken. To minimize contamination, unused sample material should be stored in closed containers or (depending on sample composition) at a low temperature.

Choices must sometimes be made regarding what to include in the sample taken for analysis. Vegetation may be found to be contaminated with dust; a decision must be made whether to remove the dust or include it in the sample. Natural water often contains suspended matter, which must be either filtered out or allowed to remain. If the particles filtered from an air stream contain volatile forms of arsenic, consideration must be given to the losses that may occur at the temperatures and air velocities to which the particles are exposed on the filter and to the duration of exposure (arsenic trioxide has a vapor pressure of 0.68 mm Hg at 200 C).[453,655]

Many authors (e.g., Portman and Riley,[652] Whitnack and Brophy,[855] Al-Sibbai and Fogg,[11] and C. Feldman, personal communication) have found that acidic, neutral, or basic solutions of inorganic arsenites and arsenates can be stored without substantial changes in concentration for several weeks. However, some arsenic compounds present in natural water are said to disappear rapidly from solution after collection of the sample (R. S. Braman, personal communication). The investigator must always be aware of the possibility of losing some of the species of interest through adsorption on vessel walls or on suspended matter or through volatilization.

Large liquid samples can be properly divided into aliquots only if homogeneous, i.e., if the species of interest does not adhere to the vessel walls and if suspended matter is uniformly distributed before division. Large solid samples of a mineral nature may, of course, be subdivided by conventional crushing or impact treatment followed by mixing and quartering or riffling. Large samples of biologic tissues can be homogenized in a blender (with the addition of water, if necessary). If the density of the resulting slurry can be stabilized long enough, the sample can be subdivided in this manner. Alternatively, the slurry can be centrifuged and proportionate amounts of residue and supernatant liquid taken for analysis. Another possibility is lyophilization of the slurry; the cake obtained is easily pulverized, and the resulting powder is homogeneous.[247] If volatile species are to be determined, the lyophilization technique may not be appropriate. The amount of handling must always be minimized, in order to minimize contamination.

PRETREATMENT AND DISSOLUTION OF SAMPLES

If organic arsenic compounds are to be determined, the species in question must be isolated.[99,779] If total arsenic is to be determined, the

Appendix C: Traces of Arsenic in Natural Materials

arsenic must be brought into solution and, if necessary, converted to inorganic form. Regardless of the dissolution procedure used, care must be taken to ensure that no arsenic is lost by the volatilization of trivalent arsenic halides. Loss can usually be prevented by boiling the sample with concentrated nitric acid under reflux early in the procedure.[778]

The following sample-preparation procedures are typical of those used in environmental work.

Coal is heated to fumes with concentrated sulfuric acid and treated with successive small portions of concentrated nitric acid until degradation essentially ceases. Destruction of the remaining nitrogenous compounds is completed by small additions of fuming concentrated perchloric acid. The latter step is essential if the arsine generation–arc emission procedure is to be used for the final determination step.[99]

The arsenic in fly ash is usually assumed to exist as a surface coating. All this arsenic can be dissolved with fuming sulfuric acid, as is shown by comparison with analyses of the same material by neutron-activation analysis.[245] Refluxing such material in boiling water for 1 h recovers only 13% of the arsenic present (C. Feldman, personal communication). If the arsenic was deposited from the vapor phase, it may have been thinly covered by other substances deposited later.

Coal slag is a highly refractory glass and usually contains only small amounts of arsenic. The arsenic that it does contain cannot be leached out with ordinary acids. Treatment with hydrofluoric acid in the usual way would be of dubious value—on the one hand, this reagent may contain substantial amounts of impurities; on the other, arsenic trifluoride and especially arsenic pentafluoride are rather volatile, so both contamination and losses might occur. Attack of the slag by fusion is open to similar objections.

Quartz can be attacked without metallic contamination by vapor-phase treatment with hydrofluoric acid and nitric acid in a closed system.[891] This approach was therefore tried with slag, albeit with some misgivings regarding the volatility of arsenic fluorides. No losses or contamination seem to have occurred, however, inasmuch as the results obtained on fly ash agreed well with those obtained with neutron activation and sulfuric acid leaching.[245]

Procedures for digesting plant or animal tissues for determining total arsenic must completely convert the arsenic to inorganic form (preferably arsenate) and must eliminate any substances that would interfere with the particular procedure to be used in later determination. Only the more widely used digestion methods will be mentioned here; others have been reviewed elsewhere.[778] Small samples can be charred with concentrated sulfuric acid and then subjected to repeated small additions of concentrated nitric acid[150] or 30%[700] or 50% hydrogen peroxide. In the latter case, trivalent arsenic will be lost if chloride is present.[212] Ordinary and fatty tissue weighing up to 5 g can be safely wet-ashed in a volumetric flask by refluxing under a short air condenser with appropriate mixtures of sulfuric, nitric, and perchloric acid, with potassium dichromate as a catalyst.[246]

PRECONCENTRATION OF ARSENIC SPECIES

To increase the sensitivity and accuracy of analysis, the arsenic-bearing species is often isolated from its matrix and concentrated. The principal preconcentration procedures used are coprecipitation, liquid–liquid extraction, and volatilization.

Coprecipitation with ferric hydroxide, $Fe(OH)_3$, has long been known to collect pentavalent arsenic quantitatively from solution at concentrations as low as 2 ng/ml.[643,652] The hydroxides of cerium and zirconium appear to be as effective as ferric hydroxide in this regard.[649] Thionalide can collect arsenic efficiently from comparatively large amounts of seawater,[652] but this reagent apparently does not function well at low salt concentrations.[779]

Trivalent arsenic can readily be extracted from 6 N hydrochloric acid with mixtures of ketone and carbon tetrachloride.[276] At lower acidities (pH, 2–6), it can be precipitated with ammonium pyrrolidine dithiocarbamate, and the precipitate can be extracted.[568] If the arsenic is originally present in the pentavalent state, this fact can be turned to advantage: While the arsenic is still pentavalent, other potentially interfering metals that are extracted under the same conditions can be extracted and discarded; the arsenic can then be reduced and extracted without the metals that would otherwise have accompanied it.

Arsenic can also be separated from its matrix by volatilization, as arsine (boiling point, −55 C) or a substituted arsine. The necessary reduction can be effected by using zinc and acid in the presence of stannous chloride or potassium iodide.[252,282,511] The reducing agent most commonly used, however, is sodium borohydride, $NaBH_4$. The properties of this reagent can affect analytic results, especially at low arsenic concentrations (<1 ppm), and will therefore be discussed briefly. Sodium borohydride is supplied commercially in the form of 0.20–0.25-g pellets or powder; the grade usually used for analysis is the same as that used in preparative organic chemistry. The quantity of this reagent commonly used per determination (0.25 g) often contains 10–20 ng of arsenic;[430] the amount varies from portion to portion.

Appendix C: Traces of Arsenic in Natural Materials

This degree of contamination is of little consequence if the sample aliquot used in the determination contains several hundred nanograms of arsenic. But if it does not (e.g., in natural water and small tissue specimens), both the contamination and the variability of the blank are sources of error. The kinetics of the reaction between sodium borohydride and arsenic are an additional complicating factor: if a sodium borohydride pellet is dropped into an arsenic-free acid solution, it produces a considerably higher blank arsenic reading than if the same pellet is converted to a 1% solution before being added to the acid solution. Moreover, this blank response diminishes with the age of the solution. The fading of the blank response due to arsenic in the sodium borohydride appears to result from the gradual adsorption of dissolved arsenic onto suspended impurities in the reagent solution. The adsorbed arsenic is apparently held so tightly that acidification fails to convert it to arsine. The simplest way to avoid errors from this source is to use the analytic-grade reagent, which is more expensive, but usually contains less than 0.5 ng of arsenic per portion (C. Feldman, personal communication). The efficiency of sodium borohydride in generating arsine can be impaired by the presence of other substances that react with sodium borohydride. This effect can be serious.[739]

METHODS OF DETERMINATION OF TOTAL ARSENIC

Molecular-Absorption Spectrophotometry

Molecular-absorption spectrophotometry in aqueous solution has long been one of the most reliable methods for determining small quantities of arsenic. Because of its simplicity and low cost, it will probably continue to be widely used for all but the lowest concentrations. Arsenomolybdic acid is formed when arsenate reacts with acidified molybdate. This heteropolyacid can be partially reduced to give a blue color, which develops slowly (approximately 30 min), but is stable and free from interferences.[652] The other colorimetric method in common use involves the bubbling of arsine through a 0.5% solution of the silver salt of diethyldithiocarbamate in pyridine. An intense red color is produced; absorption is measured at 533 nm.[282,375]

Atomic Absorption

Atomic absorption (nebulized sample solution plus argon–hydrogen or air–acetylene slot burner) is claimed to give sensitivities of 50–100 ng/ml.[404] In the flameless atomic-absorption method, a small volume of sample (1–50 μl) is deposited in a graphite tube or on a tantalum strip. Strong heating vaporizes the arsenic and reduces it to As^0, which is then determined by atomic absorption. The absolute and concentrational detection limits of this method are good (40 pg and 10 ng/ml, respectively) but care is required in controlling sample vaporization and in dealing with interferences.[45] The arsenic can also be introduced into a gas stream as arsine, with conversion to As^0 by a flame or a heated tube[150,430] and detection by atomic absorption. Detection limits can be reduced to 1.0 and 0.2 ng, respectively, for these two methods by accumulating the arsine in a cold trap and releasing it quickly.

Atomic-Emission Spectroscopy

Arsenic can be determined by atomic-emission spectroscopy with various types of excitation. For example, arsine can be accumulated in a cold trap[359] and then introduced into a direct-current glow discharge in helium (Braman et al.[98–100] and C. Feldman, personal communication), giving absolute and concentrational detection limits of 0.5 ng and 25 pg/ml, respectively. Other volatile forms of arsenic (e.g., triphenylarsine), introduced into a microwave discharge in argon,[779] can give an absolute detection limit of 0.02 ng of arsenic. An arsenic-bearing aerosol, introduced into an induction-coupled radiofrequency plasma, gives a concentrational detection limit of 40 ng of arsenic per milliliter.[243,429]

Neutron-Activation Analysis

Neutron-activation analysis has the advantages of being nondestructive (in the many cases in which postirradiation radiochemical separations are not necessary) and of being immune from any danger of contamination during postirradiation handling. Its absolute sensitivity is 0.1 ng for a thermal-neutron flux of 10^{12} neutrons/cm^2-s. In tissue and mineral samples, however, this sensitivity can seldom be reached. The activity induced is the 559-keV photopeak of arsenic-76. A relatively great amount of sodium-24 activity is induced in the sodium present in such samples, and, although the decay of sodium-24 (half-life, 14.96 h) is faster than that of arsenic-76 (half-life, 26.5 h), the sodium-24 activity must be allowed to decay for several days before the arsenic-76 activity can be counted. This delay does not seriously interfere with the determination of arsenic at concentrations above a few parts per million, and the elimination of all chemical treatment of the sample

Appendix C: Traces of Arsenic in Natural Materials

compensates for the inconvenience.[601] If greater sensitivity is needed or if radiochemical interferences appear (e.g., bromine or antimony activities), chemical-group separations can still be performed to isolate the arsenic-76 activity.[350,604]

Electrochemical Methods

In the electrochemical methods that have been proposed for determining traces of arsenic, the arsenic is usually first isolated by volatilization or extraction, then converted to the trivalent form and determined polarographically.[27] The most sensitive such technique is differential pulse polarography, which has a detection limit of about 0.3 ng of arsenic per milliliter and can be used in the presence of natural pollutants, such as unfiltered sludge.[571,608]

Gas Chromatography

Total arsenic can be determined by gas chromatography if the arsenic is first collected and converted to triphenylarsine. The collection–conversion procedure is somewhat long, but the absolute limit of detection is quite low (20 pg) when an atomic-emission detector is used.[777,779]

Other Methods

There are other valid methods of determining traces of arsenic, such as coulombmetry, X-ray fluorescence, atomic optical fluorescence,[788] and ordinary and isotope-dilution mass spectrometry.[778]

METHODS OF DETERMINATION OF ARSENIC COMPOUNDS

Most of the analytic work on separating and identifying arsenic compounds has been done with substituted arsines and substituted acids of arsenic (e.g., methanearsonic and cacodylic). The compounds have been isolated with paper chromatography, electrophoresis, volatilization,[99] and (after silylation[480] or conversion to the corresponding arsine[779] or iodide[749]) gas chromatography. A specific compound is identified by its retention characteristics, sometimes in combination with a specific detector for arsenic. Among the detection methods used have been autoradiography,[507] arc emission,[99] and microwave emission.[779] Absolute sensitivities have been in the picogram range.

Glossary

In formulas: R = aliphatic group or aromatic group
R' = aliphatic group
Ar = aromatic group
X = halogen atom

Acetarsone *See* 3-Acetylamino-4-hydroxyphenylarsonic acid
4-Acetylamidophenylarsonic acid *See* 4-Acetylaminophenylarsonic acid
4-Acetylaminobenzenearsonic acid *See* 4-Acetylaminophenylarsonic acid

3-Acetylamino-4-hydroxyphenylarsonic acid HO—C$_6$H$_3$(NHCOCH$_3$)—AsO$_3$H$_2$;
synonym, acetarsone

4-Acetylaminophenylarsonic acid CH$_3$—CO—HN—C$_6$H$_4$—AsO$_3$H$_2$;

synonyms, 4-acetylamidophenylarsonic acid, 4-acetylaminobenzenearsonic acid, acetylarsanilic acid

Acetylarsan *See* Diethylammonium 3-acetylamino-4-hydroxyphenylarsonate

Acetylarsanilic acid *See* 4-Acetylaminophenylarsonic acid
N-Acetyl-4-hydroxy-m-arsanilic acid, diethylamine salt *See* Diethylammonium 3-acetylamino-4-hydroxyphenylarsonate
Adamsite *See* Phenylarsazine chloride
Alkylarsine $R'AsH_2$; also used as a synonym for trimethylarsine (*q.v.*)
Alkylarsines general term for compounds of the type $R'_n AsH_{3-n}$ ($n = 1,2,3$)

Alkylarsonic acids general term for compounds of the type
$$R' - \overset{\overset{\displaystyle O}{\uparrow}}{\underset{\displaystyle OH}{As}} - OH$$

Alkylbis(organylthio)arsines general term for compounds of the type $RAs(SR')_2$
Alkyldihaloarsines general term for compounds of the type $R'AsX_2$
Alkyldihydroxyarsines general term for compounds of the type $R'As(OH)_2$
Alkylhaloarsines general term for compounds of the types $RAsX_2$ and R_2AsX; *see also* Dialkylhaloarsines and Alkyldihaloarsines
Alkylmethylarsines general term for compounds of the types $R-\overset{\overset{\displaystyle CH_3}{|}}{As}-H$ and R_2AsCH_3
Aluminum arsenate $AlAsO_4 \cdot 8H_2O$; *synonym*, aluminum *o*-arsenate
AMA *See* Dodecyl(octyl)ammonium methanearsonate
Amine methanearsonate *See* Dodecyl(octyl)ammonium methanearsonate

p-Aminoarsenobenzene $H_2N-\langle\bigcirc\rangle-As=As-\langle\bigcirc\rangle-NH_2$

p-Aminobenzenearsonic acid *See* Arsanilic acid
3-Amino-4-hydroxyphenyldichloroarsine *See* Dichlorophenarsine
p-Aminophenylarsonic acid *See* Arsanilic acid
4-Aminophenylarsonic acid *See* Arsanilic acid
3-Amino-3'-sulfinoxymethylamino-4,4'-dihydroxyarsenobenzene, sodium salt *See* Neoarsphenamine
Ammonium arsenite *See* Ammonium *m*-arsenite
Ammonium m-arsenite NH_4AsO_2; *synonym*, ammonium arsenite
Arrhenal *See* Disodium methanearsonate

2-Arsa-1,3-dithiacyclopentane
$$\begin{array}{c} H_2\;\;H_2 \\ C-C \\ \diagup\;\;\;\;\;\diagdown \\ S\;\;\;\;\;\;\;\;S \\ \diagdown\;\;\;\diagup \\ As \\ | \\ R \end{array}$$

Arsanilic acid $H_2N-C_6H_4-AsO_3H_2$; *synonyms,* p-aminobenzenearsonic acid, p-aminophenylarsonic acid, 4-aminophenylarsonic acid, atoxylic acid

Arsenamide *See* Bis(carboxymethylmercapto) (p-carbamoylphenyl)arsine, disodium salt

Arsenates salts derived from o-arsenic acid (*q.v.*) and containing the anion $H_2AsO_4^-$, $HAsO_4^{-2}$, or AsO_4^{-3}, or derived from m-arsenic acid (*q.v.*) and containing the anion AsO_3^-; o-arsenates are salts of o-arsenic acid, and m-arsenates are salts of m-arsenic acid

m-Arsenic acid $HAsO_3$

o-Arsenic acid H_3AsO_4

Arsenic acid anhydride *See* Arsenic pentoxide

Arsenic chlorides general term for $AsCl_3$ and $AsCl_5$ (which has never been isolated)

Arsenic halide general term for compounds of the types AsX_3 (X = F, Cl, Br, I) and AsX_5 (X = F)

Arsenic pentafluoride AsF_5

Arsenic pentasulfide As_2S_5 ; *synonym,* diarsenic pentasulfide

Arsenic pentoxide As_2O_5 ; *synonym,* arsenic acid anhydride

Arsenic sulfosalts compounds obtained by dissolving arsenic trisulfide (*q.v.*) or arsenic pentasulfide (*q.v.*) in alkali sulfide solutions, e.g., $As_2S_3 + 3K_2S \rightarrow 2K_3[AsS_3]$ (potassium trithioarsenite, potassium sulfoarsenite); *synonyms,* thioarsenites, thioarsenates

Arsenic trichloride $AsCl_3$; *synonyms,* arsenous chloride, butter of arsenic, fuming liquid arsenic

Arsenic trifluoride AsF_3

Arsenic trihydride *See* Arsine

Arsenic trioxide As_2O_3 ; *synonyms,* arsenous acid anhydride, white arsenic

Arsenic trisulfide As_2S_3 ; *synonyms,* yellow arsenic sulfide, orpiment

Arsenides binary compounds of arsenic with a metal, e.g., sodium arsenide (*q.v.*)

Arsenious acid arsenous acid

Arsenites salts derived from o-arsenous acid (*q.v.*) and containing the anion $H_2AsO_3^-$, $HAsO_3^{-2}$, or AsO_3^{-3}, or derived from m-arsenous acid (*q.v.*) and containing the anion AsO_2^-; o-arsenites are salts of o-arsenous acid, and m-arsenites are salts of m-arsenous acid

4,4′-Arsenobis(2-aminophenol) dihydrochloride *See* Arsphenamine

Arsenolite the cubic crystalline modification, As_4O_6, of arsenic trioxide (*q.v.*)

Arsenomolybdic acid $As_2O_5 \cdot 6MoO_3 \cdot 18H_2O$

Arsenopyrite FeAsS

Arsenosoalkanes general term for compounds of the types R'AsO and (R'AsO)$_n$

Arsenosobenzene C$_6$H$_5$AsO; *synonyms*, Arzene, oxyphenylarsine

Arsenoso compounds general term for organic compounds containing the AsO group, e.g., RAsO

m-**Arsenous acid** HAsO$_2$

o-**Arsenous acid** H$_3$AsO$_3$

Arsenous acid anhydride *See* Arsenic trioxide

Arsenous chloride *See* Arsenic trichloride

Arsenoxide general term for compounds of the type RAsO

Arsine AsH$_3$; *synonym*, arsenic trihydride

Arsines general term for compounds of the form R$_n$AsH$_{3-n}$ (n = 1,2,3), organic derivatives of arsine (*q.v.*) with one or more hydrogen atoms replaced with organic groups

Arsonates salts derived from arsonic acids (*q.v.*) and containing the anion RAsO$_3$H$^-$ or RAsO$_3$$^{-2}$

Arsonation a reaction that introduces the -AsO(OH)$_2$ group into an organic (in most cases an aromatic) molecule; the arsenic atom in the product is bonded to a carbon atom

Arsonic acids general term for compounds of the type $RAs(=O)(OH)_2$; *synonym*, organylarsonic acids

Arsphenamine HO—C$_6$H$_3$(NH$_2$·HCl)—As=As—C$_6$H$_3$(NH$_2$·HCl)—OH;

synonyms, 4,4'-arsenobis(2-aminophenol) dihydrochloride, 3,3'-diamino-4,4'-dihydroxy-arsenobenzene dihydrochloride, Salvarsan

Arylbis(organylthio)arsine general term for compounds of the form ArAs(SR)$_2$

Arzene *See* Arsenosobenzene

Atoxyl *See* Sodium arsanilate

Atoxylic acid *See* Arsanilic acid

BAL *See* British antilewisite

BAL-arsenite complex compound formed between trivalent arsenic derivatives (*q.v.*) and British antilewisite,

Glossary

Benzenearsonic acid *See* Phenylarsonic acid

Bis(carboxymethylmercapto) (*p*-carbamoylphenyl)arsine, sodium salt

$$\underset{NH_2}{\overset{O}{\overset{\|}{C}}}-\underset{}{\bigcirc}-\underset{SCH_2COONa}{\overset{SCH_2COONa}{As}}$$

synonyms, arsenamide; Caparsolate; {[(*p*-carbamoylphenyl)arsylene] dithio} diacetic acid, disodium salt; thiacetarsamide

Bis(dimethylarsine) oxide *See* Cacodyl oxide

10,10-Bis(phenoxarsine) oxide
synonym, Vinyzene

[structure: two phenoxarsine units linked: O⟨benzene⟩As—O—As⟨benzene⟩O]

Black arsenic an allotropic form of arsenic obtained by condensing arsenic vapor

Bolidensalt BIS a zinc–chromium arsenate (20% arsenic acid, 19% sodium arsenate, 16% sodium dichromate, and 43% zinc sulfate)

Bolidensalt BIS Copperized 20% arsenic acid, 19% sodium arsenate, 16% sodium dichromate, 22% zinc sulfate, and 22% copper sulfate

Bolidensalt K33 copper–chromium arsenate (34% arsenic pentoxide, 26.6% chromium trioxide, 14.8% cupric oxide, and 24.6% water)

British antilewisite $CH_2-CH-CH_2OH$; *synonyms,* BAL, dimercaprol,
$\qquad\qquad\qquad\quad\ \ |\quad\ \ |$
$\qquad\qquad\qquad\ \ SH\ \ SH$

1,2-dimercapto-3-hydroxypropane, 2,3-dimercaptopropanol, 1,2-dithioglycerol

Butter of arsenic *See* Arsenic trichloride

Cacodyl $(CH_3)_2As-As(CH_3)_2$; *synonym,* tetramethyldiarsine

Cacodylates salts of cacodylic acid (*q.v.*) containing the anion $(CH_3)_2AsO_2^-$; *synonym,* dimethylarsinates

Cacodyl hydride *See* Dimethylarsine

Cacodylic acid $(CH_3)_2AsO(OH)$; *synonyms,* dimethylarsinic acid, hydroxydimethylarsine oxide

Cacodyl oxide $(CH_3)_2As-O-As(CH_3)_2$; *synonym,* bis(dimethylarsine) oxide

Calcium arsenate $Ca_3(AsO_4)_2$; *synonym,* tricalcium *o*-arsenate; *see also* London purple

Caparsolate *See* Bis(carboxymethylmercapto) (*p*-carbamoylphenyl)arsine, disodium salt

***p*-Carbamoylaminophenylarsonic acid** *See* Carbarsone

***N*-Carbamoylarsanilic acid** *See* Carbarsone

N-(Carbamoylmethyl)arsanilic acid, monosodium salt *See* Tryparsamide

{ [*p*-Carbamoylphenyl)arsylene] dithio } diacetic acid, disodium salt. *See* Bis(carboxymethylmercapto) (*p*-carbamoylphenyl)arsine, disodium salt

Carbarsone $H_2N-\overset{\overset{O}{\|}}{C}-NH-\langle\bigcirc\rangle-AsO_3H_2$; *synonyms*, *p*-carbamoylaminophenylarsonic acid, *N*-carbamoylarsanilic acid, *p*-ureidobenzenearsonic acid, *p*-ureidophenylarsonic acid, 4-ureidophenylarsonic acid

10-Chloro-5-aza-10-arsa-5,10-dihydroanthracene *See* Phenylarsazine chloride

10-Chloro-5,10-dihydrophenarsazine *See* Phenylarsazine chloride

2-Chlorovinyldichloroarsine *See* Lewisite

β-Chlorovinyldichloroarsine *See* Lewisite

Chlorpicrin *See* Diphenylchloroarsine

Chromated copper arsenate a mixture of copper arsenate (*q.v.*) and chromium arsenate (*q.v.*) used in wood preservation

Chromium arsenate $CrAsO_4$

Claudetite the monoclinic crystalline modification of arsenic trioxide (*q.v.*)

Cobalt arsenide sulfide CoAsS

Cobalt diarsenide $CoAs_2$

Copper acetoarsenite $Cu(CH_3COO)_2 \cdot 3Cu(AsO_2)_2$; *synonyms*, cupric acetoarsenite, Paris green, Schweinfurt green

Copper arsenate $Cu_3(AsO_4)_2 \cdot 4H_2O$; *synonym*, copper *o*-arsenate

Copper *o*-arsenate *See* Copper arsenate

Copper arsenide sulfide CuAsS

Copper(II) *m*-arsenite *See* Cupric arsenite

Cupric acetoarsenite *See* Copper acetoarsenite

Cupric arsenite $Cu(AsO_2)_2$, $CuHAsO_3$; *synonyms*, copper(II) *m*-arsenite, Scheele's green, Swedish green

DA *See* Diphenylchloroarsine

DC *See* Diphenylcyanoarsine

Dialkylarsines general term for compounds of the type R'_2AsH

Dialkylarsinic acids general term for compounds of the type $R'_2AsO(OH)$

Dialkylhaloarsines general term for compounds of the type R'_2AsX

3,3'-Diamino-4,4'-dihydroxyarsenobenzene dihydrochloride *See* Arsphenamine

2-[*p*-(4,6-Diamino-*s*-triazin-2-ylamino)phenyl]-4,5-dicarboxy-1,3-dithia-2-arsacyclopentane *See* Melarsonyl

2-[4-(4,6-Diamino-1,3,5-triazin-2-ylamino)phenyl]-4,5-dicarboxy-1,3,2-dithiaarsolan *See* Melarsonyl

2-[*p*-(4,6-Diamino-*s*-triazin-2-ylamino)phenyl]-4-hydroxymethyl-1,3-dithia-2-arsacyclopentane *See* Melarsoprol

Diarsenic pentasulfide *See* Arsenic pentasulfide

Dichloro(2-chlorovinyl)arsine *See* Lewisite
Dichloro(β-chlorovinyl)arsine *See* Lewisite

Dichlorophenarsine HO–C$_6$H$_3$(NH$_2$)–AsCl$_2$; *synonym*, 3-amino-4-hydroxyphenyldichloroarsine

Diethylamine acetarsone *See* Diethylammonium 3-acetylamino-4-hydroxyphenylarsonate

Diethylammonium 3-acetylamino-4-hydroxyphenylarsonate

[(C$_2$H$_5$)$_2$NH$_2$]$^+$ [HO–C$_6$H$_3$(NHCOCH$_3$)–As(=O)(OH)(O)]$^-$; *synonyms*, Acetylarsan; N-acetyl-4-hydroxy-*m*-arsanilic acid, diethylamine salt; diethylamine acetarsone

5,10-Dihydrophenarsazine chloride *See* Phenylarsazine chloride
Dimercaprol *See* British antilewisite
1,2-Dimercapto-3-hydroxypropane *See* British antilewisite
2,3-Dimercaptopropanol *See* British antilewisite
Dimethylarsinates *See* Cacodylates
Dimethylarsine (CH$_3$)$_2$AsH; *synonym*, cacodyl hydride
Dimethylarsinic acid *See* Cacodylic acid
[(Dimethylarsino)oxy]sodium *See* Sodium cacodylate
Dimethylhydroxyarsine (CH$_3$)$_2$AsOH
Diorganylarsinic acids general term for compounds of the type R$_2$As(=O)–OH
Diphenylamine chlorarsine *See* Phenylarsazine chloride
Diphenylaminocyanoarsine NH(C$_6$H$_4$)$_2$AsCN
Diphenylchlorarsine *See* Diphenylchloroarsine
Diphenylchloroarsine (C$_6$H$_5$)$_2$AsCl; *synonyms*, chlorpicrin, DA, diphenylchlorarsine
Diphenylcyanoarsine (C$_6$H$_5$)$_2$As–CN; *synonym,* DC
Dipotassium hydrogen arsenate K$_2$HAsO$_4$
Disodium arsenate *See* Sodium arsenate
Disodium hydrogen arsenate *See* Sodium arsenate
Disodium methanearsonate (CH$_3$)$_2$As(=O)–ONa; *synonyms*, Arrhenal, disodium methylarsonate, DSMA

| ONa

Disodium methylarsonate *See* Disodium methanearsonate
1,2-Dithioglycerol *See* British antilewisite
DM *See* Phenylarsazine chloride

Dodecyl(octyl)ammonium methanearsonate
synonyms, AMA, amine

$$\left[C_{12}H_{25} - \overset{\overset{C_8H_{17}}{|}}{\underset{H}{N}} H \right]^+ \left[CH_3 - \overset{\overset{O}{\uparrow}}{\underset{O}{As}} - OH \right]^-;$$

methanearsonate, dodecyl(octyl)ammonium methylarsonate

Dodecty(octyl)ammonium methylarsonate *See* Dodecyl(octyl)ammonium methanearsonate
DSMA *See* Disodium methanearsonate
ED *See* Ethyldichloroarsine
Ethylarsine dichloride *See* Ethyldichloroarsine
Ethyldichlorarsine *See* Ethyldichloroarsine
Ethyldichloroarsine $C_2H_5AsCl_2$; *synonyms*, ED, ethylarsine dichloride, ethyldichlorarsine
Fluor chrome arsenate phenol an arsenic-containing wood preservative; *synonym*, osmose
Fowler's solution potassium arsenite solution, containing arsenic trioxide, potassium bicarbonate, and alcohol in water
Fuming liquid arsenic *See* Arsenic trichloride
Gallium arsenide GaAs

Glycobiarsol $HOCH_2-\overset{\overset{O}{\|}}{C}-HN-\langle\bigcirc\rangle-AsO_3^{-2}\ BiOH^{+2}$; *synonym*, oxo(hydrogen *N*-glycoloylarsanilate)bismuth

***p-N*-Glycoloylarsanilate** $HOCH_2-\overset{\overset{O}{\|}}{C}-NH-\langle\bigcirc\rangle-AsO_3^{-2}$; *synonym, p-N-*glycolylarsanilate
***p-N*-Glycolylarsanilate** *See p-N-*Glycoloylarsanilate
Gosio gas *See* Trimethylarsine
Hydroxydimethylarsine oxide *See* Cacodylic acid
4-Hydroxy-3-nitrobenzenearsonic acid *See* 3-Nitro-4-hydroxyphenylarsonic acid
Indium arsenide InAs
Iron arsenate $Fe_3(AsO_4)_2 \cdot 6H_2O$; *synonym*, iron *o*-arsenate; *see also* Scorodite
Iron diarsenide $FeAs_2$
Iron disulfide *See* Pyrite
Lead arsenate mixture of $PbHAsO_4$ and $Pb_3(AsO_4)_2$

Glossary

Lead *m*-arsenate $Pb(AsO_3)_2$
Lead arsenite $Pb(AsO_2)_2$
Lewisite $ClCH=CH-AsCl_2$; *synonyms,* 2-chlorovinyldichloroarsine, β-chlorovinyldichloroarsine, dichloro(2-chlorovinyl)arsine, dichloro(β-chlorovinyl)arsine, Ml
London purple a waste product used as an insecticide; it usually contains about 40% arsenic trioxide (*q.v.*) and 25% calcium carbonate, the rest being iron and aluminum oxides and dyestuff
Ml *See* Lewisite
MAA *See* Methanearsonic acid
Magnesium ammonium arsenate $MgNH_4AsO_4 \cdot 6H_2O$
Magnesium arsenate $Mg_3(AsO_4) \cdot MgO \cdot H_2O$
Manganese arsenate $MnHAsO_4$; *synonym,* manganese hydrogen arsenate
Manganese hydrogen arsenate *See* Manganese arsenate
MD *See* Methyldichloroarsine

Melarsonyl

[structure: 4,6-diamino-s-triazin-2-ylamino linked via NH to phenyl-As with dithiolane bearing two CH–COOH groups]

synonyms, 2-[*p*-(4,6-diamino-*s*-triazin-2-ylamino)phenyl]-4,5-dicarboxy-1,3-dithia-2-arsacyclopentane, 2-[4-(4,6-diamino-1,3,5-triazin-2-ylamino)phenyl]-4,5-dicarboxy-1,3,2-dithiaarsolan

Melarsonyl potassium dipotassium salt of Melarsonyl,

[structure: same as Melarsonyl with COOK groups in place of COOH]

Melarsoprol

[structure: 4,6-diamino-s-triazin-2-ylamino linked via NH to phenyl-As with dithiolane bearing CH₂ and CH–CH₂OH]

synonym, 2-[*p*-(4,6-diamino-*s*-triazin-2-ylamino)phenyl]-4-hydroxymethyl-1,3-dithia-2-arsacyclopentane

Methanearsonates salts of methanearsonic acid containing the anion $CH_3AsO_3H^-$ or $CH_3AsO_3^{-2}$; *synonym,* methylarsonates

Methanearsonic acid $CH_3-\overset{\overset{\displaystyle O}{\uparrow}}{\underset{\displaystyle OH}{As}}-OH$; *synonyms*, MAA, methylarsonic acid

Methylarsine CH_3AsH_2
Methylarsines general term for compounds of the type $(CH_3)_n AsH_{3-n}$ ($n = 1,2,3$)
Methylarsonates *See* Methanearsonates
Methylarsonic acid *See* Methanearsonic acid
Methylbis(alkylthio)arsine $CH_3As(SR')_2$
Methyldichloroarsine CH_3AsCl_2; *synonym*, MD
Methyldihydroxyarsine $CH_3As(OH)_2$
Monohydrogen sodium *o*-arsenate *See* Sodium arsenate
Monolead *o*-arsenate $PbH_4(AsO_4)_2 = PbHAsO_4 \cdot H_3AsO_4$

Monosodium methanearsonate $CH_3-\overset{\overset{\displaystyle O}{\uparrow}}{\underset{\displaystyle OH}{As}}-ONa$; *synonyms*, MSMA, sodium
acid methanearsonate, sodium acid methylarsonate, sodium hydrogen methane arsonate

MSMA *See* Monosodium methanearsonate

Neoarsphenamine HO—⟨◯⟩—As = As—⟨◯⟩—OH ;
 synonyms, 3-   NH₂   NH—CH₂OSO₂Na
amino-3′-sulfinoxymethylamino-4,4′-dihydroxyarsenobenzene, sodium salt; Neosalvarsan; sodium { 5-[(3-amino-4-hydroxyphenyl)arseno]-2-hydroxyanilino } methanol sulfoxylate

Neosalvarsan *See* Neoarsphenamine
Nickel arsenide NiAs
Nickel diarsenide $NiAs_2$
3-Nitro-4-hydroxybenzenearsonic acid *See* 3-Nitro-4-hydroxyphenylarsonic acid
3-Nitro-4-hydroxyphenylarsonic acid HO—⟨◯⟩—AsO_3H_2 ;
                                                   NO₂
synonyms, 4-hydroxy-3-nitrobenzenearsonic acid, 3-nitro-4-hydroxybenzenearsonic acid, Roxarsone
4-Nitrophenylarsonic acid O_2N—⟨◯⟩—AsO_3H_2

Glossary

3-Nitro-4-ureidophenylarsonic acid $H_2NC(=O)-NH-C_6H_3(NO_2)-AsO_3H_2$

Organylarsonic acids *See* Arsonic acids

Organylbis(alkylthio)arsines general term for compounds of the type $RAs(SR')_2$

2-Organyl-4-(4'-carboxybutyl)-1,3,2-dithiaarsacyclohexane

(structure: 1,3,2-dithiaarsacyclohexane ring with $-CH-CH_2CH_2CH_2CH_2-COOH$ substituent, As bearing R)

2-Organyl-4-hydroxymethyl-1,3,2-dithiaarsacyclopentane

(structure: 1,3,2-dithiaarsacyclopentane ring with $-CH-CH_2OH$ substituent, As bearing R)

Orpiment *See* Arsenic trisulfide

Osmosalts a wood preservative containing 25% sodium arsenate (*q.v.*)

Osmose *See* Fluor chrome arsenate phenol

Oxo(hydrogen *N*-glycoloylarsanilate)bismuth *See* Glycobiarsol

Oxyphenylarsine *See* Arsenosobenzene

Paris green *See* Copper acetoarsenite

Pentaorganyl arsenic general term for compounds of the type R_5As

Phenylarsazine chloride (structure: phenarsazine with Cl on As-10, NH at 5, numbered 1–9); *synonyms*, adamsite, 10-chloro-5-aza-10-arsa-5,10-dihydroanthracene, 10-chloro-5,10-dihydrophenarsazine, 5,10-dihydrophenarsazine chloride, diphenylamine chlorarsine, DM

Phenylarsonates salts derived from phenylarsonic acid (*q.v.*) or substituted phenylarsonic acids (*q.v.*) and containing the anion $ArAsO_3H_2^-$ or $ArAsO_3^{-3}$

Phenylarsonic acid $C_6H_5AsO_3H_2$; *synonym*, benzenearsonic acid

Phenylarsonic acids general term for compounds of the type $ArAsO_3H_2$, with Ar representing the C_6H_5 or a substituted phenyl group

Phenylarsonic compounds compounds with a phenyl or substituted phenyl group bonded to an arsonic group, e.g., phenylarsonic acid (*q.v.*)

Phenylarsonic formulation a mixture of substances in which one ingredient is a phenylarsonic compound, e.g., 4-aminophenylarsonic acid (*q.v.*) in poultry feed

Phenyldichloroarsine $C_6H_5AsCl_2$

Potassium arsenate KH_2AsO_4; *synonym*, potassium dihydrogen arsenate

Potassium *m*-arsenate $(KAsO_3)_n$

Potassium arsenite $KAsO_2$; *synonym*, potassium *m*-arsenite

Potassium *m*-arsenite *See* Potassium arsenite

Potassium dihydrogen arsenate *See* Potassium arsenate

Pyrite FeS_2; *synonym*, iron disulfide

Realgar *See* Tetraarsenic tetrasulfide

Roxarsone *See* 3-Nitro-4-hydroxyphenylarsonic acid

Salvarsan *See* Arsphenamine

Scheele's green *See* Cupric arsenite

Schweinfurt green *See* Copper acetoarsenite

Scorodite natural ferric arsenate, $Fe_2O_3 \cdot As_2O_5 \cdot 4H_2O$; *see also* Iron arsenate

Sodium acid methanearsonate *See* Monosodium methanearsonate

Sodium acid methylarsonate *See* Monosodium methanearsonate

Sodium {5-[(3-amino-4-hydroxyphenyl)arseno]-2-hydroxyanilino} methanol sulfoxylate *See* Neoarsphenamine

Sodium arsanilate sodium hydrogen 4-aminophenylarsonate; *synonym*, Atoxyl

Sodium arsenate Na_2HAsO_4; *synonyms*, disodium arsenate, disodium hydrogen arsenate, monohydrogen sodium *o*-arsenate

Sodium arsenide Na_3As

Sodium arsenite $NaAsO_2$; *synonym*, sodium *m*-arsenite

Sodium *m*-arsenite *See* Sodium arsenite

Sodium cacodylate $(CH_3)_2\overset{\overset{O}{\uparrow}}{As}-ONa \cdot 3H_2O$; *synonyms*, [(dimethylarsino)oxy] sodium, sodium dimethylarsinate

Sodium dimethylarsinate *See* Sodium cacodylate

Sodium *p-N*-glycoloylarsanilate HOCH$_2$—C(=O)—NH——As(=O)(OH)(ONa) ; *synonym*, sodium *p-N*-glycolylarsanilate

Sodium *p-N*-glycolylarsanilate *See* Sodium *p-N*-glycoloylarsanilate

Sodium hydrogen 4-aminophenylarsonate *See* Sodium arsanilate

Sodium hydrogen methane arsonate *See* Monosodium methanearsonate

Sodium methane arsonate *See* Sodium methanearsonate

Glossary

Sodium methanearsonate CH$_3$As(=O)(OH)(ONa) · 6H$_2$O;

synonyms, sodium methane arsonate, sodium methylarsonate

Sodium methylarsonate *See* Sodium methanearsonate

Sodium N-phenylglycinamide-p-arsonate *See* Tryparsamide

p-Sulfamylphenylarsonic acid H$_2$N–S(=O)$_2$–C$_6$H$_4$–AsO$_3$H$_2$

p-Sulfophenylarsonic acid HO$_3$S–C$_6$H$_4$–As$_3$O$_3$H$_2$

Swedish green *See* Cupric arsenite

Tetraarsenic tetrasulfide As$_4$S$_4$; *synonym*, realgar

Tetradodecylammonium methanearsonate [(C$_{12}$H$_{25}$)$_4$N]$^+$CH$_3$AsO$_3$H$^-$

Tetramethyldiarsine *See* Cacodyl

Tetraoctylammonium methanearsonate [(C$_8$H$_{17}$)$_4$N]$^+$CH$_3$AsO$_3$H$^-$

Tetraorganylarsonium salts general term for compounds of the type [R$_4$As]$^+$X$^-$

Tetrapotassium diarsenate K$_4$As$_2$O$_7$

Thiacetarsamide *See* Bis(carboxymethylmercapto)(p-carbamoylphenyl)arsine, disodium salt

Thioarsenates *See* Arsenic sulfosalts

Thioarsenites *See* Arsenic sulfosalts

TMA *See* Trimethylarsine

Tricalcium arsenate Ca$_3$(AsO$_4$)$_2$

Tricalcium o-arsenate *See* Calcium arsenate

Trilead arsenate Pb$_3$(AsO$_4$)$_2$

Trimethylarsine (CH$_3$)$_3$As; *synonyms*, Gosio gas, TMA

Trimethylarsine oxide (CH$_3$)$_3$AsO

Triorganyl arsenate general term for neutral esters of arsenic acid of the type (RO)$_3$AsO

Triorganyl arsenite general term for neutral esters of arsenous acid of the type (RO)$_3$As

Triorganylarsine general term for compounds of the type R$_3$As

Triphenylarsine (C$_6$H$_5$)$_3$As

Trivalent arsenic derivatives compounds containing an arsenic atom that has formed three bonds with other groups or atoms, e.g., arsenic trichloride (*q.v.*), arsenic trioxide (*q.v.*), and triorganylarsines (*q.v.*)

Tryparsamide $H_2N-\underset{\underset{O}{\|}}{C}-CH_2-HN-C_6H_4-\underset{\underset{ONa}{|}}{\overset{\overset{O}{\uparrow}}{As}}-OH \cdot \tfrac{1}{2}H_2O$;
  synonyms, *N*-(carbamoylmethyl)arsanilic acid, monosodium salt; sodium *N*-phenyl-glycinamide-*p*-arsonate

p-**Ureidobenzenearsonic acid** *See* Carbarsone

p-**Ureidophenylarsonic acid** *See* Carbarsone

4-Ureidophenylarsonic acid *See* Carbarsone

Vinyzene *See* 10,10-Bis(phenoxarsine) oxide

White arsenic *See* Arsenic trioxide

Wolman salts a mixture of three parts sodium chromate, two parts sodium fluoride, two parts sodium arsenate (*q.v.*), and one part dinitrophenol or equivalent

Yellow arsenic sulfide *See* Arsenic trisulfide

Zinc arsenate $Zn_3(AsO_4)_2$

Zinc arsenite *See* Zinc *m*-arsenite

Zinc *m*-arsenite $Zn(AsO_2)_2$; *synonyms*, zinc arsenite, ZMA

Zinc fluoroarsenate $ZnFAsO_4$

ZMA *See* Zinc *m*-arsenite

References

1. Abbott, O. J., H. R. Bird, and W. W. Cravens. Effects of dietary arsanilic acid on chicks. Poult. Sci. 33:1245–1253, 1954.
2. Abernethy, F. R., M. J. Peterson, and F. H. Gibson. Spectrochemical Analysis of Coal Ash for Trace Elements. Bureau of Mines Report of Investigations 7281. Washington, D.C.: U.S. Department of the Interior, 1969. 30 pp.
3. Ahr, W. M. Long-lived pollutants in sediments from the Laguna Atoscosa National Wildlife Refuge, Texas. Geol. Soc. Amer. Bull. 84:2511–2516, 1973.
4. Ahrens, J. F., and A. R. Olson. Prevention and Control of Crabgrass in Lawns. Connecticut Agricultural Experiment Station Bulletin 642. New Haven, 1961. 8 pp.
5. Albert, A. Resistance to drugs and other agents, pp. 129–138. In Selective Toxicity and Related Topics. (4th ed.) London: Methuen & Co., Ltd., 1968.
6. Albert, W. B. Arsenic solubility in soils. South Carolina Agric. Exp. Sta. Ann. Rep. 47:45–46, 1934.
7. Albert, W. B., and C. H. Arndt. The concentration of soluble arsenic as an index of arsenic toxicity to plants. South Carolina Agric. Exp. Sta. Ann. Rep. 44:47–48, 1931.
8. Alderdice, D. F., and J. R. Brett. Toxicity of sodium arsenite to young chum salmon. Prog. Rep. Pacific Coast Sta. Fish. Res. Bd. Can. 108:27–29, 1957.
9. Aldrich, C. J. Leuconychia striata arsenicalis transversus. With report of three cases. Amer. J. Med. Sci. 127:702–709, 1904.
10. Allaway, W. H. Agronomic controls over the environmental cycling of trace elements. Adv. Agron. 20:235–274, 1968.
11. Al-Sibaai, A. A., and A. G. Fogg. Stability of dilute standard solutions of antimony, arsenic, iron and rhenium used in colorimetry. Analyst 98:732–738, 1973.

12. Al-Timimi, A. A., and T. W. Sullivan. Safety and toxicity of dietary organic arsenicals relative to performance of young turkeys. I. Arsanilic acid and sodium arsanilate. Poult. Sci. 51:111–116, 1972.
13. Amor, A. J., and P. Pringle. A review of selenium as an industrial hazard. Bull. Hyg. 20:239–241, 1945.
14. Anastasia, F. B., and W. J. Kender. The influence of soil arsenic on the growth of lowbush blueberry. J. Environ. Qual. 2:335–337, 1973.
15. Andersen, O. Studies on the absorption and translocation of amitrol (3-amino-1,2,4-triazole) by nutgrass (*Cyperus rotundus* L.). Weeds 6:370–385, 1958.
16. Anderson, N. P. Bowen's precancerous dermatosis and multiple benign superficial epithelioma. Arch. Derm. Syphilol. 26:1052–1064, 1932.
17. Andren, A. W., J. A. C. Fortescue, G. S. Henderson, D. E. Reichle, and R. I. Van Hook. Environmental monitoring of toxic materials in ecosystems, pp. 61–119. In Ecology and Analysis of Trace Contaminants. Progress Report, June 1972–January 1973. Oak Ridge National Laboratory ORNL-NSF-EATC-1. Oak Ridge, Tenn.: U.S. Atomic Energy Commission, 1973.
18. Angino, E. E., L. M. Magnuson, T. C. Waugh, O. K. Galle, and J. Bredfeldt. Arsenic in detergent: Possible danger and pollution hazard. Science 168:389–390, 1970.
19. Anke, M., M. Grun, and M. Partshefeld. The essentiality of arsenic for animals. In D. D. Hemphill, Ed. Trace Substances in Environmental Health—X. Proceedings of University of Missouri's 10th Annual Conference on Trace Substances in Environmental Health held June 8–10, 1976. Columbia: University of Missouri, 1977.
20. Ansul Company. Comments in Support of Continued Registration of Organic Arsenical Herbicides. In Response to the Federal Register Arsenic and Lead Notice 36 FR 12709. Marinette, Wisconsin: The Ansul Company, August 31, 1971. 55 pp.
21. Applegate, V. C., J. H. Howell, A. E. Hall, Jr., and M. A. Smith. Toxicity of 4,346 Chemicals to Larval Lampreys and Fishes. Fish and Wildlife Service Special Scientific Report—Fisheries No. 207. Washington, D.C.: U.S. Department of the Interior, 1957. 157 pp.
22. Apted, F. I. C. Four years' experience of melarsenoxide/BAL in the treatment of late Rhodesian sleeping sickness. Trans. Roy. Soc. Trop. Med. Hyg. 51:75–86, 1957.
23. Aras, N. K., W. H. Zoller, and G. E. Gordon. Instrumental photon activation analysis of atmospheric particulate material. Anal. Chem. 45:1481–1490, 1973.
24. Arguello, R. A., D. D. Cenget, and E. E. Tello. Cancer y arsenicismo regional endemico en Cordoba. Rev. Argentina Dermatosifilol. 22(4th part):461–487, 1938.
25. Arima, K., and M. Beppu. Induction and mechanisms of arsenite resistance in *Pseudomonas pseudomallei*. J. Bacteriol. 88:143–150, 1964.
26. Arle, H. F., and K. C. Hamilton. Topical applications of DSMA and MSMA in irrigated cotton. Weed Sci. 19:545–547, 1971.
27. Arnold, J. P., and R. M. Johnson. Polarography of arsenic. Talanta 16:1191–1207, 1969.
28. Arnott, J. T., and A. L. Leaf. The determination and distribution of toxic levels of arsenic in a silt loam soil. Weeds 15:121–124, 1967.
29. Arsenic, pp. 234–235. In W. H. Ranking, Ed. The Half-yearly Abstract of the Medical Sciences. Vol. 11. London: John Churchill, 1850.
30. Arsenic-eaters. Boston Med. Surg. J. 51:189–195, 1854.

References

31. Arsenic in beer. Lancet 1:496, 1901.
32. Arsen(III)-oxyd As_2O_3, pp. 236–273. In Gmelins Handbuch der Anorganischen Chemie. Achte Auflage. Arsen. System-Nummer 17. Weinheim: Verlag Chemie GMBH, 1952.
33. Arsen und Schwefel, pp. 415–462. In Gmelins Handbuch der Anorganischen Chemie. Achte Auflage. Arsen. System-Nummer 17. Weinheim: Verlag Chemie GMBH, 1952.
34. Arsenverbindungen des Calciums, pp. 256–263. In Gmelins Handbuch der Anorganischen Chemie. Achte Auflage. Calcium. Teil B—Lieferung 1. System-Nummer 28. Weinheim: Verlag Chemie GMBH, 1956.
35. Ashton, F. M., and A. S. Crafts. Mode of Action of Herbicides. New York: Wiley-Interscience Publishers, 1973. 504 pp.
36. Askerov, A. A., S. D. Kerimova, and R. B. Khalilova. Stimulation effect of some chemical preparations on the fattening of silkworm caterpillars. Mater. Nauch. Konf., Azerb. Nauch.-Issled. Inst. Zhivetnovod. 179–181, 1967. (in Russian)
37. Aston, B. C. Chemistry section, pp. 60–65. In New Zealand Department of Agriculture Annual Report 1934–1935.
38. Aston, S. R., I. Thornton, and J. S. Webb. Arsenic in stream sediments and waters of south west England. Sci. Total Environ. 4:347–358, 1975.
39. Auger, V. Action des alcalis sur les acides mono- et diméthyl-arsiniques et sur leur dérivés iodo-substitués. C. R. Acad. Sci (D) 146:1280–1282, 1908.
40. Ayres, S., Jr., and N. P. Anderson. Cutaneous manifestations of arsenic poisoning. Arch. Derm. Syphilol. 30:33–43, 1934.
41. Baca, E. J., Jr. Thermodynamics of Proton Ionization in Dilute Aqueous Solution at 25°. Ph.D. Thesis. Albuquerque: University of New Mexico, 1969. 188 pp.
42. Bado, A. A. Composition of water and interpretation of analytical results. J. Amer. Water Works Assoc. 31:1975–1977, 1939. (abstract)
43. Baetjer, A. M., A. M. Lilienfeld, and M. L. Levin. Cancer and occupational exposure to inorganic arsenic, p. 393. In Abstracts. 18th International Congress on Occupational Health, Brighton, England, 14–19 September, 1975.
44. Bailey, E. M. The twenty-fourth report on food products and the twelfth report on drug products, 1919. Part 1, pp. 213–259. In Connecticut Agricultural Experiment Station Bulletin 219. New Haven: University of Connecticut, 1919.
45. Baird, R. B., and S. M. Gabrielian. A tantalum foil-lined graphite tube for the analysis of arsenic and selenium by atomic absorption spectroscopy. Appl. Spectrosc. 28:273–274, 1974.
46. Baker, R. S., H. F. Arle, J. H. Miller, and J. T. Holstun, Jr. Effects of organic arsenical herbicides on cotton response and chemical residues. Weed Sci. 17:37–40, 1969.
47. Ball, R. C., and F. H. Hooper. The use of [74]-tagged sodium arsenite in a study of effects of a herbicide on pond ecology, pp. 146–163. In Isotopes in Weed Research. Proceedings of a Symposium, Vienna, 1965. Vienna: International Atomic Energy Agency, 1966.
48. Barber, H. J. The hydrolysis of arylthioarsinites. J. Chem. Soc. 1932:1365–1369.
49. Barela, C., and G. Pezzeri. Sulla origine dell'arsenico cosiddetto fisiologico. Indagini sul contenuto in arsenico degli alimenti. Zacchia 41 (Vol. 2, Ser. 3):447–461, 1966.
50. Barnard, H. E. Some poisons found in food. Pure Products 7:145–148, 1911.
51. Baron, R. R. The use of arsenicals in feeding stuffs, pp. 1–7. In The Use of

Arsenicals in Feedingstuffs. Proceedings of a Seminar held at the Criterion, Lower Regent Street, London, March 20, 1969. London: Salisbury Laboratories, 1969.
52. Baroni, C., G. J. van Esch, and U. Saffiotti. Carcinogenesis tests of two inorganic arsenicals. Arch. Environ. Health 7:668–674, 1963.
53. Barry, K. G., and E. G. Herndon, Jr. Electrocardiographic changes associated with acute arsenic poisoning. Med. Ann. D. C. 31:25–27, 65–66, 1962.
54. Bartlett, J. M. Blueberries [arsenic content of], pp. 2–3. In Maine Agriculture Experiment Station Official Inspections 151. Orono, Maine, 1934.
55. Batjer, L. P., and N. R. Benson. Effect of metal chelates in overcoming arsenic toxicity to peach trees. Proc. Amer. Soc. Hort. Sci. 72:74–78, 1958.
56. Baud, E. Sur l'acide dimethylpyroarsinique. C. R. Acad. Sci. (D) 139:411–413, 1904.
57. Beaudoin, A. R. Teratogenicity of sodium arsenate in rats. Teratology 10:153–158, 1974.
58. Becker, C. D., and T. O. Thatcher. Arsenates and arsenites, pp. C1–C11. In Toxicity of Power Plant Chemicals to Aquatic Life. U.S. Atomic Energy Commission WASH 1249. Richland, Wash.: Battelle Memorial Institute, Pacific Northwest Laboratories, 1973.
59. Becker, K. A., K. Plieth, and I. N. Stranski. The polymorphic modifications of arsenic trioxide. Prog. Inorg. Chem. 4:1–72, 1962.
60. Beer poisoning epidemic. Lancet 1:570, 1901.
61. Bencko, V. Arsenic in the hair of nonprofessionally exposed population. Cesk. Hyg. 11:539–543, 1966. (in Czech)
62. Bencko, V. Hygienic problems of atmospheric pollution with arsenic. Gig. Sanit. 38(10):85–87, 1973. (in Russian)
63. Bencko, V. Oxygen consumption by mouse liver homogenate during drinking water arsenic exposure. Part II. J. Hyg. Epidemiol. Microbiol. Immunol. 16:42–46, 1972.
64. Bencko, V., V. Cmarko, and Š. Palan. The cumulation dynamics of arsenic in the tissues of rabbits exposed in the area of the ENO plant. Cesk. Hyg. 13:18–22, 1968. (in Czech, summary in English)
65. Bencko, V., V. Dvorak, and K. Symon. Organ retention of parenterally administered arsenic (labelled with ^{74}As) in mice preliminarily exposed to the element in drinking water. A study in arsenic tolerance. J. Hyg. Epidemiol. Microbiol. Immunol. 17:165–168, 1973.
66. Bencko, V., and Z. Šimáne. The effect of chronical intake of arsenic on the liver tissue respiration in mice. Experientia 24:706, 1968.
67. Bencko, V., and K. Symon. Dynamics of arsenic cumulation in hairless mice after peroral administration. J. Hyg. Epidemiol. Microbiol. Immunol. 13:248–253, 1969.
68. Bencko, V., and K. Symon. Suitability of hairless mice for experimental work and their sensitivity to arsenic. J. Hyg. Epidemiol. Microbiol. Immunol. 13:1–6, 1969.
69. Bencko, V., and K. Symon. The cumulation dynamics in some tissue of hairless mice inhaling arsenic. Atmos. Environ. 4:157–161, 1970.
70. Bennett, R. L., and M. H. Malamy. Arsenate resistant mutants of *Escherichia coli* and phosphate transport. Biochem. Biophys. Res. Commun. 40:496–503, 1970.
71. Benson, N. R. Can profitable orchards be grown on old orchard soils? Wash. State Hort. Assoc. Proc. 64:109–115, 1968.
72. Beppu, M., and K. Arima. Decreased permeability as the mechanism of arsenite resistance in *Pseudomonas pseudomallei*. J. Bacteriol. 88:151–157, 1964.
73. Bergoglio, R. M. Mortalidad por cáncer en zonas de aguas arsenicales de la Provincia de Córdoba, República Argentina. Prensa Med. Argent. 51:994–998, 1964.

References

74. Bespalov, A. I., V. N. Bolovina, and F. P. Kosorotova. Certain data on atmospheric pollution with arsenic from the gas electric power stations of the Rostovskaya Oblast. Gig. Sanit. 34(10):111–112, 1969. (in Russian)
75. Billeter, O., and E. Marfurt. De la teneur normale en arsenic dans le corps humain. Helv. Chim. Acta 6:780–784, 1923.
76. Bird, H. R., A. C. Groschke, and M. Rubin. Effect of arsonic acid derivatives in stimulating growth of chickens. J. Nutr. 37:215–226, 1949.
77. Bird, M. L., F. Challenger, P. T. Charlton, and J. O. Smith. Studies on biological methylations. II. The action of moulds on inorganic and organic compounds of arsenic. Biochem. J. 43:78–83, 1948.
78. Birmingham, D. J. Arsenic, pp. 1046–1047. In T. Fitzpatrick, K. A. Arndt, W. H. Clark, Jr., A. Z. Eisen, E. J. van Scott, and J. H. Vaughan, Eds. Dermatology in General Medicine. New York: McGraw-Hill Book Company, 1971.
79. Birmingham, D. J., M. M. Key, D. A. Holaday, and V. B. Perone. An outbreak of arsenical dermatosis in a mining community. Arch. Derm. 91:457–464, 1965.
80. Bishop, R. F., and D. Chisholm. Arsenical spray residues on apples and in some apple products. Can. J. Plant Sci. 46:225–231, 1966.
81. Blakeslee, P. A. Monitoring considerations for municipal wastewater effluent and sludge application to the land, pp. 183–198. In Proceedings of the Joint Conference on Recycling Municipal Sludges and Effluent on Land. Champaign, Illinois, July 1973. Washington, D.C.: National Association of State Universities and Land-Grant Colleges, 1973.
82. Blanchard, E. Les arsenicaux en arboriculture fruitière. C. R. Acad. Agric. France 19:183–186, 1933.
83. Blei und Arsen, pp. 887–905. In Gmelins Handbuch der Anorganischen Chemie. Achte Auflage. Blei. Teil C 3. System-Nummer 47. Weinheim: Verlag Chemie GMBH, 1970.
84. Boischot, P., and M. Tyszkiewicz. Absorption de l'arsenic par les plantes. C. R. Acad. Agric. France 35:678–679, 1949.
85. Bolton, N. E., R. I. Van Hook, W. Fulkerson, W. S. Lyon, A. W. Andren, J. A. Carter, and J. F. Emery. Trace Element Measurements at the Coal-Fired Allen Steam Plant. Progress Report June 1971–January 1973. Oak Ridge National Laboratory Report ORNL-NSF-EP-43. Oak Ridge, Tenn.: U.S. Atomic Energy Commission, 1973. 83 pp.
86. Borgono, J. M., and R. Greiber. Epidemiological study of arsenicism in the city of Antofagasta, pp. 13–24. In D. D. Hemphill, Ed. Trace Substances in Environmental Health—V. Proceedings of University of Missouri's 5th Annual Conference on Trace Substances in Environmental Health. Held June 29–July 1, 1971. Columbia: University of Missouri, 1972.
87. Borst Pauwels, G. W. F., J. K. Peter, S. Jager, and C. C. B. Wijffels. A study of the arsenate uptake by yeast cells compared with phosphate uptake. Biochim. Biophys. Acta 94:312–314, 1965.
88. Boschetti, M. M., and T. F. McLoughlin. Toxicity of sodium arsenite to minnows. Sanitalk 5(4):14–18, 1957.
89. Boström, K., and S. Valdes. Arsenic in ocean floors. Lithos 2:351–360, 1969.
90. Bounds, G. I. Use of selective weed control for municipalities. South. Weed Conf. Proc. 21:280–281, 1968.
91. Boutwell, R. K. A carcinogenicity evaluation of potassium arsenite and arsanilic acid. J. Agric. Food Chem. 11:381–385, 1963.
92. Bowen, H. J. M. Trace Elements in Biochemistry. New York: Academic Press, 1966. 241 pp.

93. Boyce, A. P., and I. J. Verme. Toxicity of Arsenite Debarkers to Deer in Michigan. Report No. 2025. Presented at the 16th Midwest Wildlife Conference, St. Louis, Missouri, Dec. 1954. 9 pp.
94. Boyle, R. W., and I. R. Jonasson. The geochemistry of arsenic and its use as an indicator element in geochemical prospecting. J. Geochem. Explor. 2:251–296, 1973.
95. Boylen, G. W., Jr., and H. L. Hardy. Distribution of arsenic in nonexposed persons (hair, liver, and urine). Amer. Ind. Hyg. Assoc. J. 28:148–150, 1967.
96. Bradicich, R., N. E. Foster, F. E. Hons, M. T. Jeffus, and C. T. Kenner. Residues in food and feed. Arsenic in cottonseed products and various commodities. Pest. Monit. J. 3:139–141, 1969.
97. Braman, R. S. Arsenic in the environment, pp. 108–123. In E. A. Woolson, Ed. Arsenical Pesticides. ACS Symposium Series 7. Washington, D.C.: American Chemical Society, 1975.
98. Braman, R. S., and A. Dynako. Direct current discharge spectral emission-type detector. Anal. Chem. 40:95–106, 1968.
99. Braman, R. S., and C. C. Foreback. Methylated forms of arsenic in the environment. Science 182:1247–1249, 1973.
100. Braman, R. S., L. L. Justen, and C. C. Foreback. Direct volatilization–spectral emission type detection system for nanogram amounts of arsenic and antimony. Anal. Chem. 44:2195–2199, 1972.
101. Braun, W. Carcinoma of the skin and the internal organs caused by arsenic: Delayed occupational lesions due to arsenic. German Med. Monthly 3:321–324, 1958.
102. Briski, B., and Z. Klepić. Additives as sources of contamination of food with heavy metals and arsenic. Farm. Glas. 24:49–60, 1968. (in Croatian)
103. Britton, H. T. S., and P. Jackson. Physicochemical studies of complex formation involving weak acids. Part X. Complex formation between tartaric acid and (a) arsenic acid, (b) arsenious acid, (c) antimonous hydroxide, in acid and alkaline solutions. The dissociation constants of arsenious and arsenic acids. Part XI. Complex formation between tartaric acid and (a) molybdic acid, (b) tungstic acid. J. Chem. Soc. 1934:1048–1055.
104. Brock, R. Death of Napoleon. Nature 195:841–842, 1962.
105. Brock, R. Napoleon's death. Lancet 1:272, 1962. (letter)
106. Brown, A. W. A. Insect Control by Chemicals. New York: John Wiley & Sons, Inc., 1951. 817 pp.
107. Brown, E. R., J. J. Hazdra, L. Keith, I. Greenspan, J. B. G. Kwapinski, and P. Beamer. Frequency of fish tumors found in a polluted watershed as compared to nonpolluted Canadian waters. Cancer Res. 33:189–198, 1973.
108. Brumm, M. C., and A. L. Sutton. The effect of arsenic on swine growth and swine waste composition, pp. 11–13. In Proceedings of Purdue Swine Day, September 4, 1975. West Lafayette, Indiana: Purdue University, Cooperative Extension Service, Agricultural Experiment Station, 1975.
109. Buchanan, W. D. Toxicity of Arsenic Compounds. New York: Elsevier Publishing Company, 1962. 155 pp.
110. Buck, W. B. Diagnosis of feed-related toxicoses. J. Amer. Vet. Med. Assoc. 156:1434–1443, 1970.
111. Buck, W. B. Hazardous arsenical residues associated with the use of a lawn crabgrass control preparation. Vet. Toxic. 15:25–27, 1973.
112. Buck, W. B. Laboratory toxicologic tests and their interpretation. J. Amer. Vet. Med. Assoc. 155:1928–1941, 1969.

References

113. Buck, W. B. Pesticides and economic poisons in the food chain. U.S. Anim. Health Assoc. Proc. 73:221–226, 1969.
114. Buck, W. B. Untoward reactions encountered with medicated feeds, pp. 196–217. In The Use of Drugs in Animal Feeds. Proceedings of a Symposium. NAS Publ. 1679. Washington, D.C.: National Academy of Sciences, 1969.
115. Buck, W. B., G. D. Osweiler, and G. A. Van Gelder. Clinical and Diagnostic Veterinary Toxicology. Dubuque, Iowa: Kendall-Hunt Publishing Co., 1973. 287 pp.
116. Buechley, R. W. Epidemiological consequences of an arsenic-lung cancer theory. Amer. J. Public Health 53:1229–1232, 1963.
117. Bunsen, R. Untersuchungen über die Kakodylreihe. Ann. Chem. Pharm. 46:1–48, 1843.
118. Burgess, S. G. The analysis of trade-waste waters, pp. 65–84. In P. C. G. Isaac, Ed. Treatment of Trade-Waste Waters and the Prevention of River Pollution. The Proceedings of a Course held in the Department of Civil Engineering, King's College, Newcastle upon Tyne, 1–12 April 1957. Newcastle upon Tyne: University of Durham, King's College, 1957.
119. Burleson, C. A., and N. R. Page. Phosphorus and zinc interactions in flax. Soil Sci. Soc. Amer. Proc. 31:510–513, 1967.
120. Burrus, R. P., Jr., and D. M. Sargent. Technical and Microeconomic Analysis of Arsenic and Its Compounds. EPA 560/6-76-016. Springfield, Va.: Versar, Inc., 1976. 242 pp.
121. Butzengeiger, K. H. Über die chronische Arsenvergiftung. I. EKg-Veränderung und andere Erscheinungen am Herzen und Gefässsystem. II. Schleim hautsymptome und Pathogenese. Dtsch. Arch. Klin. Med. 194:1–16, 1949.
122. Butzengeiger, K. H. Über periphere Zinkulationsstörungen bei chronischer Arsenvergiftung. Klin. Wochenschr. 19:523–527, 1940.
123. Byron, W. R., G. W. Bierbower, J. B. Brouwer, and W. H. Hansen. Pathologic changes in rats and dogs from two-year feeding of sodium arsenite and sodium arsenate. Toxicol. Appl. Pharmacol. 10:132–147, 1967.
124. Calabrese, A., R. S. Collier, D. A. Nelson, and J. R. MacInnes. The toxicity of heavy metals to embryos of the American oyster *Crassostrea virginica*. Mar. Biol. 18:162–166, 1973.
125. Calesnick, B., A. Wase, and L. R. Overby. Availability during human consumption of the arsenic in tissue of chicks fed arsanilic-^{74}As acid. Toxicol. Appl. Pharmacol. 9:27–30, 1966.
126. Calvert, C. C. Feed additive residues in animal manure processed as feed. Feedstuffs 45(17):32–33, 1973.
127. Calvery, H. O., E. P. Laug, and H. J. Morris. The chronic effects on dogs of feeding diets containing lead acetate, lead arsenate, and arsenic trioxide in varying concentrations. J. Pharmacol. Exp. Ther. 64:364–387, 1938.
128. Cannon, A. B. Chronic arsenical poisoning. Symptoms and sources. N.Y. State J. Med. 36:219–241, 1936.
129. Cardiff, I. D. Observations with reference to arsenic on apples and other foodstuffs. Washington State Hort. Assoc. Proc. 33:153–168, 1937.
130. Carlson, C. W., E. Guenthner, W. Kohlmeyer, and O. E. Olson. Some effects of selenium, arsenicals, and vitamin B_{12} on chick growth. Poult. Sci. 33:768–774, 1954.
131. Castro, J. A. Effects of alkylating agents on human plasma cholinesterase. The role of sulfhydryl groups in its active center. Biochem. Pharmacol. 17:295–303, 1968.
132. Cawadias, A. P. Napoleon's death. Lancet 1:101, 1962. (letter)

133. Cawse, P. A., and D. H. Peirson. An Analytical Study of Trace Elements in the Atmospheric Environment. United Kingdom Atomic Energy Authority Research Group Report HERE R 7134. Harwell, Berkshire: Atomic Energy Research Establishment, Health Physics and Medical Division, 1972. 34 pp.
134. Cevey, F. L'arsenic au Point de l'Hygiène et sa Recherche par la Methode Biologique de Gosio. Lausanne: A. Borgeaud, 1902. 48 pp.
135. Challenger, F. Biological methylation. Adv. Enzymol. 12:429–491, 1951.
136. Challenger, F. Biological methylation. Chem. Rev. 36:315–361, 1945.
137. Challenger, F., and L. Ellis. The formation of organo-metalloidal compounds by micro-organisms. Part III. Methylated alkyl- and dialkyl-arsines. J. Chem. Soc. 1935:396–400.
138. Challenger, F., and C. Higginbottom. The production of trimethylarsine by *Penicillium brevicaule* (*Scopulariopsis brevicaulis*). Biochem. J. 29:1757–1778, 1935.
139. Challenger, F., C. Higginbottom, and L. Ellis. The formation of organo-metalloidal compounds by micro-organisms. Part I. Trimethylarsine and dimethylethylarsine. J. Chem. Soc. (London) 1933:95–101.
140. Challenger, F., and A. A. Rawlings. The formation of organo-metalloidal compounds by micro-organisms. Part IV. Dimethyl-n-propylarsine and methylethyl-n-propylarsine. J. Chem. Soc. 1936:264-267, 1936.
141. Chamberlain, W., and J. Shapiro. On the biological significance of phosphate analysis: Comparison of standard and new methods with a bioassay. Limn. Oceanogr. 14:921–927, 1969.
142. Chan, T.-L., B. R. Thomas, and C. L. Wadkins. Formation and isolation of an arsenylated component of rat liver mitochondria. J. Biol. Chem. 244:2883–2890, 1969.
143. Chapman, A. C. On the presence of compounds of arsenic in marine crustaceans and shell fish. Analyst 51:548–563, 1926.
144. Chappellier, A., and M. Raucourt. Les traitements insecticides arsenicaux. Sont-ils dangereux pour le gibier et pour les animaux de la ferme? Ann. Ephiphyt. Phytogenet. II(2):191–239, 1936.
145. Chattopadhyay, A., L. G. I. Bennett, and R. E. Jervis. Activation analysis of environmental pollutants. Can. J. Chem. Eng. 50:189–193, 1972.
146. Chisholm, D. Lead, arsenic, and copper content of crops grown on lead arsenate-treated and untreated soils. Can. J. Plant Sci. 52:583–588, 1972.
147. Chisholm, D., and A. W. MacPhee. Persistence and effects of some pesticides in soil. J. Econ. Entomol. 65:1010–1013, 1972.
148. Chisolm, J. J. Poisoning due to heavy metals. Pediatr. Clin. North Amer. 17:591–615, 1970.
149. Chorley, J. K., and R. McChlery. Experiments on the toxicity to fowls of arsenate of soda and poisoned locusts. Rhodesia Agric. J. 32:322–326, 1935.
150. Chu, R. C., G. P. Barrow, and P. A. W. Baumgarner. Arsenic determination at sub-microgram levels by arsine evolution and flameless atomic absorption spectrophotometric technique. Anal. Chem. 44:1476–1479, 1972.
151. Chukhlantsev, V. G. Solubility products of a series of arsenates. Zh. Anal. Khim. 11:529–535, 1956. (in Russian)
152. Chukhlantsev, V. G. Solubility products of a series of arsenates. Zh. Neorg. Khim. 1:1975–1982, 1956. (in Russian)
153. Clarke, E. G. C., and M. L. Clarke. Arsenic, pp. 44–54. In Garner's Veterinary Toxicology. (3rd ed.) Baltimore: Williams & Wilkins Company, 1967.
154. Clemens, H. P., and K. E. Sneed. Lethal Doses of Several Commercial Chemicals for Fingerling Channel Catfish. U.S. Fish and Wildlife Service Special Scientific

Report—Fisheries No. 316. Washington, D.C.: U.S. Department of the Interior, 1959. 10 pp.
155. Clemente, G. F., G. G. Mastinu, and G. P. Santaroni. Trace element concentrations in some Italian underground waters, determined by neutron activation analysis, pp. 213–227. In Comparative Studies of Food and Environmental Contamination. IAEA Proceedings Series, Otaniemi, Finland, Aug. 27-31, 1973. Vienna: International Atomic Energy Agency, 1974.
156. Clements, H. F., and J. Munson. Arsenic toxicity studies in soil and in culture solution. Pacific Sci. 1:151–171, 1947.
157. Clendenning, W. E., J. B. Block, and I. C. Radde. Basal cell nevus syndrome. Arch. Derm. 90:38–53, 1964.
158. Colagrande, O. Microdetermination of arsenic content of wines. Riv. Viticolt. Enol. (Conegliano) 13:379–385, 1960. (in Italian)
159. Colbourn, P., B. J. Alloway, and I. Thornton. Arsenic and heavy metals in soils associated with regional geochemical anomalies in south-west England. Sci. Total Environ. 4:359–363, 1975.
160. Collins, W. D. Arsenic in sulfured food products. J. Ind. Eng. Chem. 10:360–364, 1918.
161. Commissioner of Public Health, Queensland, Australia. Annual Report for the year ending June 30, 1929. U.S. Public Health Engineering Abstracts 10(PHA):3, Mar. 8, 1930. (abstract)
162. Cook, D. Chemi-peeling and wildlife. New York State Conservationist 7(6):8, 1953.
163. Cooper, H. P., W. R. Paden, E. E. Hall, W. B. Albert, W. B. Rogers, and J. A. Riley. Effect of calcium arsenate on the productivity of certain soil types. South Carolina Agric. Exp. Sta. Ann. Rep. 44:28–36, 1931.
164. Cooper, H. P., W. R. Paden, E. E. Hall, W. B. Albert, W. B. Rogers, and J. A. Riley. Soils differ markedly in their response to additions of calcium arsenate. South Carolina Agric. Exp. Sta. Ann. Rep. 45:23–27, 1932.
165. Cope, O. B. Contamination of the freshwater ecosystem by pesticides. J. Appl. Ecol. 3(Suppl):33–44, 1966.
166. Corneliussen, P. E. Pesticide residues in total diet samples. V. Pest. Monit. J. 4:89–105, 1970.
167. Costa, M. R. M., and M. I. C. Da Fonseca. The amount of natural arsenic in shellfish. Rev. Port. Farm. 17:1–19, 1967. (in Portuguese, summary in English)
168. Costa, M. R. M., M. I. C. Da Fonseca, and N. M. Do Paço. Arsenic content of meat and viscera in chickens. Rev. Port. Farm. 20:1–7, 1970. (in Portuguese)
169. Cotton, F. A., and G. Wilkinson. Arsenic, p. 401. In Advanced Inorganic Chemistry. (3rd ed.) New York: Interscience Publishers, 1972.
170. Cotton, F. A., and G. Wilkinson. Oxo acids and anions of phosphorus, pp. 394–400. In Advanced Inorganic Chemistry. (3rd ed.) New York: Interscience Publishers, 1972.
171. Coulson, E. J., R. E. Remington, and K. M. Lynch. Metabolism in the rat of the naturally occurring arsenic of shrimp as compared with arsenic trioxide. J. Nutr. 10:255–270, 1935.
172. Coulson, E. J., R. E. Remington, and K. M. Lynch. Toxicity of naturally occurring arsenic in foods. Science 80:230–231, 1934.
172a. Coutant, R. W., J. S. McNulty, and R. D. Giammar. Final Report on Determination of Trace Elements in a Combustion System. Columbus, Ohio: Battelle Columbus Laboratories, 1975. 32 pp.
173. Cowell, B. C. The effects of sodium arsenite and silvex on the plankton populations in farm ponds. Trans. Amer. Fish. Soc. 94:371–377, 1965.

174. Cox, D. P., and M. Alexander. Effect of phosphate and other anions on trimethylarsine formation by *Candida humicola*. Appl. Microbiol. 25:408–413, 1973.
175. Cox, D. P., and M. Alexander. Production of trimethylarsine gas from various arsenic compounds by three sewage fungi. Bull. Environ. Contam. Toxicol. 9:84–88, 1973.
176. Cox, H. E. On certain new methods for the determination of small quantities of arsenic and its occurrence in urine and in fish. Analyst 50:3–13, 1925.
177. Cox, H. E. Tests available for the identification of small quantities of the war gases. Analyst 64:807–813, 1939.
178. Crafts, A. S., H. D. Bruce, and R. N. Raynor. Plot Tests with Chemical Soil Sterilants in California. California Agriculture Experiment Station Bulletin 648. Berkeley: University of California, 1941. 25 pp.
179. Crafts, A. S., and P. B. Kennedy. The physiology of *Convolvulus arvensis* (morning-glory or bindweed) in relation to its control by chemical sprays. Plant Physiol. 5:329–344, 1930.
180. Crafts, A. S., and H. G. Reiber. Studies of the activation of herbicides. Hilgardia 16:487–500, 1945.
181. Crafts, A. S., and R. S. Rosenfels. Toxicity studies with arsenic in eighty California soils. Hilgardia 12:177–200, 1939.
182. Crane, R. K., and F. Lipmann. The effect of arsenate on aerobic phosphorylation. J. Biol. Chem. 201:235–243, 1953.
183. Crawford, T. B. B., and G. A. Levvy. Changes undergone by phenylarsenious acid and phenylarsonic acid in the animal body. Biochem. J. 41:333–336, 1947.
184. Crawford, T. B. B., and I. D. E. Storey. Quantitative micro-method for the separation of inorganic arsenite from arsenate in blood and urine. Biochem. J. 38:195–198, 1944.
185. Crecelius, E. A. Chemical Changes in Arsenic Following Ingestion by Man. Paper Presented at the Fifteenth Annual Hanford Life Sciences Symposium, Richland, Washington, Sept. 29–Oct. 1, 1975. ERDA CONF-750929.
186. Crecelius, E. A., M. H. Bothner, and R. Carpenter. Geochemistries of arsenic, antimony, mercury, and related elements in sediments of Puget Sound. Environ. Sci. Technol. 9:325–333, 1975.
187. Crecelius, E. A., and R. Carpenter. Arsenic distribution in waters and sediments of the Puget Sound region, pp. 615–625. In Proceedings of First Annual NSF Trace Contaminants Conference, Oak Ridge National Laboratory, August 8–10, 1973. Oak Ridge, Tenn.: U.S. Atomic Energy Commission, 1974.
188. Crecelius, E. A., C. J. Johnson, and G. C. Hofer. Contamination of soils near a copper smelter by arsenic, antimony, and lead. Water Air Soil Pollut. 3:337–342, 1974.
189. Crosby, D. G., and R. K. Tucker. Toxicity of aquatic herbicides to *Daphnia magna*. Science 154:289–291, 1966.
190. Cuffe, S. T., and R. W. Gerstle. Emissions from Coal-Fired Power Plants: A Comprehensive Summary. PHS Publ. No. 999-AP-35. Cincinnati: U.S. Department of Health, Education, and Welfare, Public Health Service, National Center for Air Pollution Control, 1967. 30 pp.
191. Currie, A. N. The role of arsenic in carcinogenesis. Brit. Med. Bull. 4:402–405, 1947.
192. Czajka, J., and A. Pietrzykowa. Classification of fruit products in regard to

References

quantitative content of arsenic, lead, and copper. Ann. Univ. Mariae-Skłodowska Lublin-Polonia Sect. D. 10:345–358, 1955. (in Polish, summary in English)

193. Da Costa, E. W. B. Variation in the toxicity of arsenic compounds to microorganisms and the suppression of the inhibitory effects by phosphate. Appl. Microbiol. 23:46–53, 1972.
194. Damsgaard, E., K. Heydorn, N. H. Larsen, and B. Nielsen. Simultaneous Determination of Arsenic, Manganese, and Selenium in Human Serum by Neutron Activation Analysis. Risø Report No. 271. Roskilde: Danish Atomic Energy Commission, 1973. 35 pp.
195. Daris, B. T., C. Papadopoulou, J. Kleperis, and A. P. Grimanis. Herbicide influence on the arsenic uptake of grapes. A study by neutron activation analysis. Proc. Brit. Weed Control Conf. 10(1):429–433, 1971.
196. Davis, W. E., & Associates. National Inventory of Sources of Emissions. Arsenic, Beryllium, Manganese, Mercury and Vanadium. 1968. Arsenic: Section I. Leawood, Kansas: W. E. Davis & Associates, 1971. 51 pp.
197. de Groot, A. J., K. H. Zschuppe, M. de Bruin, J. Houtman, and P. A. Singgih. Activation analysis applied to sediments from various river deltas. National Bureau of Standards (U.S.) Special Publication No. 312:62–71, 1969.
198. Dehn, W. M. Primary arsines. Amer. Chem. J. 33:101–153, 1905.
199. Dehn, W. M. Reactions of the arsines. Amer. Chem. J. 40:88–127, 1908.
200. Dehn, W. M., and B. B. Wilcox. Secondary arsines. Amer. Chem. J. 35:1–54, 1906.
201. Delavault, R. E., and R. J. Manson. Spectroscopic determination of arsenic in geochemical samples, pp. 552–553. In Geochemical Exploration. Proceedings of 3rd International Symposium on Geochemical Exploration, 1971.
202. Del Vecchio, V., P. Valori, A. M. Alasia, and G. Gualdi. La determinazione dell'arsencio nei molluschi (*Mytilus* Linn). Ig. Sanità Pubblica 18:18–30, 1962.
203. Dick, J., and L. I. Pugsley. The arsenic, lead, tin, copper, and iron content of canned clams, oysters, crabs, lobsters, and shrimps. Can. J. Res. Sect. F. Tech. 28:199–201, 1950.
204. Dickens, R., and A. E. Hiltbold. Movement and persistence of methanearsonates in soil. Weeds 15:299–304, 1967.
205. Dickinson, J. O. Toxicity of the arsenical herbicide monosodium acid methanearsonate in cattle. Amer. J. Vet. Res. 33:1889–1892, 1972.
206. Dietrich, L. E. Treatment of canine lungworm infection with thiacetarsamide. J. Amer. Vet. Med. Assoc. 140:572–573, 1962.
207. Dixon, M., and E. C. Webb. Enzymes. New York: Academic Press, Inc., 1958. 782 pp.
208. Dobson, R. L., M. R. Young, and J. S. Pinto. Palmar keratoses and cancer. Arch. Derm. 92:553–556, 1965.
209. Domonkos, A. N. Neutron activation analysis of arsenic in normal skin, keratoses, and epitheliomas. A.M.A. Arch. Derm. 80:672–677, 1959.
210. Done, A. K., and A. J. Peart. Acute toxicities of arsenical herbicides. Clin. Toxicol. 4:343–355, 1971.
211. Doudoroff, M., H. A. Barker, and W. Z. Hassid. Studies with bacterial sucrose phosphorylase. III. Arsenolytic decomposition of sucrose and of glucose-1-phosphate. J. Biol. Chem. 170:147–150, 1947.
212. Down, J. L., and T. T. Gorsuch. The recovery of trace elements after the oxidation of organic material with 50 per cent hydrogen peroxide. Analyst 92:298–402, 1967.

213. Drobiz, F. D. Concentration of arsenic in the blood and the dynamics of its elimination for the organism in syphilis therapy by osarsol. Vestnik Dermatol. Venerol. 1:15–19, 1947. (in Russian)
214. Drudge, J. H. Arsenamide in the treatment of canine filariasis. Amer. J. Vet. Res. 13:220–235, 1952.
215. Duble, R. L., and E. C. Holt. Effect of AMA on synthesis and utilization of food reserves in purple nutsedge. Weed Sci. 18:174–179, 1970.
216. Duble, R. L., E. C. Holt, and G. C. McBee. The translocation of two organic arsenicals in purple nutsedge. Weed Sci. 16:421–424, 1968.
217. Duble, R. L., E. C. Holt, and G. C. McBee. Translocation and breakdown of disodium methanearsonate (DSMA) in coastal bermudagrass. J. Agric. Food Chem. 17:1247–1250, 1969.
218. Dubois, K. P., A. L. Moxon, and O. E. Olson. Further studies on the effectiveness of arsenic in preventing selenium poisoning. J. Nutr. 19:477–482, 1940.
219. Dubois, L., T. Teichman, and J. L. Monkman. The "normal" value of arsenic in human hair. Proc. Can. Soc. Forensic Sci. 4:217–231, 1965.
220. Ducoff, H. S., W. B. Neal, R. L. Straube, L. O. Jacobson, and A. M. Brues. Biological studies with arsenic. II. Excretion and tissue localization. Proc. Soc. Exp. Biol. Med. 69:548–554, 1948.
221. Duke, B. O. L. The effects of drugs on *Onchocerca volvulus*. 4. Trials of melarsonyl potassium. Bull. WHO 42:115–127, 1970.
222. Dunlap, L. G. Perforations of the nasal septum due to inhalation of arsenous oxide. J.A.M.A. 76:568–569, 1921.
223. Dupree, H. K. The arsenic content of water, plankton, soil and fish from ponds treated with sodium arsenite for weed control, pp. 132–137. In Proceedings of the Fourteenth Annual Conference, Southeastern Association of Game and Fish Commissioners, October 23–26, 1960. Biloxi, Mississippi. Columbia, S.C.: Southeastern Association of Game and Fish Commissioners, 1960.
224. Durum, W. H., J. D. Hem, S. G. Heidel. Reconnaissance of Selected Minor Elements in Surface Waters of the United States, October 1970. Geological Survey Circular 643. Washington, D.C.: U.S. Department of the Interior, 1971. 49 pp.
225. Dyke, K. G. H., M. T. Parker, and M. H. Richmond. Penicillinase production and metal-ion resistance in *Staphylococcus aureus* cultures isolated from hospital patients. J. Med. Microbiol. 3:125–136, 1970.
226. Eagland, J. S. Bee mortality in the orchard. The effect of arsenical sprays. J. Dept. Agric. Victoria 34:299–301, 1936.
227. Eagle, H., and G. O. Doak. The biological activity of arsenosobenzenes in relation to their structure. Pharmacol. Rev. 3:107–143, 1951.
228. Eckert, J. E., and H. W. Allinger. Relation of airplane dusting to beekeeping. J. Econ. Entomol. 29:885–895, 1936.
229. Ehman, P. J. Residues in cottonseed from weed control with methanearsonates. Proc. South. Weed Conf. 19:540–541, 1966.
230. Eipper, A. W. Effects of five herbicides on farm pond plants and fish. N.Y. Fish Game J. 6:46–56, 1959.
231. Ellis, M. M. Arsenic storage in game fish. Copeia 1934(2):97.
232. Ellis, M. M. Detection and measurement of stream pollution. Bull. Bur. Fish. 48:365–437, 1940.
233. Ellis, M. M., B. A. Westfall, and M. D. Ellis. Arsenic in fresh-water fish. Ind. Eng. Chem. 33:1331–1332, 1941.
234. Englund, B. Die Reaktion zwischen mehrwertigen Alkoholen oder Phenolen und

References

Arsenverbindungen, speziell Arsonessigsäure II. J. Prakt. Chem. 124:191–208, 1930.
235. Epidemic of arsenical poisoning in beer-drinkers in the north of England during the year 1900. Lancet 1:98–100, 1901.
236. Epps, E. A., and M. B. Sturgis. Arsenic compounds toxic to rice. Soil Sci. Soc. Amer. Proc. 4:215–218, 1939.
237. Evans, R. J., and S. Bandemer. Determination of arsenic in biologic materials. Anal. Chem. 26:595–598, 1954.
238. Evans, R. J., S. L. Bandemer, D. A. Libby, and A. C. Groschke. The arsenic content of eggs from hens fed arsanilic acid. Poult. Sci. 32:743–744, 1953.
239. Everett, C. F. Effect of Phosphorus on the Phytotoxicity of Tricalcium Arsenate as Manifested by Bluegrass and Crabgrass. Ph.D. Thesis. New Brunswick, N.J.: Rutgers University, 1962. 104 pp.
240. Fabre, J. H., and E. Bremond. L'arsenic dans les mouts de raisins et les vins. Ann. Falsifications Fraudes 31:149–157, 1938.
241. Fairhall, L. T. Toxic contaminants in drinking water. New Engl. Water Works Assoc. J. 55:400–410, 1941.
242. Fan, C.-I., and W.-F. Yang. Arsenic removal from well water by rapid filtration. K'uo Li Taiwan Ta Hsueh Kung Cheng Hsueh Kan 13:95–112, 1969. (in Chinese)
243. Fassel, V. A., and R. N. Kniseley. Inductively coupled plasma—optical emission spectroscopy. Anal. Chem. 46:1110A–1120A, 1974.
244. Feinglass, E. J. Arsenic intoxication from well water in the United States. New Engl. J. Med. 288:828–830, 1973.
245. Feldman, C. Determination of arsenic in ecological microcosms, pp. 6–7. In Analytical Chemistry Division Annual Progress Report, period ending Nov. 30, 1975. ORNL 5100. Oak Ridge, Tenn.: Oak Ridge National Laboratory, 1975.
246. Feldman, C. Perchloric acid procedure for wet-ashing organics for the determination of mercury (and other metals). Anal. Chem. 46:1606–1609, 1974.
247. Feldman, C., J. A. Carter, and L. C. Bate. Measuring mercury. Environment 14(6):48, 1972. (letter)
248. Ferenčik, M., B. Havelka, and M. Halåsa. Effect of arsenic wastes on agricultural products. Cesk. Hyg. 12:73–81, 1967. (in Czech, summary in English)
249. Ferguson, J. F., and J. Gavis. A review of the arsenic cycle in natural waters. Water Res. 6:1259–1274, 1972.
250. Ferm, V. H., and S. J. Carpenter. Malformation induced by sodium arsenate. J. Reprod. Fertil. 17:199–201, 1968.
251. Ferm, V. H., A. Sakon, and B. M. Smith. The teratogenic profile of sodium arsenate in the golden hamster. Arch. Environ. Health 22:557–560, 1971.
252. Fernandez, F. J., and D. C. Manning. The determination of arsenic at submicrogram levels by atomic absorption spectrophotometry. Atom. Absorpt. Newslett. 10:86–88, 1971.
253. Fierz, U. Katamnestische Untersuchungen über die Nebenwirkungen der Therapie mit anorganischem Arsen bei Hautkrankheiten. Dermatologica 131:41–58, 1965.
254. Fitch, L. W. N., R. E. R. Grimmett, and E. M. Wall. Occurrence of arsenic in the soils and waters of the Waiotapu Valley and its relation to stock health. II. Feeding experiments at Wallaceville. N. Z. J. Sci. Tech. Sect. A 21:146A–149A, 1939.
255. Flaubert, G. Madame Bovary. (Translated by F. Steegmuller) New York: The Modern Library, 1957. 396 pp.
256. Flis, I. E., K. P. Mishchenko, and T. A. Tumanova. Dissociation of arsenic acid. Russ. J. Inorg. Chem. 4:120–124, 1959.

257. Fluharty, A. L., and D. R. Sanadi. On the mechanism of oxidative phosphorylation. II. Effect of arsenite alone and in combination with 2,3-dimercaptopropanol. J. Biol. Chem. 236:2772–2778, 1961.
258. Fontenot, J. P., K. E. Webb, Jr., B. W. Harmon, R. E. Tucker, and W. E. C. Moore, Studies of processing, nutritional value and palatability of broiler litter for ruminants, pp. 301–304. In Livestock Waste Management and Pollution Abatement. Proceedings of an International Symposium on Livestock Wastes, Columbus, Ohio, 1971. St. Joseph, Mich.: American Society of Agricultural Engineers, 1971.
259. Forshufvud, S., H. Smith, and A. Wassén. Arsenic content of Napoleon I's hair probably taken immediately after his death. Nature 192:103–105, 1961.
260. Forshufvud, S., H. Smith, and A. Wassén. Napoleon's illness 1816–1821 in the light of activation analyses of hairs from various dates. Arch. Toxikol. 20:210–219, 1964.
261. Forstner, G. E. The occurrence of metallic contaminants in foods. Chem. Ind. (London) 1948:499–501.
262. Frank, F. J., and N. A. Johnson. Selected Ground-Water Data in the Eugene–Springfield Area, Southern Willamette Valley, Oregon. Oregon State Engineer Ground Water Report No. 14, 1970. 70 pp.
263. Franke, K. W., and A. L. Moxon. A comparison of the minimum fatal doses of selenium, tellurium, arsenic, and vanadium. J. Pharmacol. Exp. Ther. 58:454–459, 1936.
264. Franke, K. W., A. L. Moxon, W. E. Poley, and W. C. Tully. Monstrosities produced by the injection of selenium salts into hens' eggs. Anat. Rec. 65:15–22, 1936.
265. Frans, R. Organic arsenical herbicides. Weeds Today 3(2):6,13, 1972.
266. Franseen, C. C., and G. W. Taylor. Arsenical keratoses and carcinomas. Amer. J. Cancer 22:287–307, 1934.
267. Fraumeni, J. F., Jr. Respiratory carcinogenesis: An epidemiologic appraisal. J. Nat. Cancer Inst. 55:1039–1046, 1975.
268. Frost, D. V. Arsenicals in biology—retrospect and prospect. Fed. Proc. 26:194–208, 1967.
269. Frost, D. V. Consideration on the safety of arsanilic acid for use in poultry feeds. Poult. Sci. 32:217–227, 1953.
270. Frost, D. V. NACA Industry Task Force for Agricultural Arsenical Pesticides. Washington, D.C.: National Agricultural Chemicals Association, 1971. 37 pp.
271. Frost, D. V. Recent advances in trace elements: Emphasis on interrelationships, pp. 31–40. In Proceedings of the Cornell Nutrition Conference for Feed Manufactures, 1967.
272. Frost, D. V., L. R. Overby, and H. C. Spruth. Studies with arsanilic acid and related compounds. J. Agric. Food Chem. 3:235–243, 1955.
273. Frost, D. V., H. S. Perdue, B. T. Main, J. A. Kolar, I. D. Smith, R. J. Stein, and L. R. Overby. Further considerations on the safety of arsanilic acid for feed use, pp. 234–237. In Proceedings, 12th World's Poultry Congress, Sydney, Australia, 1962. Section Papers.
274. Frost, D. V., and H. C. Spruth. Arsenicals in feeds, pp. 136–149. In H. Welch and F. Marti-Ibanez, Eds. Proceedings of the Symposium on Medicated Feeds, 1956. New York: Medical Encyclopedia, Inc., 1956.
275. Frozen breaded shrimp. Consumer Rep. 37(1):27–32, 1972.
276. Gagliardi, E., and H. P. Wöss. Metallextraktion mit aliphatischen Ketonen. Anal. Chim. Acta 48:107–114, 1969.

References

277. Gainer, J. H. Effects of arsenicals on interferon formation and action. Amer. J. Vet. Res. 33:2579–2586, 1972.
278. Gainer, J. H., and T. W. Pry. Effects of arsenicals on viral infections in mice. Amer. J. Vet. Res. 33:2299–2307, 1972.
279. Ganther, H. E., and C. A. Baumann. Selenium metabolism. I. Effects of diet, arsenic, and cadmium. J. Nutr. 77:210–216, 1962.
280. Ganther, H. E., and C. A. Baumann. Selenium metabolism. II. Modifying effects of sulfate. J. Nutr. 77:408–414, 1962.
281. Garratt, D. C., and W. W. Taylor. Arsenic in dried parsley. Analyst 70:48–49, 1945.
282. Gastiner, E. Zur spektralphotometrischen Arsenbestimmung mit Silberdiäthyldithiocarbamidat. Mikrochim. Acta 1972:526–543.
283. Gates, M., J. W. Williams, and J. A. Zapp. Arsenicals, pp. 83–114. In Chemical Warfare Agents, and Related Chemical Problems. Parts I–II. Summary Technical Report of Division 9, NDRC. Vol. 1. Washington, D.C.: Office of Scientific Research and Development, National Defense Research Committee, 1946.
284. Geisman, J. R., W. E. Carey, W. A. Gould, and E. K. Alban. Distribution of arsenic residues by activation analysis. J. Food Sci. 34:295–298, 1969.
285. Gentilini, L. L'arsenico e il piombo nei vini. Annuar. Staz. Sper. Viticolt. Enol. (Conegliano) 12:251–267, 1944–45.
286. George, G. M., L. J. Frahm, and J. P. McDonnell. Recovery of arsenic by dry ashing from animal tissue fortified with organoarsenicals or arsenic trioxide. J. Assoc. Off. Anal. Chem. 56:1304–1305, 1973.
287. Gerin, C., and C. de Zorzi. The arsenic content in the organs of the human body. Zacchia 36(Vol. 24, Ser. 2):1–19, 1961.
288. Geyer, L. Über die chronischen Hautveränderungen beim Arsenicismus und Betrachtungen über die Massenerkrankungen in Reichenstein in Schlesien. Arch. Derm. Syphilol. 43:221–280, 1898.
289. Gilderhus, P. Sodium arsenite and bluegills at LaCrosse, Wis., pp. 31–32. In Pesticide-Wildlife Studies, 1963. A Review of Fish and Wildlife Service Investigations during the Calendar Year. Fish and Wildlife Service Circular 199. Washington, D.C.: U.S. Department of the Interior, 1964. 130 pp.
290. Gilderhus, P. A. Some effects of sublethal concentrations of sodium arsenite on bluegills and the aquatic environment. Trans. Amer. Fish. Soc. 95:289–296, 1966.
291. Ginsburg, J. M. Renal mechanism for excretion and transformation of arsenic in the dog. Amer. J. Physiol. 208:832–840, 1965.
292. Ginsburg, J. M., and W. D. Lotspeich. Interrelations of arsenate and phosphate transport in the dog kidney. Amer. J. Physiol. 205:707–714, 1963.
293. Glazener, F. S., J. G. Ellis, and P. K. Johnson. Electrocardiographic findings with arsenic poisoning. Calif. Med. 109:158–162, 1968.
294. Goldblatt, E. L., A. S. van Denburgh, and R. A. Marsland. The Unusual and Widespread Occurrence of Arsenic in Well Waters of Lane County, Oregon. Oregon Department of Health, 1963. 24 pp.
295. Goldschmidt, V. M. Arsenic, pp. 468–475. In A. Muir, Ed. Geochemistry. Oxford: Clarendon Press, 1954.
296. Goldsmith, J. R., M. Deane, J. Thom, and G. Gentry. Evaluation of health implications of elevated arsenic in well water. Water Res. 6:1133–1136, 1972.
297. Gomes, L. G. Port wine and the presence of arsenic. Rev. Port. Farm. 13:159–162, 1963. (in Portuguese, summary in English)
298. Goodman, L. S., and A. Gilman, Eds. Inorganic arsenic, pp. 950–956. In The

Pharmacological Basis of Therapeutics. (2nd ed.) New York: The Macmillan Co., 1958.
299. Gorgy, S., N. W. Rakestraw, and D. L. Fox. Arsenic in the sea. J. Marine Res. 7:22–32, 1948.
300. Gosio, B. Action de quelques moisissures sur les composes fixes d'arsenic. Arch. Ital. Biol. 18:253–265, 1893.
301. Goulden, F., E. L. Kennaway, and M. E. Urquhart. Arsenic in the suspended matter of town air. Brit. J. Cancer 6:1–7, 1952.
302. Goulden, P. D., and P. Brooksbank. Automated atomic absorption determination of arsenic, antimony, and selenium in natural waters. Anal. Chem. 46:1431–1436, 1974.
303. Graham, J. H., and E. B. Helwig. Bowen's disease and its relationship to systemic cancer. A.M.A. Arch. Derm. 80:133–159, 1959.
304. Graham, J. H., G. R. Mazzanti, and E. B. Helwig. Chemistry of Bowen's disease: Relationship to arsenic. J. Invest. Derm. 37:317–332, 1961.
305. Grantham, R. G., and C. B. Sherwood. Chemical Quality of Waters of Broward County, Florida. Florida Geological Survey, Report of Investigations No. 51. Tallahassee: State of Florida, Board of Conservation, 1968. 52 pp.
306. Gray, G. P. Tests of chemical means for the control of weeds. Report of progress. Univ. Calif. Publ. Agric. Sci. 4:67–97, 1919.
307. Greaves, J. E. The arsenic content of soils. Soil Sci. 38:355–362, 1934.
308. Greaves, J. E. The occurrence of arsenic in soils. Biochem. Bull. 2:519–523, 1913.
309. Green, S. J., and T. S. Price. The chlorovinylchloroarsines. J. Chem. Soc. Trans. 119:448–453, 1921.
310. Grigg, F. J. T. Distribution of arsenic in the body after a fatal case of poisoning by hydrogen arsenide. Analyst 54:659–660, 1929.
311. Grimmett, R. E. R. Arsenical soils of the Waiotapu Valley: Evidence of poisoning of stock at Reporoa. N. Z. J. Agric. 58:383–391, 1939.
312. Grimmett, R. E. R., and I. G. McIntosh. Occurrence of arsenic in soils and waters in the Waiotapu Valley, and its relation to stock health. N. Z. J. Sci. Tech. A. Agric. Sect. 21:137A–145A, 1939.
313. Grindley, J. Toxicity to rainbow trout and minnows of some substances known to be present in waste water discharged to rivers. Ann. Appl. Biol. 33:103–112, 1946.
314. Gualtieri, J. L. Arsenic, pp. 51–61. In D. A. Brobst and W. P. Pratt, Eds. United States Mineral Resources. Geological Survey Professional Paper No. 820. Washington, D.C.: U.S. Government Printing Office, 1973.
315. Guatelli, M. A., and N. A. Gallego Gandara de Germicola. El contenido de arsenico en el aqua de consumo de la localidad de Monte Quemado (Pcia. de Santiago del Estero, Rep. Arg.) Rev. Farm. (Buenos Aires) 112:69–73, 1970.
316. Gulbrandsen, R. A. Chemical composition of phosphorites of the Phosphoria formation. Geochim. Cosmochim. Acta 30:769–778, 1966.
317. Guthmann, H., and K. H. Henrich. Der Arsengehalt der Uterusschleimhaut und des Blutes. Arch. Gynaekol. 172:380–391, 1941.
318. Guthrie, F. E., C. B. McCants, and H. G. Small, Jr. Arsenic content of commercial tobacco, 1917–1958. Tobacco Sci. 3:62–64, 1959.
319. Hamaguchi, H., N. Ohta, N. Onuma, and K. Kawasaki. Studies on inorganic constituents in biological material. XIV. Contents of thallium, selenium, and arsenic in fish and shells from the Minamata district, Kyushu. J. Chem. Soc. Jap. (Nippon Kagaku Zasshi) 81:920–927, 1960. (in Japanese, summary in English)
320. Hamilton, E. I., and M. J. Minski. Abundance of the chemical elements in man's

diet and possible relations with environmental factors. Sci. Total Environ. 1:375–394, 1972/1973.
321. Hamilton, K. C. Johnsongrass control with organic arsenicals and dalapon. Res. Prog. Rep. West. Soc. Weed Sci. 1968:16–17.
322. Hamilton, K. C. Repeated, foliar applications of herbicides on Johnsongrass. Weed Sci. 17:245–250, 1969.
323. Hamilton, K. C. Response of Johnsongrass strains to herbicides. Res. Prog. Rep. West. Soc. Weed Sci. 1967:11–12.
324. Hamilton, K. C., and H. F. Arle. Directed applications of herbicides in irrigated cotton. Weed Sci. 18:85–88, 1970.
325. Hamimoto, E. Infant arsenic poisoning by powdered milk. Jap. Med. J. (Nihon iji Shimpo) 1649:3–12, Dec. 1955. (in Japanese)
326. Harding, J. D. J., G. Lewis, and J. T. Done. Experimental arsanilic acid poisoning in pigs. Vet. Rec. 83:560–564, 1968.
327. Harington, J. S. Contents of cystine-cysteine, glutathione, and total free sulphydryl in arsenic-resistant and sensitive strains of the blue tick, *Boophilus decoloratus*. Nature 184:1739–1740, 1959.
328. Harkins, W. D., and R. E. Swain. The determination of arsenic and other solid constituents of smelter smoke, with a study of the effects of high stacks and large condensing flues. J. Amer. Chem. Soc. 29:970–998, 1907.
329. Harrison, J. W. E., E. W. Packman, and D. D. Abbott. Acute oral toxicity and chemical and physical properties of arsenic trioxides. A.M.A. Arch. Ind. Health 17:118–123, 1958.
330. Harter, J. G., and A. M. Novitch. An evaluation of Gay's solution in the treatment of asthma. J. Allergy 40:327–336, 1967.
331. Hartzell, M. B. Epithelioma as a sequel of psoriasis and the probability of its arsenical origin. Amer. J. Med. Sci. 118:265–272, 1899.
332. Harvey, A. B., and M. K. Wilson. Vibrational spectrum of methyl arsine. J. Chem. Phys. 44:3535–3546, 1966.
333. Harvey, S. C. Arsenic, pp. 944–951. In L. S. Goodman and A. Gilman, Eds. The Pharmacological Basis of Therapeutics. (3rd ed.) New York: The Macmillan Company, 1965.
334. Harvey, S. C. Arsenic, pp. 958–965. In L. S. Goodman and A. Gilman, Eds. The Pharmacological Basis of Therapeutics. (4th ed.) New York: The Macmillan Company, 1970.
335. Hatch, R. C., and H. S. Funnell. Inorganic arsenic levels in tissues and ingesta of poisoned cattle: An eight-year study. Can. Vet. J. 10:117–120, 1969.
336. Havelka, U. D., and M. G. Merkle. Arsenic residues in cotton and Johnsongrass. South. Weed Sci. Soc. Proc. 22:51–57, 1969.
337. Hawes, A. J. Napoleon's death. Lancet 1:749, 1962. (letter)
338. Haywood, J. K. Injury to vegetation and animal life by smelter fumes. J. Amer. Chem. Soc. 29:998–1009, 1907.
339. Headden, W. P. The occurrence of arsenic in soils, plants, fruits and animals. Proc. Colorado Sci. Soc. 9:345–360, 1910.
340. Headford, D. W. R. An improved method of control of *Paspalum conjugatum* with amitrol-T and paraquat. Weed Res. 6:304–313, 1966.
341. Heath, R. G., J. W. Spann, E. F. Hill, and J. F. Kreitzer. Comparative Dietary Toxicities of Pesticides to Birds. Fish and Wildlife Service Special Scientific Report—Wildlife No. 152. Washington, D.C.: U.S. Department of the Interior, 1972. 57 pp.

342. Helminen, M. The effect on pheasants of an arsenic-containing plant protectant. Suomen Riista 12:173, 1958. (in Finnish)
343. Hemphill, F. E., M. L. Kaeberle, and W. B. Buck. Lead suppression of mouse resistance to *Salmonella typhimurium*. Science 172:1031–1032, 1971.
344. Hendrick, C., H. L. Klug, and O. E. Olson. Effect of 3-nitro, 4-hydroxyphenylarsonic acid and arsanilic acid on selenium poisoning in the rat. J. Nutr. 51:131–136, 1953.
345. Hendricks, R. L., F. B. Reisbick, E. J. Mahaffey, D. B. Roberts, and M. N. A. Peterson. Chemical composition of sediments and interstitial brine from the Atlantis II, Discovery and Chain Deeps, pp. 407–440. In E. T. Degens and D. A. Ross, Eds. Hot Brines and Recent Heavy Metal Deposits in the Red Sea. A Geochemical and Geophysical Account. New York: Springer-Verlag, Inc., 1969.
346. Hengl, F., P. Reckendorfer, and F. Beran. Use of arsenic and lead in the treatment of diseases of the vine. Wein Rebe 13:459–468, 1932. (in German)
347. Herbicide Handbook of the Weed Society of America. (1st ed.) Geneva, N.Y.: W. F. Humphrey Press, Inc., 1967. 292 pp.
348. Hermann, E. R. A toxicity index for industrial wastes. Ind. Eng. Chem. 51(4):84A–87A, 1959.
349. Herrmann, R., and H. Kretzdorn. Untersuchungen über den Arsengehalt von Weinbergsböden und die Aufnahme von Arsen aus arsenhaltigen Böden durch die Reben. Bodenk. Pflanzenernähr. 13:169–176, 1939.
350. Heydorn, K., and E. Damsgaard. Simultaneous determination of arsenic, manganese and selenium in biological materials by neutron-activation analysis. Talanta 20:1–11, 1973.
351. Heyman, A., J. B. Pheiffer, Jr., R. W. Willett, and H. M. Taylor. Peripheral neuropathy caused by arsenical intoxication. A study of 41 cases with observations on the effects of BAL (2,3,dimercapto-propanol). New Engl. J. Med. 254:401–409, 1956.
352. Hill, A. B., and E. L. Faning. Studies in the incidence of cancer in a factory handling inorganic compounds of arsenic. I. Mortality experience in the factory. Brit. J. Ind. Med. 5:1–6, 1948.
353. Hill, E. F., R. G. Heath, J. W. Spann, and J. D. Williams. Lethal Dietary Toxicities of Environmental Pollutants to Birds. Patuxent Wildlife Research Center, U.S. Fish and Wildlife Service, Special Scientific Report—Wildlife No. 191. Washington, D.C.: U.S. Department of the Interior, 1975. 61 pp.
354. Hiltbold, A. E. Behavior of organoarsenicals in plants and soils, pp. 53–69. In E. A. Woolson, Ed. Arsenical Pesticides. ACS Symposium Series 7. Washington, D.C.: American Chemical Society, 1975.
355. Hiltbold, A. E., B. F. Hajek, and G. A. Buchanan. Distribution of arsenic in soil profiles after repeated applications of MSMA. Weed Sci. 22:272–275, 1974.
356. Hiltner, R. S., and H. J. Wichmann. Zinc in oysters. J. Biol. Chem. 38:205–221, 1919.
357. Hindawi, I. J., and G. E. Neely. Soil and vegetation study, pp. 81–94. In Helena Valley, Montana Area Environmental Pollution Study. Office of Air Programs Publication AP-91. Research Triangle Park, N.C.: U.S. Environmental Protection Agency, 1972.
358. Hogan, R. B., and H. Eagle. The pharmacologic basis for the widely varying toxicity of arsenicals. J. Pharmacol. Exp. Ther. 80:93–113, 1944.
359. Holak, W. Gas-sampling technique for arsenic determination by atomic absorption spectroscopy. Anal. Chem. 41:1712–1713, 1969.

360. Holdgate, M. W., Ed. The Sea Bird Wreck in the Irish Sea—Autumn 1969. London: The Natural Environment Research Council. Publications Series C No. 4, 1971. 38 pp.
361. Holland, A. A., J. E. Lasater, E. D. Neumann, and W. E. Eldridge. Toxic Effects of Organic and Inorganic Pollutants on Young Salmon and Trout. State of Washington, Department of Fisheries Research Bulletin No. 5. 1960. 264 pp.
362. Holland, J. W. Arsenic, pp. 404–415. In F. Peterson and W. S. Haines, Eds. A Text-Book of Legal Medicine and Toxicology. Vol. 2. Philadelphia: W. B. Saunders & Company, 1904.
363. Holmberg, R. E., and V. H. Ferm. Interrelationships of selenium, cadmium, and arsenic in mammalian teratogenesis. Arch. Environ. Health 18:873–877, 1969.
364. Holmes, A. D., and R. Remmington. Arsenic content of American cod liver oil. Ind. Eng. Chem. 26:573–574, 1934.
365. Holmqvist, I. Occupational arsenical dermatitis. A study among employees at a copper ore smelting work including investigations of skin reactions to contact with arsenic compounds. Acta Derm. Venereol. 31(Suppl. 26):1–214, 1951.
366. Holt, E. C., J. L. Faubion, W. W. Allen, and C. G. McBee. Arsenic translocation in nutsedge tuber systems and its effect on tuber viability. Weeds 15:13–15, 1967.
367. Hood, R. D., and S. L. Bishop. Teratogenic effects of sodium arsenate in mice. Arch. Environ. Health 24:62–65, 1972.
368. Hood, R. D., and C. T. Pike. BAL alleviation of arsenate-induced teratogenesis in mice. Teratology 6:235–237, 1972.
369. Hoover, W. L., J. R. Melton, P. A. Howard, and J. W. Bassett, Jr. Atomic absorption spectrometric determination of arsenic. J. Assoc. Off. Anal. Chem. 57:18–21, 1974.
370. Hopewell, J. Napoleon's death. Lancet 1:914, 1962.
371. Hove, E., C. A. Elvehjem, and E. B. Hart. Arsenic in the nutrition of the rat. Amer. J. Physiol. 124:205–212, 1938.
372. Hueper, W. C. Environmental lung cancer. Ind. Med. Surg. 20:49–62, 1951.
373. Hueper, W. C., and W. W. Payne. Experimental studies in metal carcinogenesis. Chromium, nickel, iron, arsenic. Arch. Environ. Health 5:445–462, 1962.
374. Hughes, J. S., and J. T. Davis. Effects of selected herbicides on bluegill sunfish, pp. 480–482. In Proceedings of the Eighteenth Annual Conference, Southeastern Association of Game and Fish Commissioners. October 18, 19, 20 and 21, 1964. Clearwater, Florida. Columbia, S.C.: Southeastern Association of Game and Fish Commissioners, 1967.
375. Hundley, H. K., and J. C. Underwood. Determination of total arsenic in total diet samples. J. Assoc. Offic. Anal. Chem. 53:1176–1178, 1970.
376. Hunter, F. T., A. F. Kip, and J. W. Irvine, Jr. Radioactive tracer studies on arsenic injected as potassium arsenite. J. Pharmacol. Exp. Ther. 76:207–220, 1942.
377. Hutchinson, J. On some examples of arsenic-keratoses of the skin and of arseniccancer. Trans. Path. Soc. (London) 39:352–363, 1888.
378. Hwang, S. W., and L. S. Schanker. Absorption of organic arsenical compounds from the rat small intestine. Xenobiotica 3:351–355, 1973.
379. International Agency for Research on Cancer. IARC Monographs on the Evaluation of the Carcinogenic Risk of Chemicals to Man. Vol. 2. Some Inorganic and Organometallic Compounds. Lyon: World Health Organization, IARC, 1973. 181 pp.
380. Ioanid, N., G. Bors, and I. Popa. Beiträge zur Kenntnis des normalen Arsengehaltes von Nägeln und des Gehaltes in den Fällen von Arsenpolyneuritis. Dtsch. Z. Gesamte Gerichtl. Med. 52:90–94, 1961.

381. Ireland, F. A. Reactions following the administration of the arsphenamines and methods of prevention. Amer. J. Syphilol. 16:22–38, 1932.
382. Irvine, H. G., and D. D. Turnacliff. Study of a group of handlers of arsenic tri-oxide. Arch. Derm. Syphilol. 33:306–312, 1936.
383. Isensee, A. R., P. C. Kearney, E. A. Woolson, G. E. Jones, and V. P. Williams. Distribution of alkyl arsenicals in model ecosystem. Environ. Sci. Technol. 7:841–845, 1973.
384. Ito, S., and Y. Izumi. On the quantity of adhered arsenic on summer orange (*Citrus natsudaidai*) fruits sprayed with lead arsenate. J. Food Sci. Technol. (Nippon Shokuhin Kogyo Gakkai Shi) 13:486–488, 1966. (in Japanese)
385. Ivancévić, I., and D. Tomić. Über Speicherung von Eisen und Arsen aus Mineralwässern im Tierkörper. Arch. Physik. Ther. 8:349–357, 1956.
386. Jackson, R. F. Two-day treatment with thiacetarsamide for canine heartworm disease. J. Amer. Vet. Med. Assoc. 142:23–26, 1963.
387. Jacobs, L. W., D. R. Keeney, and L. M. Walsh. Arsenic residue toxicity to vegetable crops grown on Plainfield sand. Agron. J. 62:588–591, 1970.
388. Jadin, F., and A. Astruc. L'arsenic et le manganèse dans quelques produits végétaux servant d'aliments aux animaux. C. R. Acad. Sci. (Paris) 159:268–270, 1914.
389. Jadin, F., and A. Astruc. Sur la présence de l'arsenic dans quelques plantes parasites et parasitées. C. R. Acad. Sci. (Paris) 155:291–295, 1912.
390. James, L. F., V. A. Lazar, and W. Binns. Effects of sublethal doses of certain minerals on pregnant ewes and fetal development. Amer. J. Vet. Res. 27:132–135, 1966.
391. Japanese Pediatric Society. Morinaga Arsenic-tainted Powdered Milk Poisoning Investigation Special Committee. Summary of Report of Activities of the Morinaga Arsenic-tainted Powdered Milk Poisoning Investigation. May 26, 1973. (English translation from Japanese, TR-124-74, EPA)
392. Jesensky, J., and L. Ondrejcak. Incidence of arsenic in the atmosphere in the (pyrometallurgial) production of copper. Pracovni Lekar. 17:203–206, 1965. (in Czech, summary in English)
393. Johnson, D. L. Bacterial reduction of arsenate in sea water. Nature 240:44–45, 1972.
394. Johnson, F. A. A Reconnaissance of the Winyah Bay Estuarine Zone, South Carolina. South Carolina Water Resources Commission Report No. 4, 1970. 36 pp.
395. Johnson, L. R., and A. E. Hiltbold. Arsenic content of soil and crops following use of methanearsonate herbicides. Soil Sci. Soc. Amer. Proc. 33:279–282, 1969.
396. Johnston, J. Ueber den amphoteren Charakter der Kakodylsäure. Ber. Dtsch. Chem. Ges. 37:3625–3627, 1904.
397. Johnstone, R. M. Sulfhydryl agents: Arsenicals, pp. 99–118. In R. M. Hochster, and J. H. Quastel, Eds. Metabolic Inhibitors. A Comprehensive Treatise. Vol. 2. New York: Academic Press, 1963.
398. Jones, A. J. The arsenic content of some of the marine algae. Pharm. J. 109:86–87, 1922.
399. Jones, C. R., and E. C. Dawson. The arsenic content of grain dried directly with flue gas. Analyst 70:256–257, 1945.
400. Jones, J. R. E. Fish and river pollution, pp. 254–310. In L. Klein, Ed. River Pollution. Vol. 2. Causes and Effects. London: Butterworths, 1962.
401. Jones, J. S., and M. B. Hatch. Spray residues and crop assimilation of arsenic and lead. Soil Sci. 60:277–288, 1945.

402. Jones, L. M. Veterinary Pharmacology and Therapeutics. (3rd ed.) Ames: Iowa State University Press, 1965. 1037 pp.
403. Josephson, C. J., S. S. Pinto, and S. J. Petronella. Arsine: Electrocardiographic changes produced in acute human poisoning. A.M.A. Arch. Ind. Hyg. Occup. Med. 4:43–52, 1951.
404. Kahn, H. L., and J. E. Schallis. Improvement of detection limits for arsenic, selenium, and other elements with an argon-hydrogen flame. Atom. Absorpt. Newslett. 7:5–8, 1968.
405. Kanamori, S., and K. Sugawara. Geochemical study of arsenic in natural waters. I. Arsenic in rain and snow. J. Earth Sci. Nagoya Univ. 13(1):23–35, 1965.
406. Kanisawa, M., and H. A. Schroeder. Life term studies on the effect of trace elements on spontaneous tumors in mice and rats. Cancer Res. 29:892–895, 1969.
407. Kapanadze, P. I. Microelements (trace elements) and their content in vegetable food sources. Gig. Sanit. 13(11):35–38, 1948. (in Russian)
408. Kaplan, I. R., R. E. Sweeney, and A. Nissenbaum. Sulfur isotope studies on Red Sea geothermal brines and sediments, pp. 474–498. In E. T. Degens and D. A. Ross, Eds. Hot Brines and Recent Heavy Metal Deposits in the Red Sea. A Geochemical and Geophysical Account. New York: Springer-Verlag, Inc., 1969.
409. Katsura, K. Medicolegal studies on arsenic poisoning. Report 1. Arsenic contents in the visceral organs, bone, and hair of normal human individuals. Shikoku Acta Med. (Shikoku Igaku Zasshi) 11:439–444, 1957. (in Japanese, summary in English)
410. Kawashiro, I., and T. Kondo. Determination of trace amounts of poisonous metals in foods. II. The content of arsenic, cadmium, copper, manganese, and mercury in rice, wheat flour, and soybeans. Bull. Nat. Inst. Hyg. Sci. (Tokyo) (Eisei Shikenjo Hokoku) 80:75, 1962. (in Japanese)
411. Kawashiro, I., T. Okada, and T. Kondo. Determination of trace amounts of poisonous metals in food. I. The arsenic content of commercial cow milk. Bull. Nat. Hyg. Lab. (Eisei Shikenjo Hokoku) 76:329–330, 1958. (in Japanese)
412. Kearney, P. C., and E. A. Woolson. Chemical distribution and persistence of ^{14}C-cacodylic acid in soil, Abstract PEST No. 28. In Abstracts of Papers. 162nd National Meeting of the American Chemical Society, Washington, Sept. 12–17, 1971.
413. Keeley, P. E., and R. J. Thullen. Control of nutsedge with organic arsenical herbicides. Weed Sci. 19:601–606, 1971.
414. Keeley, P. E., and R. J. Thullen. Cotton response to temperature and organic arsenicals. Weed Sci. 19:297–300, 1971.
415. Keeley, P. E., and R. J. Thullen. Vitality of tubers of yellow nutsedge treated with arsenical herbicides. Weed Sci. 18:437–439, 1970.
416. Kekin, N. A., V. E. Marincheva. Spectrographic method for determining arsenic in coals and cokes. Zavod. Lab. 36:1061–1063, 1970. (in Russian)
417. Kempen, H. M. A Study of Monosodium Acid Methanearsonate in Plants. M.S. Thesis. Davis: University of California, 1970.
418. Kempen, H. M. The seasonal response of hardstem bulrush to methanearsonate herbicides. Res. Prog. Rep. West. Soc. Weed Sci. 1968:91–92.
419. Kempen, H. M., D. E. Bayer, R. Russell, and C. E. Davis. Methane arsonates on Johnsongrass in California, pp. 7–8. In Abstracts. 1966 Meeting of the Weed Society of America, St. Louis, Missouri, Feb. 7–10, 1966.
420. Kennaway, E. L. A contribution of the mythology to cancer research. Lancet 2:769–772, 1942.

421. Kennedy, M. V., B. J. Stofanovic, and F. L. Shuman, Jr. Chemical and thermal methods for disposal of pesticides. Residue Rev. 29:89–104, 1969.
422. Kerr, K. B., J. W. Cavett, and O. L. Thompson. Toxicity of an organic arsenical, 3-nitro-4-hydroxyphenylarsonic acid. I. Acute and subacute toxicity. Toxicol. Appl. Pharmacol. 5:507–525, 1963.
423. Kesselring, J. Arsenic and Old Lace. New York: Dramatists Play Service, 1968. 96 pp.
424. King, H., and R. J. Ludford. The relation between the constitution of arsenicals and their action on cell division. J. Chem. Soc. 1950:2086–2088.
425. Kirk, R. E., and D. R. Othmer, Eds. Encyclopedia of Chemical Technology. Vol. 2. New York: Interscience Encyclopedia, Inc., 1948.
426. Kitamura, N., and T. Kasuyama. Arsenic poisoning due to Morinaga M.F. dried milk. 1. Arsenic content in M.F. dried milk. Okayamaken Eisei Kenkyujo Nenpo 6:42–43, 1955. (English translation from Japanese, TR-115-74, EPA)
427. Kleifeld, Y. Combined effect of trifluralin and MSMA on Johnsongrass control in cotton. Weed Sci. 18:16–18, 1970.
428. Knecht, E., and W. F. Dearden. The elimination of arsenic through the hair and its relation to arsenical poisoning. Lancet 1:854, 1901.
429. Kniseley, R. N. Analytical Applications of Inductively Coupled Plasma-Optical Emission Spectroscopy. Report No. IS-T-626. ERDA Ames Laboratory. Ames, Iowa: U.S. Energy Research and Development Agency, 1974. 89 pp.
430. Knudson, E. J., and G. D. Christian. Flameless atomic absorption determination of volatile hydrides using cold trap collection. Anal. Lett. 6:1039–1054, 1973.
431. Kodama, J., N. Kitamura, and K. Inoue. Arsenic poisoning due to Morinaga M.F. dried milk. 2. Arsenic content inside the body of infants affected with arsenic poisoning. Okayamaken Eisei Kenkyujo Nenpo 6:44–46, 1955. (English translation from Japanese, TR-115-74, EPA)
432. Kölle, W., K. Dorth, G. Smiricz, and H. Sontheimer. Aspekte der Belastung des Rheins mit Schwermetallen. Vom Wasser 38:183–196, 1971.
433. Koller, L. D., and S. Kovacic. Decreased antibody formation in mice exposed to lead. Nature 250:148–150, 1974.
434. Konopik, N., and O. Leberl. Dissoziationskonstanten sehr schwacher Säuren. Monatsh. Chem. 80:655–669, 1949.
435. Kopp, J. F., and R. C. Kroner. Trace Metals in Waters of the United States. A Five Year Summary of Trace Metals in Rivers and Lakes of the United States. (Oct. 1, 1962–Sept. 30, 1967). Cincinnati: U.S. Department of the Interior, Federal Water Pollution Control Administration, 1969. 212 pp.
436. Kopp, J. F., and R. C. Kroner. Tracing water pollution with an emission spectrograph. J. Water Pollut. Control Fed. 39(Part 1): 1659–1668, 1967.
437. Kosta, L., V. Zelenko, V. Ravnik, M. Levstek, M. Dermeij, and A. R. Byrne. Trace elements in human thyroid, with special reference to the observed accumulation of mercury following long-term exposure, pp. 541–550. In Comparative Studies of Food and Environmental Contamination. IAEA Proceedings Series, Otaniemi, Finland, Aug. 27–31, 1973. Vienna: International Atomic Energy Agency, 1974.
438. Krantz, B. A., and A. L. Brown. When and how to fertilize with micronutrients. Agrichem. West 8(3):16, 27, 29, 30, 32, 1965.
439. Kraybill, H. F., and M. B. Shimkin. Carcinogenesis related to foods contaminated by processing and fungal metabolites. Adv. Cancer Res. 8:191–248, 1964.
440. Kroes, R., M. J. van Logten, J. M. Berkvens, T. de Vries, and G. J. van Esch. Study on the carcinogenicity of lead arsanate and sodium arsenate and on the

possible synergistic effect of diethylnitrosamine. Food Cosmet. Toxicol. 12:671–679, 1974.
441. Kuhs, M. L., B. J. Longley, and A. L. Tatum. Development of tolerance to organic arsenicals in laboratory animals. J. Pharmacol. Exp. Ther. 66:312–217, 1939.
442. Kume, S., and I. Ohishi. Observations on the chemotherapy of canine heartworm infections with arsenicals. J. Amer. Vet. Med. Assoc. 131:476–480, 1957.
443. Kuratsune, M., S. Tokudome, T. Shirakusa, M. Yoshida, Y. Tokumitsu, T. Hayano, and M. Seita. Occupational lung cancer among copper smelters. Int. J. Cancer 13:552–558, 1974.
444. Kuschner, M., and S. Laskin. Interaction of atmospheric agents with carcinogens from other sources, pp. 37–46. In R. L. Clark, R. W. Cumley, J. E. McCay, and M. M. Copeland, Eds. Oncology 1970. Vol. V. Proceedings of the Tenth International Cancer Congress. Chicago: Year Book Publications, Inc., 1971.
445. Kvashnevskaya, N. V., and E. I. Shablovskaya. Study of content of ore elements in suspensions of a river system. Dokl. Akad. Nauk sssr 151:426–429, 1963. (in Russian)
446. Lakso, J. U., and Peoples, S. A. Methylation of inorganic arsenic by mammals. J. Agric. Food Chem. 23:674–676, 1975.
447. Lakso, J. U., S. A. Peoples, and D. E. Bayer. Simultaneous determinations of MSMA and arsenic acid in plants. Weed Sci. 21:166–169, 1973.
448. Lancaster, R. J., M. R. Coup, and J. W. Hughes. Toxicity of arsenic present in lakeweed. N. Z. Vet. J. 19:141–145, 1971.
449. Lander, H., P. R. Hodge, and C. S. Crisp. Arsenic in hair and nails. Its significance in acute arsenic poisoning. J. Forensic Med. 12:52–67, 1965.
450. Lange, A. H. Phytotoxicity of eight herbicides applied as foliar sprays on peach and plum rootstocks. Res. Prog. Rep. West. Soc. Weed Sci. 1968:51.
451. Lansche, A. M. Arsenic, pp. 75–80. In Bureau of Mines. Mineral Facts and Problems. 1965 ed. Bureau of Mines Bulletin 630. Washington, D.C.: U.S. Department of the Interior, 1965.
452. Lanz, H., Jr., P. W. Wallace, and J. G. Hamilton. The metabolism of arsenic in laboratory animals using As^{74} as a trace. Univ. Calif. Pub. Pharmacol. 2:263–282, 1950.
453. Lao, R. C., R. S. Thomas, T. Teichman, and L. Dubois. Efficiency of collection of arsenic trioxide in high volume sampling. Sci. Total Environ. 2:373–379, 1974.
454. Laurin, R. E., and R. A. Dever. The effect of spraying date on *Avena fatua* control with methanearsonates. Res. Prog. Rep. Canada Weed Comm. West. Sect. 13:77–78, 1966.
455. Lawrence, J. M. Recent investigations on the use of sodium arsenite as an algicide and its effects on fish production in ponds, pp. 281–287. In Proccedings of 11th Annual Conference, Southeastern Association of Game and Fish Commissioners, October 20–23, 1957, Mobile, Alabama. Columbia, S.C.: Southeastern Association of Game and Fish Commissioners, 1958.
456. Leatherland, T. M., and J. D. Burton. The occurrence of some trace metals in coastal organisms with particular reference to the Solent region. J. Mar. Biol. Assoc. U.K. 54:457–468, 1974.
457. LeBlanc, F., G. Robitaille, and D. N. Rao. Biological response of lichens and bryophytes to environmental pollution in the Murdochville copper mine area, Quebec. J. Hattori Bot. Lab. 38:405–433, 1974.

458. Ledet, A. E. Clinical, Toxicological and Pathological Aspects of Arsanilic Acid Poisoning in Swine. Ph.D. Thesis. Ames: Iowa State University, 1970. 110 pp.
459. Ledet, A. E., J. R. Duncan, W. B. Buck, and R. K. Ramsey. Clinical, toxicological, and pathological aspects of arsanalic acid poisoning in swine. Clin. Toxicol. 6:439–457, 1973.
460. Lee, A. M., and J. F. Fraumeni, Jr. Arsenic and respiratory cancer in man: An occupational study. J. Nat. Cancer Inst. 42:1045–1052, 1969.
461. Lerner, A. B. Enzymes and vesication, p. 571. In S. Rothman. Physiology and Biochemistry of the Skin. Chicago: University of Chicago Press, 1954.
462. Levan, A. Cytological reactions induced by inorganic salt solutions. Nature 156:751–752, 1945.
463. Levander, O. A., and C. A. Baumann. Selenium metabolism. V. Studies on the distribution of selenium in rats given arsenic. Toxicol. Appl. Pharmacol. 9:98–105, 1966.
464. Levander, O. A., and C. A. Baumann. Selenium metabolism. VI. Effect of arsenic on the excretion of selenium in the bile. Toxicol. Appl. Pharmacol. 9:106–115, 1966.
465. Lewis, E. A., L. D. Hansen, E. J. Baca, and D. J. Temer. Effects of alkyl chain length on the thermodynamics of protein ionization from arsonic and arsinic acid. J. Chem. Soc. Perkin Trans. II 1976:125–128.
466. Lewis, T. R. Effects of air pollution on livestock and animal products, pp. 113–124. In Helena Valley, Montana Area Environmental Pollution Study. Office of Air Programs Publication AP-91. Research Triangle Park, N.C.: U.S. Environmental Protection Agency, 1972.
467. Lewis, W. L., and G. A. Perkins. The beta-chlorovinyl chloroarsines. Ind. Eng. Chem. 15:290–295, 1923.
468. Liebig, G. F., Jr., G. R. Bradford, and A. P. Vanselow. Effects of arsenic compounds on citrus plants in solution culture. Soil Sci. 88:342–348, 1959.
469. Liebscher, K., and H. Smith. Essential and nonessential trace elements. A method of determining whether an element is essential or nonessential in human tissue. Arch. Environ. Health 17:881–890, 1968.
470. Lilly, J. G. The effect of arsenical grasshopper poisons upon pheasants. J. Econ. Entomol. 33:501–505, 1940.
471. Lindemann, H. Der Arsengehalt des Hopfens bestimmt der Arsengehalt der Brauereihefe. Wochschr. Brau. 49:257–259, 1932.
472. Lindner, R. C. Arsenic injury of peach trees. Proc. Amer. Soc. Hort. Sci. 42:275–279, 1943.
473. Lindner, R. C., and E. R. Reeves. Arsenic injury of peach trees: A disorder sometimes confused with Western X-disease. Washington State Hort. Assoc. Proc. 38:37–40, 1942.
474. Lis, S. A., and P. K. Hopke. Anomalous arsenic concentrations in Chautauqua Lake. Environ. Lett. 5:45–51, 1973.
475. Lisella, F. S., K. R. Long, and H. G. Scott. Health aspects of arsenicals in the environment. J. Environ. Health 34:511–518, 1972.
476. Lissack, S. E., and M. J. Huston. Arsenic content of commercial tobaccos. Can. Pharm. J. (Sci. Sect.) 92:89–90, 1959.
477. Liverpool Medical Institution. Report on the outbreak of arsenical poison in Liverpool amongst beer-drinkers. Appendicitis. Lancet 1:672–673, 1901.
478. Livingston, D. A. Data of Geochemistry. (6th ed.) Chapter G. Chemical Composition of Rivers and Lakes. U.S. Geological Survey Professional Paper 440-G. Washington, D.C.: U.S. Government Printing Office, 1963. 64 pp.

References

479. Lockemann, G. Über den Arsengehalt von Honig und Bienen nach Verstäubung arsenhaltiger Schädlingsbekämpfungsmittel. Z. Untersuch. Lebensmitt. 69:80, 1935.
480. Lodmell, J. D. The Development and Utilization of a Wavelength-Selective Multielement Flame-Spectrometric Detector for the Gas Chromatograph. Ph.D. Thesis. Knoxville: University of Tennessee, 1973. 119 pp.
481. Loehr, T. M., and R. A. Plane. Raman spectra and structures of arsenious acid and arsenites in aqueous solution. Inorg. Chem. 7:1708–1714, 1968.
482. Long, J. A., W. W. Allen, and E. C. Holt. Control of nutsedge in Bermuda grass turf. Weeds 10:285–287, 1962.
483. Long, J. A., and E. C. Holt. Selective and non-selective performance of several herbicides for the control of southern nutgrass (*Cyperus rotundus*). South. Weed Conf. Proc. 12:195, 1959. (abstract)
484. Long, J. W., and W. J. Ray, Jr. Kinetics and thermodynamics of the formation of glucose arsenate. Reaction of glucose arsenate with phosphoglucomutase. Biochemistry 12:3932–3937, 1973.
485. Long, T. A., J. W. Bratzler, and D. E. H. Frear. The value of hydrolyzed and dried poultry waste as a feed for ruminant animals, pp. 98–104. In Animal Waste Management. Conference on Agricultural Waste Management, Syracuse, New York. Ithaca, N.Y.: Cornell University, 1969.
486. Lovern, J. A. Fat metabolism in fishes. VI. The fats of some plankton crustacea. Biochem. J. 29:847–849, 1935.
487. Low, D. G. Arsenic poisoning, pp. 138–139. In R. W. Kirk, Ed. Current Veterinary Therapy. V. Small Animal Practice. Philadelphia: W. B. Saunders Company, 1974.
488. Lowry, O. H., F. T. Hunter, A. F. Kip, and J. W. Irvine, Jr. Radioactive tracer studies on arsenic injected as potassium arsenite. II. Chemical distribution in tissues. J. Pharmacol. Exp. Ther. 76:221–225, 1942.
489. Loy, H. W., S. S. Schiaffino, and W. B. Savchuck. Determination of arsenic valence by microbiological assay. Anal. Chem. 33:283–285, 1961.
490. Lunde, G. Activation analysis of trace elements in fishmeal. J. Sci. Food Agric. 19:432–434, 1968.
491. Lunde, G. Analysis of arsenic and bromine in marine and terrestrial oils. J. Amer. Oil Chem. Soc. 49:44–47, 1972.
492. Lunde, G. Analysis of arsenic and selenium in marine raw materials. J. Sci. Food Agric. 21:242–247, 1970.
493. Lunde, G. Analysis of arsenic in marine oils by neutron activation. Evidence of arseno organic compounds. J. Amer. Oil Chem. Soc. 45:331–332, 1968.
494. Lunde, G. Analysis of organically bound elements (As, Se, Br) and phosphorus in raw, refined, bleached, and hydrogenated marine oils produced from fish of different quality. J. Amer. Oil Chem. Soc. 50:26–28, 1973.
495. Lunde, G. Analysis of trace elements in seaweed. J. Sci. Food Agric. 21:416–418, 1970.
496. Lunde, G. Separation and analysis of organic-bound and inorganic arsenic in marine organisms. J. Sci. Food Agric. 24:1021–1027, 1973.
497. Lunde, G. The analysis of arsenic in the lipid phase from marine and limnetic algae. Acta Chem. Scand. 26:2642–2644, 1972.
498. Lunde, G. The synthesis of fat and water soluble arseno organic compounds in marine and limnetic algae. Acta Chem. Scand. 27:1586–1594, 1973.
499. Lunde, G. Trace metal contents of fish meal and of the lipid phase extracted from fish meal. J. Sci. Food Agric. 24:413–419, 1973.

500. Lunde, G. Water soluble arseno-organic compounds in marine fishes. Nature 224:186–187, 1969.
501. Luzanski, N. Arsenic content of marine foodstuffs. Tids. Kjemi Bergvesen 15:154, 1935. (in Norwegian)
502. Luzanski, N. Arsenic content of samples of Norwegian cod-liver oil. Tids. Kjemi Bergvesen 16:56–59, 1936. (in Norwegian)
503. Machlis, L. Accumulation of arsenic in the shoots of Sudan grass and bush bean. Plant Physiol. 16:521–543, 1941.
504. MacInnes, J. R., and R. P. Thurberg. Effects of metals on the behaviour and oxygen consumption of the mud snail. Mar. Pollut. Bull. 4:185–186, 1973.
505. Mackay, N. J., M. N. Kazacos, R. J. Williams, and M. I. Leedow. Selenium and heavy metals in black marlin. Mar. Pollut. Bull. 6:57–61, 1975.
506. Mackay, N. J., R. J. Williams, J. L. Kacprzac, M. N. Kazacos, A. J. Collins, and E. H. Auty. Heavy metals in cultivated oysters (*Crassostrea commercialis* = *Saccostrea cucullata*) from the estuaries of New South Wales. Austral. J. Mar. Freshwater Res. 26:31–46, 1975.
507. Maclagan, C. On the arsenic eaters of Styria. Edinburgh Med. J. 10:200–207, 1864.
508. Maclagan, R. C. Arsenic eaters of Styria. Edinburgh Med. J. 21:526–528, 1875.
509. MacPhee, A. W., D. Chisholm, and C. R. MacEachern. The persistence of certain pesticides in the soil and their effect on crop yields. Can. J. Soil Sci. 40:59–62, 1960.
510. Maddox, R. N., and M. D. Burns. Liquid absorption-oxidation processes show much promise. Oil Gas J. 66(20):100–103, 1968.
511. Madsen, R. E., Jr. Atomic absorption determination of arsenic subsequent to arsenic reaction with 0.01 M silver nitrate. Atom. Absorpt. Newslett. 10:57–58, 1971.
512. Maegraith, B. G. Adams & Maegraith: Clinical Tropical Diseases. (5th ed.) Oxford: Blackwell Scientific Publications, 1971. 578 pp.
513. Mamuro, T., Y. Matsuda, and A. Mizohata. Identification of an air pollution source by instrumental neutron activation analysis. Radioisotopes 21:183–185, 1972. (in Japanese)
514. Mamuro, T., Y. Matsuda, A. Mizohata, and T. Matsunami. Activation analysis of airborne dust. Radioisotopes 21:164–169, 1972. (in Japanese, summary in English)
515. Mamuro, T., Y. Matsuda, A. Mizohata, T. Takeuchi, and A. Fujita. Neutron activation analysis of airborne dust. Ann. Rep. Radiat. Center Osaka Prefect. 11:1–13, 1970.
516. Manceau, P., H. Griffon, and R. Nicolas. Sur l'arsenic introduit dans l'organisme. Ann. Falsifications Fraudes 31:262–281, 1938.
517. Mandel, H. G., J. S. Mayersak, and M. Riis. The action of arsenic on *Baccillus cereus*. J. Pharm. Pharmacol. 17:794–804, 1965.
518. Manuelidis, E. E., D. H. H. Robertson, J. M. Amberson, M. Polak, and W. Haymaker. *Trypanosoma rhodesiense* encephalitis. Clinicopathological study of five cases of encephalitis and one case of Mel B hemorrhagic encephalopathy. Acta Neuropath. 5:176–204, 1965.
519. Marcelet, H. L'arsenic et le manganèse dans quelques végétaux marins. Bull. Sci. Pharmacol. 20:271–275, 1913.
520. Mark, H. F., J. J. McKetta, Jr., and D. F. Othmer, Eds. Kirk-Othmer Encyclopedia of Chemical Technology. Vol. 2. (2nd ed.) New York: Interscience Publishers, 1963.

References

521. Marshall, S. P., F. W. Hayward, and W. R. Meagher. Effects of feeding arsenic and lead upon their secretion in milk. J. Dairy Sci. 46:580–581, 1963.
522. Martin, P. A. The estimation of arsenic in beer and malt. J. Inst. Brew. 77:365–368, 1971.
523. Martin, R. J., and R. E. Duggan. Pesticide residues in total diet samples. (III). Pest. Monit. J. 1(4):11–20, 1968.
524. Martin, W. E., and P. R. Nickerson. Mercury, lead, cadmium, and arsenic residues in starlings—1971. Pest. Monit. J. 7:67–72, 1973.
525. Masahiko, O., and A. Hideyasu. Epidemiological studies on the Morinaga powdered milk poisoning incident: Final report of the joint project team from Hiroshima and Okayama Universities for survey of the Seno area. Jap. J. Hyg. (Nihon Eiseigaku Zasshi) 27:500–531, 1973. (in Japanese)
526. Mathies, J. C. X-ray spectrographic microanalysis of human urine for arsenic. Appl. Spectroscopy 28:165–170, 1974.
527. McBride, B. C., and R. S. Wolfe. Biosynthesis of dimethylarsine by methanobacterium. Biochemistry 10:4312–4317, 1971.
528. McChesney, E. W., J. O. Hoppe, J. P. McAuliff, and W. F. Banks, Jr. Toxicity and physiological disposition of sodium p-N-glycolylarsanilate. I. Observations in the mouse, cat, rat, and man. Toxicol. Appl. Pharmacol. 4:14–23, 1962.
529. McDonough, W. T. Arsenite-BAL as an inhibitor of germination. Physiol. Plant. 20:455–462, 1967.
530. McGeorge, W. T. Fate and effect of arsenic applied as a spray for weeds. J. Agric. Res. (Washington, D.C.) 5:459–463, 1915.
531. McKee, J. E., and H. W. Wolf, Eds. Water Quality Criteria. (2nd ed.) The Resources Agency of California. State Water Resources Control Board Publication No. 3-A. (Revised 1963). 548 pp.
532. McLean, H. C., A. L. Weber, and J. S. Joffe. Arsenic content of vegetables grown in soil treated with lead arsenate. J. Econ. Entomol. 37:315–316, 1944.
533. McNally, W. D. Retention of arsenic in the organs. J. Amer. Chem. Soc. 39:826–828, 1917.
534. McWhorter, C. G. Growth and control of Johnsongrass ecotypes, pp. 36–37. In Abstracts. 1967 Meeting of the Weed Society of America, Washington, D.C., Feb. 13–16, 1967.
535. McWhorter, C. G. Toxicity of DSMA to Johnsongrass. Weeds 14:191–194, 1966.
536. Mealey, J., Jr., G. L. Brownell, and W. H. Sweet. Radioarsenic in plasma, urine, normal tissues, and intracranial neoplasms. Arch. Neurol. Psychiatry 81:310–320, 1959.
537. Mees, R. A. Nails with arsenical polyneuritis. J.A.M.A. 72:1337, 1919. (abstract)
538. Meinck, F., H. Stooff, and H. Kohlschütter. Industrie-Abwässer. (2nd ed.) Stuttgart: Gustov Fisher Verlag, 1956. 527 pp.
539. Menges, R. W., L. D. Kintner, L. A. Selby, R. W. Stewart, and C. J. Marienfeld. Arsanilic acid blindness in pigs. Vet. Med. Small Anim. Clin. 65:565–568, 1970.
540. Messer, J. W., J. Lovett, G. K. Murthy, A. J. Wehby, M. L. Schafer, and R. B. Read, Jr. An assessment of some public health problems resulting from feeding poultry litter to animals. Microbiological and chemical parameters. Poult. Sci. 50:874–881, 1971.
541. Miesch, A. T., and C. Huffman, Jr. Abundance and distribution of lead, zinc, cadmium, and arsenic in soils, pp. 65–80. In Helena Valley, Montana Area Environmental Pollution Study. Office of Air Programs Publication AP-91. Research Triangle Park, N.C.: U.S. Environmental Protection Agency, 1972.

542. Miescher, G. Statische Angaben aus der Krebsstatistik der dermatologischen Klinik Zürich. Dermatol. Wochenschr. 98:420–425, 1934.
543. Milham, S., Jr., and T. Strong. Human arsenic exposure in relation to a copper smelter. Environ. Res. 7:176–182, 1974.
544. Miller, R. L., I. P. Bassett, and W. W. Yothers. Effect of Lead Arsenate Insecticides on Orange Trees in Florida. U.S. Department of Agriculture Technical Bulletin 350. Washington, D.C.: U.S. Department of Agriculture, 1933. 20 pp.
545. Millhollon, R. W. Control of Johnsongrass on drainage ditchbanks in sugarcane. Weed Sci. 17:370–373, 1969.
546. Milner, J. E. The effect of ingested arsenic on methylcholanthrene-induced skin tumors in mice. Arch. Environ. Health 18:7–11, 1969.
547. Minguzzi, C., and K. M. Naldoni. Supposed traces of arsenic in wood: Its determination in the wood of some trees. Atti Soc. Toscana Sci. Nat. (Pisa) Mem. 57, Ser. A.:38–48, 1950. (in Italian)
548. Mintz, M. Hazards of arsenic in shrimp disputed. Washington Post, December 30, 1971. p. A3, col. 1-4.
549. Mitchell, R. A., B. F. Chang, C. H. Huang, and E. G. DeMaster. Inhibition of mitochondrial energy-linked functions of arsenate. Evidence for a nonhydrolytic mode of inhibitor action. Biochemistry 10:2049–2054, 1971.
550. Mizuta, N., M. Mizuta, F. Ito, T. Ito, H. Uchida, Y. Watanabe, H. Akama, T. Murakami, F. Hayashi, K. Nakamura, T. Yamaguchi, W. Mizuia, S. Oishi, and H. Matsumura. An outbreak of acute arsenic poisoning caused by arsenic contaminated soy-sauce (shōyu): A clinical report of 220 cases. Bull. Yamaguchi Med. Sch. 4(2,3):131–150, 1956.
551. Moenke, H. Untersuchung zur Geochemie des Arsens am Quellwasser und Eisenoxydhydratabsätzen der Saalfelder "Feengrotten." Chem. Erde 18:89–91, 1956.
552. Molokhia, M. M., and H. Smith. Trace elements in the lung. Arch. Environ. Health 15:745–750, 1967.
553. Montagna, W., and P. E. Parakkal. The Structure and Function of Skin. (3rd ed.) New York: Academic Press, 1974. 433 pp.
554. Montgomery, H. Arsenic as an etiologic agent in certain types of epithelioma. Differential diagnosis from, and further studies regarding, superficial epitheliomatosis and Bowen's disease. Arch. Derm. Syphilol. 32:218–236, 1935.
555. Moody, J. P., and R. T. Williams. The fate of arsanilic acid and acetylarsanilic acid in hens. Food Cosmet. Toxicol. 2:687–693, 1964.
556. Moody, J. P., and R. T. Williams. The fate of 4-nitrophenylarsonic acid in hens. Food Cosmet. Toxicol. 2:695–706, 1964.
557. Moody, J. P., and R. T. Williams. The metabolism of 4-hydroxy-3-nitrophenylarsonic acid in hens. Food Cosmet. Toxicol. 2:707–715, 1964.
558. Morehouse, N. F. Accelerated growth in chickens and turkeys produced by 3-nitro-4-hydroxyphenylarsonic acid. Poult. Sci. 28:375–384, 1949.
559. Morehouse, N. F., and O. J. Mayfield. The effect of some aryl arsonic acids on experimental coccidiosis infection in chickens. J. Parasitol. 32:20–24, 1946.
560. Morgareidge, K. Metabolism of two forms of dietary arsenic by the rat. J. Agric. Food Chem. 11:377–378, 1963.
561. Morris, H. P., E. P. Laug, H. J. Morris, and R. L. Grant. The growth and reproduction of rats fed diets containing lead acetate and arsenic trioxide and the lead and arsenic content of newborn and suckling rats. J. Pharmacol. Exp. Ther. 64:420–445, 1938.

References

562. Morrison, J. L. Distribution of arsenic from poultry litter in broiler chickens, soil, and crops. J. Agric. Food Chem. 17:1288–1290, 1969.
563. Moutschen, J., and N. Degraeve. Influence of thiol-inhibiting substances on the effects of ethyl methane sulphonate (EMS) on chromosomes. Experientia 21:200–202, 1965.
564. Moxham, J. W., and M. R. Coup. Arsenic poisoning of cattle and other domestic animals. N. Z. Vet. J. 16:161–165, 1968.
565. Moxon, A. L. The effect of arsenic on the toxicity of seleniferous grains. Science 88:81, 1938.
566. Moxon, A. L., and K. P. DuBois. The influence of arsenic and other elements on the toxicity of seleniferous grains. J. Nutr. 18:447–457, 1939.
567. Moyana, C. S. Contenido de arsénico en algunos mariscos de la costa peruana. Bol. Soc. Quim. Peru 22:5–16, 1956.
568. Mulford, C. E. Solvent extraction techniques for atomic absorption spectroscopy. Atom. Absorpt. Newslett. 5:88–90, 1966.
569. Murphy, H. J., and M. J. Goven. Arsenic residues in potato soils and tubers. Maine Farm Res. 14(3):4–8, 1966.
570. Muth, O. H., P. D. Whanger, P. H. Weswig, and J. E. Oldfield. Occurrence of myopathy in lambs of ewes fed added arsenic in a selenium-deficient ration. Amer. J. Vet. Res. 32:1621–1623, 1971.
571. Myers, D. J., and J. Osteryoung. Determination of arsenic (III) at the parts-per-billion level by differential pulse polarography. Anal. Chem. 45:267–271, 1973.
572. Myers, G. A., and D. K. Wunderlich. Shale oil treatment. U.S. Patent 3,804,750, April 16, 1974.
573. Nadkarni, R. A., W. D. Ehmann, and D. Burdick. Investigations on the relative transference of trace elements from cigaret tobacco into smoke condensate. Tobacco Sci. 14:37–39, 1970.
574. Nagai, H., R. Okuda, H. Nagami, A. Yagi, C. Mori, and H. Wada. Subacute-chronic "arsenic" poisoning in infants—subsequent clinical observations. Ann. Pediatr. (Shōnika Kiyō) 2(2):124–132, 1956. (in Japanese)
575. Nakagawa, Y., and Y. Iibuchi. On the follow-up investigation of Morinaga milk arsenic poisoning. Footsteps Med. (Igaku no Ayumi) 74(1):1–3, 1970. (in Japanese)
576. Nakao, M. A study of the arsenic content in daily food consumption in Japan. J. Osaka City Med. Center (Osaka Shiritsu Daigaku Igakubu Zasshi) 9:541–571, 1960. (in Japanese, summary in English)
577. Napoleon's death. Lancet 2:1395–1396, 1961.
578. National Academy of Sciences. National Academy of Engineering. Environmental Studies Board. Water Quality Criteria 1972. A Report of the Committee on Water Quality Criteria. Washington, D.C.: U.S. Government Printing Office, 1974. 594 pp.
579. National Cotton Council of America. Statement in Support of Continued Registration of the Methanearsonate Herbicides and Arsenic Acid Desiccant for Use on Cotton. Memphis, Tenn.: National Cotton Council of America, Aug. 31, 1971. 22 pp.
580. Natusch, D. F. S., J. R. Wallace, and C. A. Evans, Jr. Toxic trace elements: Preferential concentration in respirable particles. Science 183:202–204, 1974.
581. Naude, C. P., and J. P. van Zijl. The toxicity of pastures after treatment with locust poison. Part I. Toxicity of treated pastures, pp. 5–13. In Union of South Africa

Department of Agriculture Science Bulletin No. 326. Pretoria: Government Printer, 1952.
582. Navarrete, M., L. Galvez, E. Tzontlimatzin, and A. Ley. Estudio de la contaminacion del aire en la Ciudad de Mexico, pp. 91–102. In Comparative Studies of Food and Environmental Contamination. IAEA Proceedings Series, Otaniemi, Finland, Aug. 27–31, 1973. Vienna: International Atomic Energy Agency, 1974.
583. Neal, P. A., W. C. Dreessen, T. I. Edwards, W. H. Reinhart, S. H. Webster, H. T. Castberg, and L. T. Fairhall. A Study of the Effect of Lead Arsenate Exposure on Orchardists and Consumers of Sprayed Fruit. Public Health Bulletin 267. Washington, D.C.: U.S. Public Health Service, Federal Security Agency, 1941. 181 pp.
584. Nelson, W. C., M. H. Lykins, J. Mackey, V. A. Newill, J. F. Finklea, and D. I. Hammer. Mortality among orchard workers exposed to lead arsenate spray: A cohort study. J. Chron. Dis. 26:105–118, 1973.
585. Neubauer, O. Arsenical cancer: A review. Brit. J. Cancer 1:192–251, 1947.
586. Nielsen, F. H., S. H. Givand, and D. R. Myron. Evidence of a possible requirement for arsenic by the rat. Fed. Proc. 34:923, 1975. (abstract)
587. 1975 Feed Additive Compendium. Vol. 13. Minneapolis: The Miller Publishing Company, 1974. 330 pp.
588. Noguchi, K., and R. Nakagawa. Arsenic in the waters and deposits of Osoreyama Hot Springs, Aomori Prefecture. Nippon Kagaku Zasshi (Chem. Soc. Jap. J., Pure Chem. Sect.) 91:127–131, 1970. (in Japanese, summary in English)
589. Nose, Y. Epidemiological observations of the poisoning incident caused by soy sauce with admixtures of arsenic. From the soy sauce poisoning to its recognition. Public Health (Koshu Eisei) 21(3):29–43, 1957. (in Japanese)
590. Notzold, R. A., D. E. Becker, F. B. Adamstone, S. W. Terrill, and A. H. Jensen. The tolerance of swine to dietary levels of p-aminophenyl arsonic acid. J. Anim. Sci. 15:1234, 1956. (abstract)
591. Novick, R. P., and C. Roth. Plasmid-linked resistance to inorganic salts in *Staphylococcus aureus*. J. Bacteriol. 95:1335–1342, 1968.
592. Nusbaum, R. E., E. M. Butt, T. C. Gilmour, and S. L. DiDio. Relation of air pollutants to trace metals in bone. Arch. Environ. Health 10: 227–232, 1965.
593. Obermeyer, B. D., I. S. Palmer, O. E. Olson, and A. W. Halverson. Toxicity of trimethylselenonium chloride in the rat with and without arsenite. Toxicol. Appl. Pharmacol. 20:135–146, 1971.
594. Oehme, F. W. British anti-lewisite (BAL), the classic heavy metal antidote. Clin. Toxicol. 5:215–222, 1972.
595. O'Gara, P. J. Presence of arsenic in fruit sprayed with arsenate of lead. Science 33:900–901, 1911.
596. Okamura, K., T. Ota, K. Horiuchi, H. Hiroshima, T. Takai, Y. Sakurane, and T. Baba. Symposium on arsenic poisoning by powdered milk. (2). Diagnos. Ther. (Shinryo) 9:155–162, 1956. (in Japanese)
597. Okamura, K., T. Ota, K. Horiuchi, H. Hiroshima, T. Takai, Y. Sakurane, and T. Baba. Symposium on arsenic poisoning by powdered milk. (2). Diagnos. Ther. (Shinryo) 9:240–249, 1956. (in Japanese)
598. Oliver, W. T., and C. K. Roe. Arsanilic acid poisoning in swine. J. Amer. Vet. Med. Assoc. 130:177–178, 1957.
599. Olson, O. E., B. M. Schulte, E. I. Whitehead, and A. W. Halverson. Selenium toxicity. Effect of arsenic on selenium metabolism in rats. J. Agric. Food Chem. 11:531–534, 1963.

600. Olson, O. E., L. L. Sisson, and A. L. Moxon. Absorption of selenium and arsenic by plants from soils under natural conditions. Soil Sci. 50:115–118, 1940.
601. Ondov, J. M., W. H. Zoller, I. Olmez, N. K. Aras, G. E. Gordon, L. A. Rancitelli, K. H. Abel, R. H. Filby, K. R. Shab, and R. C. Ragaini. Elemental concentrations in the National Bureau of Standards environmental coal and fly ash standard reference materials. Anal. Chem. 47:1102–1109, 1975.
602. Onishi, H. Arsenic, Chapter 33. In K. H. Wedepohl, Ed. Handbook of Geochemistry. Berlin: Springer-Verlag, 1969.
603. Onishi, H., and E. B. Sandell. Geochemistry of arsenic. Geochim. Cosmochim. Acta 7:1–33, 1955.
604. Orvini, E., T. E. Gills, and P. D. LaFleur. Method for determination of selenium, arsenic, zinc, cadmium, and mercury in environmental matrices by neutron activation analysis. Anal. Chem. 46:1294–1297, 1974.
605. Osburn, H. S. Cancer of the lung in Gwanda. Central African J. Med. 3:215–223, 1957.
606. Osburn, H. S. Lung cancer in a mining district in Rhodesia. S. Afr. Med. J. 43:1307–1312, 1969.
607. Osswald, H., and Kl. Goerttler. Leukosen bei der Maus nach diaplacentarer und postnataler Arsenik-Applikation. Dtsch. Gesamte Path. 55:289–293, 1971.
608. Osteryoung, J. G., and R. A. Osteryoung. Adventures in pulse voltammetry. Oral presentation at Federation of Analytical Chemistry and Spectroscopy Societies, Second National Meeting, Indianapolis, Indiana, Oct. 7, 1975.
609. Ott, M. G., B. B. Holder, and H. L. Gordon. Respiratory cancer and occupational exposure to arsenicals. Arch. Environ. Health 29:250–255, 1974.
610. Ottinger, R. S., J. L. Blumenthal, D. F. Dal Porto, G. I. Gruber, M. J. Santy, and C. C. Shih. Arsenic compounds, pp. 67–141. In Recommended Methods of Reduction, Neutralization, Recovery or Disposal of Hazardous Waste. Vol. 6. National Disposal Site Candidate Waste Stream Constituent Profile Reports. Mercury, Arsenic, Chromium and Cadmium Compounds. EPA-670/2-73-053-f. Redondo Beach, Calif.: TRW Systems Group, 1973.
611. Otto, G. F., and T. H. Maren. Studies on the chemotherapy of filariasis. Part V. Studies on the pharmacology of arsenamide and related arsenicals. Amer. J. Hyg. 51:353–370, 1950.
612. Otto, G. F., and T. H. Maren. Studies on the chemotherapy of filariasis. Part VII. Comparative review of the possible therapeutic agents available for canine and human filariasis. Amer. J. Hyg. 51:385–395, 1950.
613. Overby, L. R., and R. L. Fredrickson. Metabolic stability of radioactive arsanilic acid in chickens. J. Agric. Food Chem. 11:378–381, 1963.
614. Overby, L. R., and R. L. Fredrickson. Metabolism of arsanilic acid. II. Localization and type of arsenic excreted and retained by chickens. Toxicol. Appl. Pharmacol. 7:855–867, 1965.
615. Overby, L. R., and D. V. Frost. Nonavailability to the rat of the arsenic in tissues of swine fed arsanilic acid. Toxicol. Appl. Pharmacol. 4:38–43, 1962.
616. Overby, L. R., and L. Straube. Metabolism of arsanilic acid. I. Metabolic stability of double labeled arsanilic acid in chickens. Toxicol. Appl. Pharmacol. 7:850–854, 1965.
617. Oyanguren, H., and E. Pérez. Poisoning of industrial origin in a community. Arch. Environ. Health 13:185–189, 1966.
618. Palmer, A. W. Dimethylarsin. Ber. Dtsch. Chem. Ges. 27:1378–1379, 1894.
619. Palmer, A. W., and M. W. Dehn. Ueber primäre Arsine. Ber. Dtsch. Chem. Ges. 34:3594–3599, 1901.

620. Paton, G. R., and A. C. Allison. Chromosome damage in human cell cultures induced by metal salts. Mutation Res. 16:332–336, 1972.
621. Patterson, E. L., R. Milstrey, and E. L. R. Stokstad. Effect of selenium in preventing exudative diathesis in chicks. Proc. Soc. Exp. Biol. Med. 95:617–620, 1957.
622. Pattison, E. S. Arsenic and water pollution hazard. Science 170:870, 1970.
623. Peardon, D. L. Efficacy of p-ureidobenzenearsonic acid against blackhead in chickens. Poult. Sci. 46:1108–1112, 1967.
624. Pemberton, C. E. Entomology, pp. 19–26. In Report of the Committee in Charge of the Experiment Station. Proceedings 54th Annual Meeting Hawaiian Sugar Planters' Association for the Year Ending Sept. 30, 1934.
625. Peoples, S. A. Arsenic toxicity in cattle. Ann. N.Y. Acad. Sci. 111:644–649, 1964.
626. Peoples, S. A. Review of arsenical pesticides, pp. 1–12. In E. A. Woolson, Ed. Arsenical Pesticides. ACS Symposium Series 7. Washington, D.C.: American Chemical Society, 1975.
627. Peoples, S. A. The failure of methanearsonic acid to cross the blood–mammary barrier when administered orally to lactating cows. Fed. Proc. 28:359, 1969. (abstract)
628. Peoples, S. A. The mechanisms of action of arsenicals in feed on performance and health of animals, pp. 77–86. In The Use of Drugs in Animal Feeds. Proceedings of a symposium. NAS Publ. 1679. Washington, D.C.: National Academy of Sciences, 1969.
629. Peoples, S. A., J. Lakso, and T. Lais. The simultaneous determination of methyl arsonic acid and inorganic arsenic in urine. Proc. West. Pharmacol. Soc. 14:178–182, 1971.
630. Pereira, J. F., and E. Echandi. Residuo de arsénico en hojas y granos de plantas de café asperjadas con arseniato de plomo. Turrialba 14:85–90, 1964.
631. Peripheral neuritis of arsenical and alcoholic origin. Lancet 1:341–342, 1901.
632. Perkons, A. K., and R. E. Jervis. Trace elements in human head hair. J. Forensic Sci. 11:50–63, 1966.
633. Perry, K., R. G. Bowler, H. M. Buckell, H. A. Druett, and R. S. F. Shilling. Studies in the incidence of cancer in a factory handling inorganic compounds of arsenic. II. Clinical and environmental investigations. Brit. J. Ind. Med. 5:6–15, 1948.
634. Peters, R. A. Biochemistry of some toxic agents. I. Present state of knowledge of biochemical lesions induced by trivalent arsenical poisoning. Bull. Johns Hopkins Hosp. 97:1–20, 1955.
635. Peters, R. A., H. Rydin, and R. H. S. Thompson. The relation of pyruvic acid in brain to certain tissue poisons. Biochem. J. 29:63–71, 1935.
636. Petigny, M. Influence des traitements arsenicaux de la vigne sur la teneur en arsenic des vins du Beaujolais conséquences toxicologiques. Ann. Falsifications Fraudes 42:281–287, 1949.
637. Petres, J., and A. Berger. Zum Einfluss anorganischen Arsens auf die DNS-Synthese menschlicher Lymphocyten in vitro. Arch. Derm. Forsch. 242:343–352, 1972.
638. Petres, J., and M. Hundeiker. "Chromosomenpulverisation" nach Arseneinwirkung auf Zellkulturen in vitro. Arch. Klin. Exp. Dermatol. 231:366–370, 1968.
639. Petres, J., K. Schmid-Ullrich, and W. Wolf. Chromsomenaberrationen an menschlichen Lymphozyten bei chronischen Arsenschäden. Dtsch. Med. Wochenschr. 95:79–80, 1970.

640. Petrovic, I. Composition and purity of polyphosphate preparations used as food additives. Tehnol. Mesa 9:342–347, 1968. (in Croatian)
641. Pezzeri, G. Sull'origine dell'arsenico cosiddeto fisiologico. Indagini sul contenuto in arsenico di carni per uso alimentare. Zacchia 45(Vol. 6, Ser. 3):45–52, 1970.
642. Pharmacopoeia of the United States of America. Tenth Decennial Revision. (U.S.P.X) By Authority of the United States Pharmacopoeial Convention held at Washington, D.C., May 11, 1920. Official from January 1, 1926. Philadelphia: J. B. Lippincott Co., 1926. 626 pp.
643. Pieruccini, R. Eine empfindliche Methode für den spektralen Nachweis und die Bestimmung des Arsens durch Adsorption in Ferrihydroxyd. Spectrochim. Acta 4:189–199, 1950.
644. Pillay, K. K. S., C. C. Thomas, Jr., and C. M. Hyche. Neutron activation analysis of some of the biologically active trace elements in fish. J. Radioanal. Chem. 20:597–606, 1974.
645. Pillsbury, D. M., W. B. Shelley, and A. M. Kligman. Dermatology. Philadelphia: W. B. Saunders Company, 1956. 1,331 pp.
646. Pinkus, H., and A. Mehregan. Decrease and increase of epidermal melanin, p. 324, and Bowen's precancerous dermatosis and erythroplasia of Queyrat, pp. 406–411. In A Guide to Dermatohistopathology. New York: Meredith Corporation, 1969.
647. Pinto, S. S., and B. M. Bennett. Effect of arsenic trioxide exposure on mortality. Arch. Environ. Health 7:583–591, 1963.
648. Pinto, S. S., and C. M. McGill. Arsenic trioxide exposure in industry. Ind. Med. Surg. 22:281–287, 1953.
649. Plotnikov, V. I., and L. P. Usatova. Coprecipitation of small amounts of arsenic with metal hydroxides. J. Anal. Chem. U.S.S.R. 19:1101–1104, 1964.
650. Pool, J. F. A. Biologic reaction for arsenic with *Monilia sitophila*, Saccardo. Pharm. Weekblad 49:878–886, 1912. (in Dutch)
651. Porázik, I., V. Legáth, K. Puchá, and I. Kratochvíl. Evaluation of exposure to atmospheric arsenic oxide from the content of arsenic in the hair. Pracovni Lekar. 18:352–356, 1966. (in Czech, summary in English)
652. Portmann, J. E., and J. P. Riley. Determination of arsenic in sea water, marine plants and silicate and carbonate sediments. Anal. Chim. Acta 31:509–519, 1964.
653. Pratt, D. R., J. S. Bradshaw, and B. West. Arsenic and selenium analyses in fish. Utah Acad. Proc. Part 1 49:23–26, 1972.
654. Presley, B. J., and J. H. Culp. Lead and Arsenic Concentrations in Some South Texas Coastal-Zone Sediments. Texas A & M Environmental Quality Note 09. College Station: Texas Agricultural and Mechanical University, 1972. 14 pp.
655. Pupp, C., and R. C. Lao. Equilibrium vapour concentrations of some polycyclic aromatic hydrocarbons, As_4O_6 and SeO_2 and the collection efficiencies of these air pollutants. Atmos. Environ. 8:915–925, 1974.
656. Radeleff, R. D. Arsenic, pp. 158–161. In Veterinary Toxicology. (2nd ed.) Philadelphia: Lea & Febiger, 1970.
657. Rahn, K. A., and J. W. Winchester. Sources of Trace Elements in Aerosols—An Approach to Clean Air. University of Michigan Technical Report ORA (Office of Research Administration) 089030. Ann Arbor, 1971. 342 pp.
658. Raiziss, G. W., and J. L. Gavron. Trivalent aliphatic arsenicals, pp. 36–68. In Organic Arsenical Compounds. New York: The Chemical Catalogue Co., Inc., 1923.
659. Ray, B. J., and D. L. Johnson. A method for the neutron activation analyses of natural waters for arsenic. Anal. Chim. Acta 62:196–199, 1972.

660. Reay, P. F. Arsenic in the Waikato River system, pp. 365–376. In Proceedings of the Pollution Research Conference, Wairakei, New Zealand, June 1973.
661. Reay, P. F. The accumulation of arsenic from arsenic-rich natural waters by aquatic plants. J. Appl. Ecol. 9:557–565, 1972.
662. Reed, J. F., and M. B. Sturgis. Toxicity from arsenic compounds to rice on flooded soils. J. Amer. Soc. Agron. 28:432–436, 1936.
663. Regelson, W., U. Kim, J. Ospina, and J. F. Holland. Hemangioendothelial sarcoma of liver from chronic arsenic intoxication by Fowler's solution. Cancer 21:514–522, 1968.
664. Remy, H. Lehrbuch der Anorganischen chemie. Vol. 1. (11th ed.) Leipzig: Akademische Verlagsgesellschaft Geest & Portig K.-G., 1960. p. 770.
665. Reynolds, E. S. An account of the epidemic outbreak of arsenical poisoning occurring in beer-drinkers in the north of England and Midland Countries in 1900. Lancet 1:166–170, 1901.
666. Richardson, F. M. Napoleon's death. Lancet 1:749, 1962. (letter)
667. Richardson, F. M. Napoleon's death. Lancet 1:1128, 1962. (letter)
668. Ridgway, L. P., and D. A. Karnofsky. The effects of metals on the chick embryo: Toxicity and production of abnormalities in development. Ann. N.Y. Acad. Sci. 55:203–215, 1952.
669. Riepma, P. Disodium methylarsonate in rubber cultivation. Proc. Brit. Weed Control Conf. 7(1):282–286, 1964.
670. Robinson, D. H. Arsenic in apples. Fertiliser Feeding Stuffs Farm Supplies J. 11:600–601, 1926.
671. Robson, A. O., and A. M. Jelliffe. Medicinal arsenic poisoning and lung cancer. Brit. Med. J. 2:207–209, 1963.
672. Rockstroh, H. Zur Ätiologie des Bronchialkrebses in arsenverarbeitenden Nickelhütten. Beitrag zur Syncarcinogenese des Berufskrebses. Arch. Geschwulstforsch 14:151–162, 1959.
673. Roscoe, H. E. On the alleged practice of arsenic-eating in Styria. Mem. Lit. Phil. Soc. Manchester, London 3xs., i., 208–221, 1862.
674. Rosehart, R. G., and J. Y. Lee. The effect of arsenic trioxide on the growth of white spruce seedlings. Water Air Soil Pollut. 2:439–443, 1973.
675. Rosenfels, R. S., and A. S. Crafts. Arsenic fixation in relation to the sterilization of soils with sodium arsenite. Hilgardia 12:203–229, 1939.
676. Rossano, A. T., Jr. Analysis and Comparison of Available Data on Air Quality Criteria in Member Countries. Preprint Dept. Civil Eng. Washington University, Seattle, Washington, 1963.
677. Rosset, M. Arsenical keratoses associated with carcinomas of the internal organs. Can. Med. Assoc. J. 78:416–419, 1958.
678. Roth, F. Arsen-Leber-Tumoren (Hämangioendotheliom). Z. Krebs. Forsch. 61:468–503, 1957.
679. Roth, F. The sequelae of chronic arsenic poisoning in Moselle vintners. German Med. Monthly 2:172–175, 1957.
680. Rothberg, S. Skin sensitization potential of the riot control agents BBC, DM, CN and CS in guinea pigs. Milit. Med. 135:552–556, 1970.
681. Rothstein, A. Interactions of arsenate with the phosphate-transporting system of yeast. J. Gen. Physiol. 46:1075–1085, 1963.
682. Roy, W. R. Studies of boron deficiency in grapefruit. Proc. Florida State Hort. Soc. 56:38–43, 1943.
683. Royal Commission on Arsenical Poisoning. Lancet 1:672–673, 753, 904–905, 1901.

684. Royal Commission on Arsenical Poisoning. Evidence of Dr. F. W. Tunnicliffe. Lancet 1:980, 1901.
685. Royal Commission on the Beer-Poisoning Epidemic. Lancet 1:414, 1901.
686. Royal Medical and Chirurgical Society. Adjourned debate on arsenical beer poisoning. Lancet 1:471–472, 1901.
687. Rozenshtein, I. S. Arsenic trioxide in the atmosphere in regions in which industrial enterprises are located. Klin. Patog. Profil. Profzabol. Khim. Etiol. Predpr. Tsvet. Chern. Met. 2:184–189, 1969. (in Russian)
688. Rozenshtein, I. S. Sanitary toxicological assessment of low concentrations of arsenic trioxide in the atmosphere. Hyg. Sanit. 35(1–3):16–22, 1970.
689. Ruch, R. R., E. J. Kennedy, and N. F. Shimp. Studies of Lake Michigan Bottom Sediments.—Number Four. Distribution of Arsenic in Unconsolidated Sediments from Lake Michigan. Illinois State Geological Survey. Environmental Geology Notes No. 37. 1970. 16 pp.
690. Ruchhoft, C. C., O. R. Placak, and S. Schott. The detection and analysis of arsenic in water contaminated with chemical warfare agents. Public Health Rep. 58:1761–1771, 1943.
691. Rudd, R. L., and R. E. Genelly. Pesticides: Their Use and Toxicity in Relation to Wildlife. State of California. Department of Fish and Game. Game Management Branch. Game Bulletin No. 7, 1956. 209 pp.
692. Rudolfs, W., G. E. Barnes, G. P. Edwards, H. Heukelekian, E. Hurwitz, C. E. Renn, S. Steinberg, and W. F. Vaughan. Review of literature on toxic materials affecting sewage treatment processes, streams, and B.O.D. determinations. Sewage Ind. Wastes 22:1157–1191, 1950.
693. Rumberg, C. B., R. E. Engel, and W. F. Meggitt. Effect of temperature on the herbicidal activity and translocation of arsenicals. Weeds 8:582–588, 1960.
694. Ruppert, D. F., Ph. K. Hopke, P. Clute, W. Metzger, and D. Crowley. Arsenic concentrations and distribution in Chautaugua Lake sediments. J. Radioanal. Chem. 23:159–169, 1974.
695. Sachs, R. M., and J. L. Michael. Comparative phytotoxicity among four arsenical herbicides. Weed Sci. 19:558–564, 1971.
696. Sadolin, E. The occurrence of arsenic in fish. Dansk. Tids. Farmaci 2:186–200, 1928. (in Danish, summary in English)
697. Sadolin, E. Untersuchungen über das Vorkommen des Arsens im Organismus der Fische. Biochem. Z. 201:323–331, 1928.
698. Safety of Paris green in mosquito control, pp. 56–57. In Wildlife Research Problems, Programs Progress—1967. Fish and Wildlife Service, Bureau of Sport Fisheries and Wildlife. Publication 74. Washington, D.C.: U.S. Government Printing Office, 1969.
699. Saffiotti, U., F. Cefis, and L. H. Kolb. A method for the experimental induction of bronchogenic carcinoma. Cancer Res. 28:104–113, 1968.
700. Samsahl, K. Radiochemical method for determination of arsenic, bromine, mercury, antimony and selenium in neutron-irradiated biological material. Anal. Chem. 39:1480–1483, 1967.
701. Sandberg, G. R., and I. K. Allen. A proposed arsenic cycle in an agronomic ecosystem, pp. 124–147. In E. A. Woolson, Ed. Arsenical Pesticides. ACS Symposium Series 7. Washington, D.C.: American Chemical Society, 1975.
702. Satake, S. Concerning the cases of arsenic poisoning caused by prepared powdered milk. Jap. J. Public Health (Nihon Koshu Eisei Shu) 2(11):22–24, 1955. (in Japanese)
703. Sautet, J., H. Ollivier, and J. Quicke. Contribution a l'étude de la fixation et de

l'élimination biologique de l'arsenic par *Mytilus edulis*. Ann. Med. Legale Crimin. Police Sci. Toxicol. 44:466–471, 1964.
704. Savchuck, W. B., H. W. Loy, and S. S. Schiaffino. Effect of arsenic on growth of mammalian cells *in vitro*. Proc. Soc. Exp. Biol. Med. 105:543–547, 1960.
705. Schauer, R. L. Substantive Amendment to the Petition for the Establishment of a Tolerance for Methanearsonic Acid in Cotton Seed. Prepared by NAC [National Agricultural Chemists Association] Industry Task Force on Tolerances for Methanearsonate. 1970. 261 pp.
706. Schramel, P., K. Samsahl, and J. Pavlu. Determination of 12 selected microelements in air particles by neutron activation analysis. J. Radioanal. Chem. 19:329–337, 1974.
707. Schrauzer, G. N., J. A. Seck, R. J. Holland, T. M. Beckham, E. M. Rubin, and J. W. Sibert. Reductive dealkylation of alkylcobaloximes, alkylcobalamins, and related compounds: Simulation of corrin dependent reductase and methyl group transfer reactions. Bioinorg. Chem. 2:93–124, 1972.
708. Schrenk, H. H., and L. Schreibeis, Jr. Urinary arsenic levels as an index of industrial exposure. Amer. Ind. Hyg. Assoc. J. 19:225–228, 1958.
709. Schroeder, H. A., and J. J. Balassa. Abnormal trace elements in man: Arsenic. J. Chron. Dis. 19:85–106, 1966.
710. Schroeder, H. A., and J. J. Balassa. Arsenic, germanium, tin, and vanadium in mice: Effects on growth, survival, and tissue levels. J. Nutr. 92:245–252, 1967.
711. Schroeder, H. A., M. Kanisawa, D. V. Frost, and M. Mitchener. Germanium, tin, and arsenic in rats: Effects on growth, survival, pathological lesions and life span. J. Nutr. 96:37–45, 1968.
712. Schroeder, H. A., and M. Mitchener. Toxic effects of trace elements on the reproduction of mice and rats. Arch. Environ. Health 23:102–106, 1971.
713. Schwartze, E. W. The so-called habituation to "arsenic." Variation in the toxicity of arsenious oxide. J. Pharmacol. Exp. Ther. 20:181–203, 1922.
714. Schwarz, K., and C. M. Foltz. Selenium as an integral part of factor 3 against dietary necrotic liver degeneration. J. Amer. Chem. Soc. 79:3292–3293, 1957. (letter)
715. Schweizer, E. E. Toxicity of DSMA soil residues to cotton and rotational crops. Weeds 15:72–76, 1967.
716. Sckerl, M. M. Translocation and Metabolism of MAA-Carbon-14 in Johnsongrass and Cotton. Ph.D. Thesis. Fayetteville: University of Arkansas, 1968. 72 pp.
717. Sckerl, M. M., and R. E. Frans. Preliminary studies on absorption and translocation of C^{14}-methanearsonates in Johnsongrass. Proc. South. Weed Conf. 20:387, 1967.
718. Sckerl, M. M., and R. E. Frans. Translocation and metabolism of MAA-^{14}C in Johnsongrass and cotton. Weed Sci. 17:421–427, 1969.
719. Sckerl, M. M., R. E. Frans, and A. E. Spooner. Selective inhibition of Johnsongrass with organic arsenicals. Proc. South. Weed Conf. 19:351–357, 1966.
720. Seydel, I. S. Distribution and circulation of arsenic through water, organisms and sediments of Lake Michigan. Arch. Hydrobiol. 71:17–30, 1972.
721. Shapiro, H. A. Arsenic content of human hair and nails. Its interpretation. J. Forensic Med. 14:65–71, 1967.
722. Sharma, K. C., B. A. Krantz, A. L. Brown, and J. Quick. Interactions of Zn and P in top and root of corn and tomato. Agron. J. 60:453–456, 1960.
723. Sharpless, G. R., and M. Metzger. Arsenic and goiter. J. Nutr. 21:341–346, 1941.
724. Shtenberg, A. I. Natural arsenic content of some vegetables and fruits. Vopr. Pitan. 10(5–6):29–33, 1941. (in Russian)

References

725. Shtenberg, A. I. The influence of arsenic on the animal organism and its transfer to tissues. Vopr. Pitan. 7(2):64–83, 1938. (in Russian)
726. Shtenberg, A. I. The national content of arsenic in meat and grain products. Vopr. Pitan. 9(4):20–27, 1940. (in Russian)
727. Shukla, S. S., J. K. Syers, and D. E. Armstrong. Arsenic interference in the determination of inorganic phosphate in lake sediments. J. Environ. Quality 1:292–295, 1972.
728. Sieczka, J. B., and D. J. Lisk. Arsenic residues in red clover. Amer. Potato J. 48:395–397, 1971.
729. Siegal, G. J., and R. W. Albers. Sodium-potassium-activated adenosine triphosphatase of *Electrophorus* electric organ. IV. Modification of responses to sodium and potassium by arsenite plus 2,3-dimercaptopropanol. J. Biol. Chem. 242:4972–4979, 1967.
730. Sihlbom, E. Arsenic in potato tubers. Sveriges Utsädesfören. Tids. 66:199–201, 1956. (in Swedish, summary in English)
731. Sihlbom, E., and L. Fredriksson. Yield and arsenic content in potatoes grown in soil with different amounts of arsenite. Sveriges Utsädesfören. Tids. 70:312–317, 1960. (in Swedish, summary in English)
732. Sillén, L. G. Arsenic, p. 574. In M. Sears, Ed. Oceanography. Invited Lectures Presented at the International Oceanographic Congress, New York, 1959. Washington, D.C.: American Association for the Advancement of Science, 1961.
733. Silver, A. S., and P. L. Wainman. Chronic arsenic poisoning following use of an asthma remedy. J.A.M.A. 150:584–585, 1952.
734. Sinclair, W. A., E. L. Stone, and C. F. Scheer, Jr. Toxicity to hemlocks grown in arsenic-contaminated soil previously used for potato production. HortScience 10:35–36, 1975.
735. Sisler, H. H. Phosphorus, arsenic, antimony and bismuth, pp. 106–152. In M. C. Sneed and R. C. Brasted, Eds. Comprehensive Inorganic Chemistry. Vol. 5. New York: D. Van Nostrand Co., Inc., 1956.
736. Skinner, J. T., and J. S. McHargue. Supplementary effects of arsenic and manganese on copper in the synthesis of hemoglobin. Amer. J. Physiol. 145:500–506, 1945–1946.
737. Small, H. G., Jr., and C. B. McCants. Determination of arsenic in flue-cured tobacco and in soils. Soil Sci. Soc. Amer. Proc. 25:346–348, 1961.
738. Small, H. G., Jr., and C. B. McCants. Residual arsenic in soils and concentration in tobacco. Tobacco Sci. 6:34–36, 1962.
739. Smith, A. E. Interferences in the determination of elements that form volatile hydrides with sodium borohydride, using atomic-absorption spectrophotometry and the argon-hydrogen flame. Analyst 100:300–306, 1975.
740. Smith, D. C., R. Leduc, and C. Charbonneau. Pesticide residues in the total diet in Canada. III-1971. Pestic. Sci. 4:211–214, 1973.
741. Smith, D. C., E. Sandi, and R. Leduc. Pesticide residues in the total diet in Canada. II-1970. Pestic. Sci. 3:207–210, 1972.
742. Smith, H. The distribution of antimony, arsenic, copper, and zinc in human tissue. Forensic Sci. Soc. J. 7:97–102, 1967.
743. Smith, H. The interpretation of the arsenic content of human hair. Forensic Sci. Soc. J. 4:192–199, 1964.
744. Smith, H., S. Forshufvud, and A. Wassén. Distribution of arsenic in Napoleon's hair. Nature 194:725–726, 1962.
745. Smith, J. D. Arsenic, antimony and bismuth, pp. 547–683. In J. C. Bailar, H. J.

Emeleus, R. Nyholm, and A. F. Trotman-Dickenson, Eds. Comprehensive Inorganic Chemistry. Vol. 2. Oxford: Pergamon Press, 1973.
746. Smith, W. C. Arsenic, pp. 94–103. In D. M. Liddell, Ed. Handbook of Nonferrous Metallurgy. Recovery of the Metals. New York: McGraw-Hill Book Company, Inc., 1945.
747. Snegireff, L. S., and O. M. Lombard. Arsenic and cancer. Observation in the metallurgical industry. A.M.A. Arch. Ind. Hyg. 4:199–205, 1951.
748. Snyder, J. C. Crops planted in pulled orchards. Washington State Hort. Assoc. Proc. 31:48–54, 1935.
749. Soderquist, C. J., D. G. Crosby, and J. B. Bowers. Determination of cacodylic acid (hydroxydimethylarsine oxide) gas chromatography. Anal. Chem. 46:155–157, 1974.
750. Solis-Cohen, S., and T. S. Githens. Arsenic, pp. 594–641. In Pharmacotherapeutics, Materia Medica and Drug Action. New York: D. Appleton and Company, 1928.
751. Sollins, L. V. Arsenic and water pollution hazard. Science 170:871, 1970.
752. Sommer, K., and M. Becke-Goehring. Über das 1,1-Äthan-diarsenoxid. Z. Anorg. Allg. Chem. 370:31–39, 1969.
753. Sommers, S. C., and R. G. McManus. Multiple arsenical cancers of the skin and internal organs. Cancer 6:347–359, 1953.
754. Sporn, M. B., N. M. Dunlop, D. L. Newton, and J. M. Smith. Prevention of chemical carcinogenesis by vitamin A and its synthetic analogs (retinoids). Fed. Proc. 35:1332–1338, 1976.
755. Stankiewicz, Z., B. Manjewska, and K. Mijal. Evaluation of some pesticide residues in fruit and fruit products. Rocz. Panstw. Zakl. Hig. 14:373–380, 1963. (in Polish)
756. Stecher, P. G., Ed. Merck Index. An Encyclopedia of Chemicals and Drugs. (8th ed.) Rahway, N.J.: Merck & Co., Inc., 1968. 1713 pp.
757. Steevens, D. R., L. M. Walsh, and D. R. Keeney. Arsenic phytotoxicity on a plainfield sand as affected by ferric sulfate or aluminum sulfate. J. Environ. Quality 1:301–303, 1972.
758. Steevens, D. R., L. M. Walsh, and D. R. Keeney. Arsenic residues in soil and potatoes from Wisconsin potato fields—1970. Pest. Monit. J. 6:89–90, 1972.
759. Stewart, J., and E. S. Smith. Some relations of arsenic to plant growth. Part 2. Soil Sci. 14:119–126, 1922.
760. Stockberger, W. W., and W. D. Collins. The Presence of Arsenic in Hops. U.S. Department of Agriculture Bulletin 568 (Professional Paper). Washington, D.C.: U.S. Government Printing Office, 1917. 7 pp.
761. Stocken, L. A. 2:3-Dimercaptopropanol ("British anti-lewisite") and related compounds. J. Chem. Soc. 1947:592–595.
762. Stocken, L. A., and R. H. S. Thompson. Reactions of British anti-lewisite with arsenic and other metals in living systems. Physiol. Rev. 29:168–194, 1949.
763. Stojanovic, B. J., F. L. Shuman, Jr., and M. V. Kennedy. Pollution problems related to pesticide containers, pp. 60–66. In Proceedings of Conference of Collaborators from Southern Agricultural Experiment Stations, Agricultural Research and Pollution. ARS 72-94, November 1971.
764. Stow, S. H. The occurrence of arsenic and the color-causing components in Florida land-pebble phosphate rock. Econ. Geol. 64:667–671, 1969.

References

765. Strunz, H. Mineralogische Tabellen. 3 Auflage. Leipzig: Akademische Verlagsgesellschaft Geest & Portig K.-G., 1957. 448 pp.
766. Study of Air Pollution in Montana July 1961–July 1962. Montana State Board of Health, Division of Disease Control, 1962. 104 pp.
767. Su, H. Colorimetric determination of arsenic residues in/on rice plants. Taiwan Agric. Q. 8(4):96–104, 1972. (in Chinese, summary in English)
768. Sugawara, K., and S. Kanamori. The spectrophotometric determination of trace amounts of arsenate and arsenite in natural waters with special reference to phosphate determination. Bull. Chem. Soc. Jap. 37:1358–1363, 1964.
769. Sullivan, B. The inorganic constituents of wheat and flour. Cereal Chem. 10:503–514, 1933.
770. Sullivan, R. J. Preliminary Air Pollution Survey of Arsenic and its Compounds. A Literature Review. National Air Pollution Control Administration Publ. APTD 69-26. Raleigh, N.C.: U.S. Department of Health, Education, and Welfare, Public Health Service, 1969. 60 pp.
771. Sulzberger, M. B. Hypersensitiveness to arsphenamine in guinea pigs: 1. Experiments in prevention and in desensitization. Arch. Derm. Syphilol. 20:669–697, 1929.
772. Surber, E. W. Control of Aquatic Plants in Ponds and Lakes. U.S. Fish and Wildlife Service Fishery Leaflet 344. Washington, D.C.: U.S. Department of the Interior, 1949. 26 pp.
773. Surber, E. W. Weed control in hard-water ponds with copper sulphate and sodium arsenate. In E. M. Quee, Ed. Transactions of the Eighth North American Wildlife Conference, 1943. Washington, D.C.: American Wildlife Institute, 1943.
774. Surber, E. W., and O. L. Meehean. Lethal concentrations of arsenic for certain aquatic organisms. Trans. Amer. Fish. Soc. 61:225–239, 1931.
775. Svoboda, J. Arsenic poisoning of bees by industrial waste gases. Rostlinna Vyroba (Czechoslovak Acad. Agric.) 35:1499–1506, 1962. (in Czech)
776. Swiggart, R. C., C. J. Whitehead, Jr., A. Curley, and F. E. Kellogg. Wildlife kill resulting from the misuse of arsenic acid herbicide. Bull. Environ. Contam. Toxicol. 8:122–128, 1972.
777. Talmi, Y., and D. T. Bostick. Determination of alkylarsenic acids in pesticide and environmental samples using gas chromatography with a microwave emission spectrometric detection system. Anal. Chem. 47:2145–2150, 1975.
778. Talmi, Y., and C. Feldman. The determination of traces of arsenic: A review, pp. 13–34. In E. A. Woolson, Ed. Arsenical Pesticides. ACS Symposium Series 7. Washington, D.C.: American Chemical Society, 1975.
779. Talmi, Y., and V. E. Norvell. Determination of arsenic and antimony in environmental samples using gas chromatography with a microwave emission spectrometric system. Anal. Chem. 47:1510–1516, 1975.
780. Tankawa, Y., and M. Nakane. Agricultural pesticide residues in several fruits. Rep. Hokkaido Instit. Public Health (Hokkaidoritsu Eisei Kenkyusho Sapporo) 19:121–123, 1969. (in Japanese, summary in English)
781. Tarrant, R. F., and J. Allard. Arsenic levels in urine of forest workers applying silvicides. Arch. Environ. Health 24:277–280, 1972.
782. Tatsuno, T., S. Nakamura, Y. Hosogai, and I. Kawashiro. Determination of harmful metals in foods. V. Contents of several kinds of trace metals in dried modified milk. Bull. Nat. Instit. Hyg. Sci. (Eisei Shikenjo Hokoku) 85:143–145, 1967. (in Japanese, summary in English)

783. Tatum, A. L. Pharmacology. II. The pharmacology of arsenicals. Ann. Rev. Physiol. 2:371–386, 1940.
784. Thom, C., and K. B. Raper. The arsenic fungi of Gosio. Science 76:548–550, 1932.
785. Thompson, A. H., and L. R. Batjer. Effect of various soil treatments for correcting arsenic injury to peach trees. Soil Sci. 69:281–290, 1950.
786. Thompson, J. T., and W. S. Hardcastle. Control of crab and Dallisgrass in narrow leaf turf. Proc. South. Weed Conf. 16:115, 1963.
787. Thompson, W. T. Agricultural Chemicals. Book 1—Insecticides (1973 ed.) Indianapolis: Thompson Publications, 1973. 300 pp.
788. Thomson, K. C. The atomic-fluorescence determination of antimony, arsenic, selenium and tellurium by using the hydride generation technique. Analyst 100:307–310, 1975.
789. Thornton, I., H. Watling, and A. Darracott. Geochemical studies in several rivers and estuaries used for oyster rearing. Sci. Total Environ. 4:325–345, 1975.
790. Thumann, M. E. Action of As-containing sewage on fish and crabs. Z. Fischerei 38:659–679, 1940. (in German)
791. Thumann, M. E. Über die Wirkung arsenhaltiger Abwässer auf Fische und Krebse. Angew. Chem. 54:500, 1941.
792. Timberlake, C. F. The content of arsenic, copper, iron, lead, and zinc in apples, juices, and ciders, pp. 160–164. In University of Bristol. The Annual Report of the Agricultural and Horticultural Research Station. Long Ashton, Bristol, 1951. Bath, England: Mendip Press, Ltd., 1951.
793. Tomatis, L., and U. Mohr, Eds. Transplacental Carcinogenesis. Proceedings of a Meeting held at the Medizinische Hochschule, Hannover, Federal Republic of Germany, 6–7 October 1971. Lyon, France: International Agency for Research on Cancer, 1973. 181 pp.
794. Tourtelot, H. A. Minor-element composition and organic carbon content of marine and nonmarine shales of Late Cretaceous age in the western interior of the United States. Geochim. Cosmochim. Acta 28:1579–1604, 1964.
795. Tourtelot, H. A., L. G. Schultz, and J. R. Gill. Stratigraphic variations in mineralogy and chemical composition of the Pierre shale in South Dakota and adjacent parts of North Dakota, Nebraska, Wyoming, and Montana, pp. B447–B452. In Geologic Survey Research 1960. Short Papers in the Geological Sciences. Geological Survey Professional Paper 400-B. Washington, D.C.: U.S. Government Printing Office, 1960.
796. Trace metals: Unknown, unseen pollution threat. Chem. Eng. News 49(29): 29–30, 33, 1971.
797. Tremearne, T. H., and K. D. Jacob. Arsenic in Natural Phosphates and Phosphate Fertilizers. U.S. Department of Agriculture Technical Bulletin 781. Washington, D.C.: U.S. Department of Agriculture, 1941. 39 pp.
798. Tseng, W. P., H. M. Chu, S. W. How, J. M. Fong, C. S. Lin, and S. Yeh. Prevalence of skin cancer in an endemic area of chronic arsenicism in Taiwan. J. Nat. Cancer Instit. 40:453–463, 1968.
799. Tucker, R. K., and D. G. Crabtree. Handbook of Toxicity of Pesticides to Wildlife. Bureau of Sport Fisheries and Wildlife. Denver Wildlife Research Center. Resource Publication No. 84, June, 1970. 131 pp.
800. Tunnicliffe, F. W., and O. Rosenheim. Selenium compounds as factors in the recent beer-poisoning epidemic. Lancet 1:318, 1901.

References

801. Underwood, E. J. Arsenic, pp. 427–431. In Trace Elements in Human and Animal Nutrition. (3rd ed.) New York: Academic Press, 1971.
802. U.S. Department of Agriculture. The Pesticide Review 1970. 46 pp.
803. U.S. Department of Agriculture. Agricultural Stabilization and Conservation Service. Wood preservatives: Usage by principal kinds, United States, 1968–1973, p. 21. In The Pesticide Review 1974. Washington, D.C.: U.S. Department of Agriculture, [not dated].
804. U.S. Department of Health, Education, and Welfare. Air Quality Data from the National Air Sampling Networks and Contributing State and Local Networks. 1966 Edition. Air Quality and Emission Data. National Air Pollution Control Administration Publication APTD 68-9. Durham, N.C.: U.S. Department of Health, Education, and Welfare, 1968. 157 pp.
805. U.S. Department of Health, Education, and Welfare. Control and Disposal of Cotton-Ginning Wastes. A Symposium, Dallas, Texas, May 3 and 4, 1966. Public Health Service Publication 999-AP-31. Cincinnati: U.S. Department of Health, Education, and Welfare, 1967. 103 pp.
806. U.S. Department of Health, Education, and Welfare. National Institute for Occupational Safety and Health. Criteria for a Recommended Standard. . . . Occupational Exposure to Inorganic Arsenic. Washington, D.C.: U.S. Department of Health, Education, and Welfare, 1973. 105 pp.
807. U.S. Department of Health, Education, and Welfare. National Institute for Occupational Safety and Health. Criteria for a Recommended Standard. . . . Occupational Exposure to Inorganic Arsenic. New Criteria—1975. HEW Publ. No. (NIOSH) 75-149. Washington, D.C.: U.S. Government Printing Office, 1975. 127 pp.
808. U.S. Department of Health, Education, and Welfare. Public Health Service Drinking Water Standards 1962. Public Health Service Publication No. 956. Washington, D.C.: U.S. Government Printing Office, 1962. 61 pp.
809. U.S. Department of Labor. Occupational Safety and Health Administration. Inorganic arsenic. Proposed exposure standard. Fed. Reg. 40:3392–3404, 1975.
810. U.S. Department of the Interior. Pesticide-Wildlife Studies, 1963. A Review of Fish and Wildlife Service Investigations during the Calendar Year. Fish and Wildlife Service Circular 199. Washington, D.C.: U.S. Department of the Interior, 1964. 130 pp.
811. U.S. Department of the Interior. Bureau of Mines. Mineral and Materials Supply/Demand Analysis. Minerals in the U.S. Economy: Ten-Year Supply–Demand Profiles for Mineral and Fuel Commodities. Washington, D.C.: U.S. Government Printing Office, 1975. 96 pp.
812. U.S. Department of the Interior. Bureau of Mines. White arsenic (arsenic trioxide): World production, by country, p. 1360. In Minerals Yearbook 1973. Vol. 1. Metals, Minerals, and Fuels. Washington, D.C.: U.S. Government Printing Office, 1975.
813. U.S. Environmental Protection Agency. Interim primary drinking water standards. Fed. Reg. 40:11990–11998, 1975.
814. Vallee, B. L. Arsenic. Air Quality Monograph 73-18. Washington, D.C.: American Petroleum Institute, 1973. 36 pp.
815. Vallee, B. L., D. D. Ulmer, and W. E. C. Wacker. Arsenic toxicology and biochemistry. A.M.A. Arch. Ind. Health 21:132–151, 1960.
816. Vandecaveye, S. C. Growth and composition of crops in relation to arsenical spray residues in the soil, pp. 217–223. In Proceedings of the Sixth Pacific

Science Congress of the Pacific Science Association, 1939. Vol. 6. Los Angeles: University of California Press, 1943.
817. Vandecaveye, S. C., G. M. Horner, and C. M. Keaton. Unproductiveness of certain orchard soils as related to lead arsenate spray accumulations. Soil Sci. 42:203–215, 1936.
818. Van Itallie, L. Arsenic content of hair. Pharm. Weekblad 69:1134–1145, 1932. (in Dutch)
819. Van Itallie, L. Arsenic content of nails. Pharm. Weekblad 69:1145–1147, 1932. (in Dutch)
820. Van Zyl, J. P. On the toxicity of arsenic to fowls, pp. 1189–1202. In Union of South Africa Department of Agriculture. 15th Annual Report of the Director of Veterinary Services, October 1929.
821. Vikhm, N. A. Content of arsenic in the teeth in health, dental caries, and alveolar pyorrhea. Stomatologiia 42(3):23–25, 1963. (in Russian)
822. Vincent, C. L. Vegetable and Small Fruit Growing in Toxic Ex-orchard Soils in Central Washington. Washington Agricultural Experiment Station Bulletin 437. Pullman: State College of Washington, 1944. 31 pp.
823. Vinogradov, A. P. Arsenic in various algae (in mg per 100 G dry matter), p. 111. In The Elementary Chemical Composition of Marine Organisms. Sears Foundation for Marine Research. Memoir II. New Haven: Yale University, 1953.
824. Vivoli, G., and G. P. Beneventi. Toxic substances in the ground water in Modena province. Inquinamento 12(5–6):21–25, 1970. (in Italian)
825. Voegtlin, C., and J. W. Thompson. Quantitative studies in chemotherapy. VI. Rate of excretion of arsenicals, a factor governing toxicity and parasiticidal action. J. Pharmacol. Exp. Ther. 20:85–105, 1923.
826. Von der Heide, C. Amount of arsenic in grapes, must and wine resulting from treatment of the vines with arsenical sprays. Wein Rebe 3:515–528, 595–596, 1922. (in German)
827. von Endt, D. W., P. C. Kearney, and D. D. Kaufman. Degradation of monosodium methanearsonate by soil microorganisms. J. Agric. Food Chem. 16:17–20, 1968.
828. von Fellenberg, T. Ueber den Arsengehalt natürlicher und mit Arsenpräparaten behandelter Lebensmittel. Mitt. Gebiete Lebesnmittelunter. Hyg. 20:338–354, 1929.
829. von Rumker, R., E. Lawless, A. Meiners, K. A. Lawrence, G. L. Kelso, and F. Horay. Production, Distribution, Use and Environmental Impact Potential of Selected Pesticides. EPA 540/1-74-001. Washington, D.C.: Council on Environmental Quality, 1974. 439 pp.
830. Vorhies, M. W., S. D. Sleight, and C. K. Whitehair. Toxicity of arsanilic acid in swine as influenced by water intake. Cornell Vet. 59:3–9, 1969.
831. Vuaflart, L. L'arsenic dans la bière, le glucose et les sulfites. Ann. Falsifications 9:272–278, 1916.
832. Wagner, S. L., and P. Weswig. Arsenic in blood and urine of forest workers. As indices of exposure to cacodylic acid. Arch. Environ. Health 28:77–79, 1974.
833. Wagoner, J. K., R. W. Miller, F. E. Lundin, Jr., J. F. Fraumeni, Jr., and M. E. Haij. Unusual cancer mortality among a group of underground metal miners. New Engl. J. Med. 269:284–289, 1963.
834. Wahlstrom, R. C., L. D. Kamstra, and O. E. Olson. The effect of arsanilic acid and 3-nitro-4-hydroxyphenylarsonic acid on selenium poisoning in the pig. J. Anim. Sci. 14:105–110, 1955.

835. Walker, G. W. R., and A. M. Bradley. Interacting effects of sodium monohydrogenarsenate and selenocystine on crossing over in *Drosophila melanogaster*. Can. J. Genet. Cytol. 11:677–688, 1969.
836. Wallace, D. C. How did Napoleon die? Med. J. Austral. 1:494–495, 1964.
837. Walsh, L. M., and D. R. Keeney. Behavior and phytotoxicity of inorganic arsenicals in soils, pp. 35–52. In E. A. Woolson, Ed. Arsenical Pesticides. ACS Symposium Series 7. Washington, D.C.: American Chemical Society, 1975.
838. Warren, H. V., R. E. Delavault, and J. Barakso. The arsenic content of Douglas fir as a guide to some gold, silver, and base metal deposits. Can. Inst. Min. Metal. Bull. 61:860–866, 1968.
839. Warrick, L. F., H. E. Wirth, and W. van Horn. Control of micro-organisms and aquatic vegetation. Water Sewage Works 95:R147–R150, 1948.
840. Watanabe, T., and S. Goto. Absorption and translocation of arsenic and lead in soil by cucumber. Noyaku Kensasho Hokoku 10:57–61, 1970. (in Japanese)
841. Waters, W. A., and J. H. Williams. Hydrolyses and derivatives of some vesicant arsenicals. J. Chem. Soc. 1950:18–22.
842. Watrous, R. M., and M. B. McCaughey. Occupational exposure to arsenic—in the manufacture of arsphenamine and related compounds. Ind. Med. 14:639–646, 1945.
843. Webb, J. L. Enzyme and Metabolic Inhibition. Vol. 2. Malonate, Analogs, Dehydroacetate, Sulfhydryl Reagent, *o*-Iodosobenzoate, Mercurials. New York: Academic Press, 1966. 1237 pp.
844. Weed Science Society of America. Herbicide Handbook. (3rd ed.) Champaign, Ill.: Weed Science Society of America, 1974. 430 pp.
845. Weeks, M. E., and H. M. Leicester. [Poem on arsenic], p. 92. In Discovery of the Elements. (7th ed.) Easton, Pa.: Journal of Chemical Education, 1968.
846. Weir, P. A., and C. H. Hine. Effects of various metals on behavior of conditioned goldfish. Arch. Environ. Health 20:45–51, 1970.
847. Weiss, H. V., and K. K. Bertine. Simultaneous determination of manganese, copper, arsenic, cadmium, antimony and mercury in glacial ice by radioactivation. Anal. Chim. Acta 65:253–259, 1973.
848. Welch, A. D., and R. L. Landau. The arsenic analogue of chlorine as a component of lecithin in rats fed arsenocholine chloride. J. Biol. Chem. 144:581–588, 1942.
849. Welter, C. J., and D. T. Clark. The efficacy of *p*-ureidobenzenearsonic acid as a preventative of histomoniasis in turkey poults. Poult. Sci. 40:144–147, 1961.
850. Wester, P. O. Concentration of 24 trace elements in human heart tissue determined by neutron activation analysis. Scand. J. Clin. Lab. Invest. 17:357–370, 1965.
851. White, D. E., J. D. Hem, and G. A. Waring. Data of Geochemistry. (6th ed.) Chapter F. Chemical Composition of Subsurface Waters. Geological Survey Professional Paper 440-F. Washington, D.C.: U.S. Government Printing Office, 1963. 67 pp.
852. White, J. C. Psoriasis—verruca—epithelioma; a sequence. Amer. J. Med. Sci. 89:163–173, 1885.
853. White, W. B. Poisonous spray residues on vegetables. Ind. Eng. Chem. 25:621–623, 1933.
854. Whitehead, F. E. The Effect of Arsenic, as Used in Poisoning Grasshoppers, upon Birds. Experiment Station Bulletin 218. Stillwater: Okalahoma Agriculture and Mechanical College, Agriculture Experiment Station, 1934. 54 pp.

855. Whitnack, G. C., and R. G. Brophy. A rapid and highly sensitive single-sweep polarographic method of analysis for arsenic (III) in drinking water. Anal. Chim. Acta 48:123–127, 1969.
856. Whorton, J. C. Insecticide spray residues and public health: 1865–1938. Bull. Hist. Med. 45:219–241, 1971.
857. Wiebe, A. H., E. G. Gross, and D. H. Slaughter. The arsenic content of largemouth black bass (*Micropterus salmoides* Lacepede) fingerlings. Trans. Amer. Fish. Soc. 61:150–163, 1931.
858. Wieber, M., and H. U. Werther. Cyclische Ester der Methanarsinsäure. Monatsh. Chem. 99:1159–1162, 1968.
859. Wilder, H. B. Investigation of the occurrence and transport of arsenic in the upper Sugar Creek Watershed, Charlotte, North Carolina, pp. D205–D210. In Geological Survey Research 1972. Chapter D. Geological Survey Professional Paper 800-D. Scientific Notes and Summaries of Investigations in Geology, Hydrology, and Related Fields. Washington, D.C.: U.S. Government Printing Office, 1972.
860. Wilkinson, D. S. Arsenic, p. 2071. In A. Rook, D. S. Wilkinson, and F. J. G. Ebling, Eds. Textbook of Dermatology. Vol. 2. (2nd ed.) Oxford: Blackwell Scientific Publications, 1972.
861. Wilkinson, R. E., and W. S. Hardcastle. Plant and soil arsenic analyses. Weed Sci. 17:536–537, 1969.
862. Willcox, W. H. An address on acute arsenical poisoning. Brit. Med. J. 2:118–124, 1922.
863. Willcox, W. H. The toxicological detection of arsenic and the influence of selenium on its tests. Lancet 1:778–779, 1901.
864. Williams, K. T., and R. R. Whetstone. Arsenic Distribution in Soils and Its Presence in Certain Plants. U.S. Department of Agriculture Technical Bulletin 732. Washington, D.C.: U.S. Department of Agriculture, 1940. 20 pp.
865. Wilson, D. J. Napoleon's death. Lancet 1:428–429, 1962. (letter)
866. Wilson, S. H., and M. Fieldes. Studies in spectrographic analysis. II. Minor elements in a sea-weed (*Macrocystis pyrifera*). N. Z. J. Sci. Tech. B. Gen. Sect. 23:47B–48B, 1941.
867. Windom, H., R. Stickney, R. Smith, D. White, and F. Taylor. Arsenic, cadmium, copper, mercury, and zinc in some species of North Atlantic finfish. J. Fish. Res. Board Can. 30:275–279, 1973.
868. Winkler, W. O. Identification and estimation of the arsenic residue in livers of rats ingesting arsenicals. J. Assoc. Off. Anal. Chem. 45:80–91, 1962.
869. Wolochow, H., E. W. Putman, M. Doudoroff, W. Z. Hassid, and H. A. Barker. Preparation of sucrose labeled with C^{14} in the glucose or fructose component. J. Biol. Chem. 180:1237–1242, 1949.
870. Wood, G. B., and F. Bache. Arsenic, pp. 126–128; Preparation of arsenic compounds, pp. 953–957. In The Dispensatory of the United States of America. (11th ed.) Philadelphia: Lippincott, 1858.
871. Wood, J. M. Biological cycles for toxic elements in the environment. Science 183:1049–1052, 1974.
872. Wood, J. M. The biochemical and environmental significance of cobalamin-dependent methyl-transfer to metals, P9. In Abstracts of Papers, Sixth International Conference on Organometallic Chemistry, August 12–17, 1973, University of Massachusetts, Amherst, Massachusetts.

References

873. Woolson, E. A. Arsenic phytotoxicity and uptake in six vegetable crops. Weed Sci. 21:524–527, 1973.
874. Woolson, E. A. Effects of fertiliser materials and combinations on the phytotoxicity, availability and content of arsenic in corn (maize). J. Sci. Food Agric. 23:1477–1481, 1972.
875. Woolson, E. A. Generation of dimethyl arsine from soil. Paper No. 218 Presented at 16th Annual Meeting of the Weed Science Society of America, 1976.
876. Woolson, E. A., J. H. Axley, and P. C. Kearney. Correlation between available soil arsenic, estimated by six methods, and response to corn (*Zea mays* L.). Soil Sci. Soc. Amer. Proc. 35:101–105, 1971.
877. Woolson, E. A., J. H. Axley, and P. C. Kearney. The chemistry and phytotoxicity of arsenic in soils. I. Contaminated field soils. Soil Sci. Soc. Amer. Proc. 35:938–943, 1971.
878. Woolson, E. A., J. H. Axley, and P. C. Kearney. The chemistry and phytotoxicity of arsenic in soils. II. Effect of time and phosphorus. Soil Sci. Soc. Amer. Proc. 37:254–259, 1973.
879. Woolson, E. A., and P. C. Kearney. Persistence and reactions of ^{14}C-cacodylic acid in soils. Environ. Sci. Tech. 7:47–50, 1973.
880. World Health Organization. International Classification of Diseases. Manual of the International Statistical Classification of Diseases, Injuries, and Causes of Death. Vol. 1. Geneva: World Health Organization, 1957. 393 pp.
881. World Health Organization. Trace Elements in Human Nutrition. Report of a WHO Expert Committee. WHO Technical Report Series No. 532. Geneva: World Health Organization, 1973. 65 pp.
882. Wu, C. Glutamine synthetase. VI. Mechanism of the dithiol-dependent inhibition by arsenite. Biochim. Biophys. Acta 96:134–147, 1965.
883. Wyllie, J. An investigation of the source of arsenic in a well water. Can. Public Health J. 28:128–135, 1937.
884. Yamashina, H., Y. Nagae, and S. Sasaki. Organoarsenic compounds. Japanese Patent 21,072 (1963) to Toa Agricultural Chemical Co., Ltd.
885. Yamashita, N., M. Doi, M. Nishio, H. Hōjō, and M. Tanaka. Current State of Kyoto children poisoned by arsenic tainted Morinaga dry milk. Jap. J. Hyg. (Nihon Eiseigaku Zasshi) 27:364–399, 1972. (in Japanese)
886. Yeh, S. Relative incidence of skin cancer in Chinese in Taiwan: With special reference to arsenical cancer. Nat. Cancer Instit. Mon. 10:81–107, 1963.
887. Yeh, S., S. W. How, and C. S. Lin. Arsenical cancer of skin. Histologic study with special reference to Bowen's disease. Cancer 21:312–339, 1968.
888. Zachariae, H., H. Søgaard, and A. Nyfors. Liver biopsy in psoriatics previously treated with potassium arsenite. Acta Derm. Venereol. (Stockh.) 54:235–236, 1974.
889. Zanetti, M., and F. Cutrufelli. Sul contenuto in arsenico di differenti tipi di tabacco italiano. Nuovi Ann. Igiene Microbiol. 12:264–269, 1961.
890. Zharkova, N. S. The experimental basis for the effect of lead and arsenic aerosols. Tr. Inst. Kraev. Patol. Kas SSR 22:85–96, 1971. (in Russian)
891. Zil'bershtein, Kh. I., O. N. Nikitina, A. V. Nenarokov, and E. S. Panteleev. Determination of impurities in special purity silicon dioxide by a spectrographic method after preliminary concentration. J. Anal. Chem. U.S.S.R. 19:907–910, 1964.
892. Zingaro, R. A., and K. J. Irgolic. The methylation of arsenic compounds. Science 187:765, 1975.

Index

Absorption of arsenic compounds
    by plants, 80–81, 218
    dermal, 116
    from gastrointestinal tract, 105–7
Acrocyanosis, from arsenic exposure, 181, 182
Adaptation to arsenic toxicity
    by laboratory animals, 136–37
    by microorganisms, 118–19
Agriculture, use of arsenic in, 26
    in desiccants, 37–38
    in herbicides, 36–37
    in pesticides, 3, 9, 33–34
    suggested research on, 231
Air, arsenic in, 27, 218. *See also* Pollution, from arsenic
    from cotton plant dust, 58
    from pesticides, 76–77
    from smelting of metals, 56–57, 224
    removal of, 56
    threshold limit for, 25–26
Air samples
    for arsenic concentration, 56–57
    suggested research on analytic techniques for, 229

Alcohol, role in arsenic poisoning, 177, 179
Algae
    arsenic concentration in, 24, 217
    arsenic metabolism in, 92–96
Alkylarsines, effect on biologic systems, 14
Alkylbis(organylthio) arsines, 15
Alkyldihaloarsines, 14, 15
Alkyldihydroxyarsines, 14, 15
Aluminum arsenate, 45
Analytic methods for arsenic
    atomic absorption, 224, 259–60
    atomic emission spectroscopy, 260
    coprecipitation, 258
    electrochemical, 224, 261
    gas chromatography, 261
    liquid–liquid extraction, 258
    molecular-absorption spectrophotometry, 259
    neutron-activation analysis, 224, 260–61
    volatilization, 258–59
Animals
    arsenic concentration in, 24–25, 243–53
    arsenic derived from tissues of, 104–5

arsenic residues in, 53–54
arsenic toxicity in domestic, 144–45
  diagnosis of, 147–48, 156–57
  factors affecting, 151–53
  from feed additives, 149–50
  symptoms of, 146–47, 153–54
  treatment of, 148–49
arsenic toxicity in laboratory
  adaptation to, 136–37
  by inhalation, 137–39
  factors influencing, 128–32
  mechanism of, 133–36
disposal of arsenic wastes from, 61–62
distribution of arsenic in, 108, 111
excretion of arsenic by, 39–40, 105–7, 108, 110, 154–55
studies on carcinogenic effects of arsenic in, 202–6
Aquatic organisms. *See* Marine organisms
Arsanilic acid
  as growth promoter, 132
  effect on swine, 155, 156, 158
  in feed additives, 149, 151
  safe dietary concentration of, 152
Arsenates
  concentration in urine, 106, 107
  effect on plants, 120
  reduction of, 11, 77
Arsenic. *See also* Arsenicals; Arsenic compounds
  as trace element, 69, 230
  beneficial effects of, 142–44
  by-product, 26
  folklore related to, 2–3
  high-purity, 42
  man-made sources of, 26, 32–33, 217
  methods for measuring, 223–24, 225–26, 259–61
  production of, 26, 28
  radioactive, 86
  recycling of, 43, 97
  supply–demand relationship of, 28–29
  vaporization of, 33
Arsenic acids
  as desiccant, 37–38
  compared with phosphoric acids, 9
  disposal of, 59
  effect on thiols, 13
  esterified, 12
  formation of, 7–8

Arsenicals
  agricultural uses of organic, 34
  aliphatic, 132
  as chemotherapeutics, 2, 189
  as toxicant to domestic animals, 144–49
  criminal abuses of, 3
  for resistance to infection, 139–141
  imports of, by class, 31
  interaction between nutrients and, 125–26
  phytotoxicity of organic, 120–125
  toxicity of synthetic, 129, 132
  transformation of, in soil, 78
  volatile, 77
Arsenic chloride, burns caused by, 14–15
Arsenic–chlorine bond, 15
Arsenic compounds. *See also* Pentavalent arsenic compounds; Trivalent arsenic compounds
  absorption by plants, 80–81
  as pesticides, 34
  biochemical response to, 119–20
  environmental importance of, 4
  hydrolytic instability of, 9
  imports of, 26, 31
  inorganic, 11
  methods for determining, 261
  methods for disposing of, 67–68
  methylation of, 11–12
  mutagenic effects of, 193–95
  organic, 10–11
  plant translocation of, 81–88
  suggested research for analyzing, 229
  teratogenic effects of, 191–93
  toxic and no-effect doses of, 128, 130–31, 132–33
  toxicity of
    adaptation to, 136–37
    factors influencing, 128–32
    mechanism of, 133–36
    of trivalent versus pentavalent, 133–36
  used as feed additives, 149–52
  vaporization of, 33
  war and riot-control uses for, 41
Arsenic cycle, 46, 218
  for total environment, 68, 70
  importance of change in, 79
  in agronomic ecosystem, 68–69
  in terrestrial ecosystem, 69
Arsenic halide, 15

Index

Arsenic–oxygen–arsenic bond, 6–7, 217
Arsenic–oxygen–carbon bond, 9
Arsenic pentasulfide, 10
Arsenic pentoxide, 6, 33, 175
Arsenic poisoning. *See also* Symptoms of arsenic toxicity; Toxicity of arsenic
  acute, 176
  arsenic residues causing, 53
  chronic, 2
  effect on hair, 113, 180, 183, 188, 189–90
  effect on skin, 114, 176, 178–79, 181–87, 188, 189–91
  from contaminated food, 55
  indicators of, 25
  in domestic animals, 144, 146
  in literature, 1
  of Napoleon, 2
  polyneuritis from, 25
  sources of, 144
  subacute, 176–84
  suggested research on mechanism responsible for, 230
  susceptibility to, 145
  treatment of, 148–49
Arsenic sulfides, 10
Arsenic–sulfur bond, 217
Arsenic trioxide
  as primary arsenic compound, 5, 216
  carcinogenicity of, 76, 205
  causticity of, 174
  dietary effects of, 112
  disposal of, 62–63
  effect on birds, 166
  effects of dissolving, 6, 7
  formation of, 6
  from coal, 66
  from smelters, 5, 81, 216
  in home-use products, 36
  medicinal use of, 174
  modifications of, 5
  solubility of, 6
  toxicity of, 128–29, 138–39
  U.S. imports of, 26, 27
Arsenic trisulfide, 4, 10
Arsenism. *See* Exposure to arsenic
Arsenites, 9
  effect on plants, 120, 126
  reduction of, 11, 77
Arsenous acids, 6–7
Arsonates, toxicity of, 127

Arsonic acids, 39–40
Arsphenamine, 2, 40
Atmosphere
  arsenic concentration in, 25–26, 27
  arsenic emission into, 26
Atom, arsenic, 5, 10
Atomic absorption, to measure arsenic, 224, 259–60
Atomic emission spectroscopy, 260

Bacteria
  arsenic metabolism in, 77, 88–89
  reduction of arsenate to arsenite by, 8
Beer, toxic amounts of arsenic in, 179, 180
Bees, arsenic concentration in, 54
Biologic effects of arsenic
  in aquatic organisms, 157–60, 161–63, 220
  in domestic animals, 144–57, 158, 220
  in laboratory animals, 128–44, 221
  in man, 173–215 *passim*, 222–23
  in microorganisms, 117–18, 221
  in plants, 119–27
  in wildlife, 160, 164–72, 220
Birds
  arsenic metabolism in, 101, 103
  arsenic toxicity to, 166–67, 169, 172
Blood, arsenic concentration, 113
Blood–mammary barrier to arsenic, 113
Bowen's disease, from arsenic exposure, 185–86
Bronchiectasis, from arsenic exposure, 181
Bronchopneumonia, from arsenic exposure, 180–81
Burns, from arsenic chloride, 14–15

Cacodylic acid
  absorption of, 116
  as desiccant, 45
  as herbicide, 36, 37, 58
  disposal of, 58–59, 64
  in algae, fish, and snails, 93, 94, 95
  reactions of, 13–14
  reduction of, 77
  translocation of, 83, 87
Calcium arsenate
  as pesticide, 9, 34
  disposal of, 59–60, 64–65
Caparsolate, 41
Carbarsone, 40, 152

Carcinogenic effects of arsenic, 3, 114
  delayed, 186
  experimental animal studies of, 202–6
  experimentally induced, 214–15
  from occupational exposure, 187, 197–201
  leukemia, 203
  liver cancer, 213–14, 223
  lung cancer, 175, 185, 197, 199, 200, 208–13, 223
  morphologic changes, 214–15
  mortality rate from, 198–99, 209–11
  population studies of, 202, 223
  skin cancer, 182, 184, 185, 186
    clinical reports of, 195–97
    evaluation of, 206–8
Catarrhal symptoms of arsenic poisoning, 177
Chemotherapeutics, 2, 189. *See also* Medicinal uses of arsenic
Children, symptoms of arsenic toxicity in, 180–81, 186–87
Chlorosis, from arsenic toxicity, 120–23, 127
Chromatographic tests, for arsenic translocation, 85
Chromosomal reaction. *See* Mutagenic effects of arsenic
Claudetite, 5
Coal
  arsenic trioxide from, 66
  emission of arsenic from burning, 73–74
Colorimetry, to measure arsenic, 224
Concentration of arsenic
  in animals, 24–25, 243–53
  in atmosphere, 25–26, 27
  in earth's crust, 16
  in man, 24–25
  in marine organisms, 25, 217
  in minerals, 16
  in plants, 24, 233–42
  in rocks, 4, 17–18
  in soils, 4, 18–19, 40, 217
  in water, 4, 20–23, 217
  systemic, 175, 176
Consumption of arsenic, 26, 217–18
  as additive metal, 41–42
  in desiccants, 37–38
  in drugs, 40–41
  in feed additives, 39–40
  in glass manufacturing, 42–43
  in herbicides, 36–37
  in pesticides, 3, 33, 34
  in semiconductor technology, 42
  in wood preservatives, 38–39
Copper
  arsenic emission from smelting, 32
  arsenic imported in, 26
Copper acetoarsenite
  as pesticide, 3, 34
  disposal of, 60, 65–66
  poisonous gas emitted by, 11
Copper arsenate, 38–39
Coprecipitation
  arsenic from solution by, 20
  in analysis of arsenic samples, 258
Corrosion, arsenic's resistance to, 42
Cotton
  arsenic acid as desiccant for, 37–38, 52, 59
  arsenic residues from production of, 45, 52–53
  effect of methanearsonates on, 50–51, 125
  use of arsenical herbicides in production of, 36–37
Crustaceans. *See* Mollusks and crustaceans
Cupric arsenite, 9, 11

Deer, arsenic poisoning of, 167–68
Desiccants
  arsenic used in, 37–38, 52, 59
  cacodylic acid as, 45
Diagnosis of arsenic poisoning
  "index of suspicion" in, 222
  in domestic animals, 147–48, 156–57
  in man, 180, 222
Dialkylarsines, 14
Dialkylhaloarsines, 15
Dialkylhydroxyarsines, 15
Dichlorophenarsine, 41
Diet
  effect of arsenic trioxide in, 112
  normal intake of arsenic in, 103–4
    from animal tissue, 104–5
    from plants, 104
    from seafood, 111
Digestive system, symptoms of arsenic poisoning in, 177

Index

See also Gastrointestinal tract
Dimethylarsine, 13, 45
Dipotassium hydrogen arsenate, 9
Disodium methanearsonate
  as herbicide, 36, 45, 217
  disposal of, 59, 64
  effect on cotton, 125
  translocation of, 83, 84–85, 87
Disposal of arsenic
  from feed additives, 61–62
  from herbicides and pesticides, 58–60
  from industrial uses, 62–66
  methods for, 67
Dissipation of arsenic, 75, 76
Distribution of arsenic
  in body, 108–16
  in environment, 16–26, 217–18
Dodecyl(octyl)ammonium methanearsonate, 83, 84
Doses, of arsenic
  suggested research on, 228
  therapeutic, 176–77
  toxic and no-effect, 128, 130–31, 132–33, 222
  toxic, in wildlife, 165
Drugs. *See* Medicinal use of arsenic
Dust, arsenic in, 26, 27, 56, 174

Earth's crust, arsenic in, 116
Ecosystem, arsenic in, 68–69, 225
Electrochemical methods, for measuring arsenic, 224, 261
Electrostatic precipitation, for removing arsenic, 63
Emission of arsenic, 26
  from coal burning, 73–74
  from mining and processing of phosphate rock, 74
  from pesticides, 76–77
  from processing of nonferrous metals, 72
  from smelters, 32, 71, 73, 224
  industrial balance for, 74, 75
Environment
  arsenic contamination of, 224–26
  arsenic cycle for, 68–79
  distribution of arsenic in
    from residues, 43–58
    from waste disposal, 58–68
    man-made sources of, 26–43
    natural sources of, 16–26
    suggested research on, 231
  effect of arsenic on, 3
Enzymes, interaction with thiol proteins, 13, 15
Epidemiologic effects of arsenic, 202, 223
  suggested research on, 227–28
Erythromelalgia, from arsenic poisoning, 178, 182
Esters
  hydrolyzed, 12, 220
  prepared from arsenous or arsenic acid, 9–10
Excretion of arsenic
  in urine, 105–7, 108, 110–11, 113, 132, 154
  through skin, 114, 116, 189, 190–91
Exposure to arsenic
  chronic, 184–87
  delayed effects of, 186–87
  effects of, 180–84
  from dust, 174
  standards for, 25–26
  systemic absorption from, 175, 176
Eyes, effect of arsenic on, 153, 154

Fallout, removal of arsenic in, 76, 77
Feed additives
  arsenic compounds used as, 149–53
  arsenic used in, 39–40, 217
  disposal of waste from, 61–62
  toxicity of, 149–50, 151, 220
Fertilizer, effect of arsenic content on soils and crops, 44, 176, 217–18
Filter–bag house operations, for removing arsenic, 63
Fish
  arsenic concentration, 54
  arsenic metabolism in, 100–101, 102, 219
  arsenic residues in, 103
  arsenic toxicity to, 159–60, 161–63
  cacodylic acid accumulation in, 93, 94, 95
  dietary intake of arsenic in, 111
Fluxing, for vaporization of arsenic, 33
Fly ash, arsenic in, 56, 73
Foods, arsenic in, 54. *See also* Diet
  human intake of, 55
  institutional diet with, 55
  monitoring of, 54
  normal intake of, 103–5, 111
  suggested research on, 229
Fungi, arsenic metabolism in, 77, 89–92

Gas chromatography, for measuring arsenic, 261
Gastrointestinal tract, arsenic absorption from, 105–7, 132, 183
Glass industry, arsenic compounds used in, 5, 42, 43, 66
Glycobiarsol, 40
Growth promotion
  by arsanilic acid, 132
  by pentavalent arsenic compounds, 230–31

Hair
  arsenic concentration, 24–25
  arsenic distribution in, 114, 115
  effect of arsenic poisoning on, 113, 180, 183, 188, 189–90
Hemiplegia, from arsenic exposure, 181
Herbicides
  arsenic residues from, 45
  dimethylarsine, 13
  effect on wildlife, 167–68
  for cotton production, 36–37
  inorganic arsenicals used as, 36, 217
  methanearsonic acid, 12
  translocation of, 82–88, 90–91
Herpes zoster, from arsenic, 179, 190
Humans. *See* Man
Hydrogen chloride, toxicity of, 15
Hydrolytic instability, 7, 9
Hyperkeratosis, from arsenic exposure, 181, 183, 189
Hyperpigmentation. *See* Melanosis

Igneous rocks, arsenic in, 17
Immune response, role of arsenic in, 190
Imports, arsenic, 26, 30, 31
Industry, use of arsenic in, 4
  disposal of, 62–66
  in glass manufacturing, 5, 42–43, 66
  material balance for emission from, 74, 75
Infection, use of arsenicals in resistance to, 139–41
Ingestion of arsenic, 179, 180, 183
Inhalation of arsenic, 37–39, 228
Insecticides. *See* Pesticides
Iron arsenate, 45
Iron ore, arsenic in, 74
Ischemia, from arsenic exposure, 181

Keratoderma, from arsenic exposure, 184
Keratoses
  from arsenic poisoning, 178–79, 182, 184, 185, 186, 188, 191
  skin cancer related to, 196, 202, 206–8

Leaching, arsenic, 44–45
Lead arsenate
  as pesticide, 9, 33–34, 58, 217
  carcinogenicity of, 205–6
  disposal of, 59–60, 64–65
  effect on humans, 58
  effect on plants, 49
  in medical drugs, 41
  residues from, 43
Leukemia, 203–4
Leukoderma, from arsenic exposure, 184, 186, 187
Lewisite, 5, 14, 175
Liquid–liquid extraction, to analyze arsenic samples, 258
Liver, arsenic-caused cancer of, 213–14, 223
Lungs, arsenic-caused cancer of, 175, 185, 197, 199, 200, 208–10, 211–12, 213, 223

Magnesium arsenate, 34
Man
  arsenic concentration, 24–25
  cacodylic acid absorption in, 116
  distribution of arsenic in, 108
  excretion of arsenic by
    in urine, 111, 113, 132
    through skin, 114, 116, 189, 190–91
  toxicity of arsenic to
    from contact, 174–76
    from exposure, 184–87
Marine organisms. *See also* Fish; Shellfish
  arsenic concentration, 25
  arsenic toxicity to, 157, 159–60, 161–63
Mass spectrometry, for measuring arsenic, 169, 261
Measurement of arsenic, methods for, 223–24, 225–26, 259–61
Medicinal use of arsenic
  diseases treated by, 40–41, 174, 194, 217
  needed reevaluation of, 190
  safety of, 2
  tolerated doses of, 176–77
  toxic reactions to, 173, 189

Index

Melanosis, from arsenic exposure, 182, 183, 186, 187, 196, 202, 206–8
Melarsonyl, 41
Merlarsoprol, 40
Metabolism
  of arsenic
    in birds, 101, 103
    in fish, 100–101, 102, 219
    in mammals, 103–15, 219
    in microorganisms, 77, 88–89, 92, 96–97, 219
    in mollusks and crustaceans, 98–100, 219
    in plants, 80–88, 120, 218–19
  of selenium, 141–42
Methanearsonates
  as herbicides, 36–37
  effect on cotton, 50–51, 125
  in plant foods, 104
  translocation of, 83–88
Methanearsonic acid
  as herbicide, 12, 45
  concentration in urine, 105–7
  conversion of, 13
  effect on cotton, 125
  reduction of, 14, 77
  translocation of, 86, 87
Methylarsines, 11
  effect on biologic systems, 14
  oxidation of, 77
Methylation of arsenic compounds, 11–12, 14, 215, 216–17
Microorganisms
  adaptation to arsenic, 118–19
  arsenic metabolism in, 88–97
    in algae, 92–96
    in bacteria, 88–89, 219
    in fungi and molds, 89, 92, 219
    in plankton, 96–97
  toxicity of arsenic to, 117–18
Military use of arsenic, 27, 32, 36, 41
Minerals, arsenic in, 16
Molds
  arsenic metabolism in, 89, 92–93
  conversion of arsenic compounds to methylated arsines by, 11, 217
Mollusks and crustaceans
  arsenic metabolism in, 98–100
  dietary intake of arsenic in, 111
Monosodium methanearsonate
  as herbicide, 36, 45, 217

disposal of, 59, 64
effect on cotton, 125
translocation of, 86, 87, 88
Mutagenic effects of arsenic, 193–95, 223
  suggested research on, 228

Nails
  arsenic concentration, 25
  effect of arsenic poisoning on, 179, 183, 189
Necrosis, from arsenic toxicity, 123, 124
Neoarsphenamine, 41
Neurologic symptoms of arsenic poisoning, 177, 178, 183
Neutron-activation analysis, to measure arsenic, 224, 260–61
Nitro-4-hydroxyphenylarsonic acid, 152, 153
Nuclear-magnetic resonance studies, 6
Nutrients, interaction between arsenicals and, 125–26

Occupational hazards of arsenic, 183–84, 222
  for vintners, 186, 188, 197, 212
  from chemical plants, 201, 208, 210, 212
  from gold mining, 213
  from sheep dip, 187, 197, 207, 210
  from smelters, 175, 187, 209–10
Ores, arsenic from smelting of nonferrous, 26–27
Oxidation
  of arsenic, 16, 19, 216
  of methylarsines, 77

Particulate matter, from metal smelters, 33
Pentavalent arsenic compounds, 10, 104
  for wood preservatives, 39
  in feed additives, 150
  reaction with thiols, 13
  suggested research on growth-promoting effect of, 230–31
  toxicity of, 8, 133–135
Pesticides
  arsenic residues from, 43, 58
  arsenic used in, 3, 9, 33–34, 35, 217
  effect on wildlife, 160, 164, 166
  hazards from arsenical, 35–36, 188
  mobile arsenic from, 76–77
  suggested assessment of effects of nonuse of, 229–30

Petroleum, arsenic content of, 74
Phenylarsonic acids
  in feed additives, 149–57, 217
  toxicity of, 156–57
Phosphate rock
  arsenic emission from mining, 74
  arsenic in, 18, 19
Phosphorus, interaction between arsenic and, 9–10, 120, 125–26
Phosphorylation, 120, 127
Phytotoxicity, arsenic
  in plants, 48, 50, 120–25, 127, 221
  in soils, 45
Plankton, arsenic in, 96
Plants
  absorption of arsenic by, 80–81
  arsenic concentration, 24, 233–42
  arsenic derived from, 104
  arsenic metabolism in, 81–88, 120
  arsenic residues in, 48–53
  arsenic toxicity in, 44, 120–25
  beneficial effects of arsenic on, 50
Pollution from arsenic
  control of, 216
  from coal-burning power plants, 137
  from smelters, 32–33, 218, 224
Polyneuritis, from arsenic poisoning, 25
Potassium arsenate, 9, 191
Potassium arsenite, 204–5
Poultry
  arsenic concentration, 53
  arsenic toxicity in, 154, 157
  safe concentration of arsenic for, 152
Production of arsenic, 26, 28
Psoriasis
  arsenic therapy for, 194
  skin cancer realted to, 196

Radioactive isotopes, to study arsenic distribution, 108, 109
Rain, removal of arsenic from atmosphere by, 76
Raman spectral studies, 6
Raynaud's syndrome, from arsenic exposure, 181, 182
Recycling of arsenic, 43, 67, 218
Research suggestions for assessing environmental effects of arsenic, 227–231
Residues of arsenic, 218
  in air, 56–58
  in animals, 53–54
  in fish, 103
  in foods, 54–55, 225
  in plants, 48–53
  in soils, 43–46, 103
  in water, 46–48, 103
  suggested guidelines for disposal of, 230
Respiratory tract, arsenic-caused cancer of, 199–201, 210, 212
Riot control, arsenical compounds used for, 41
Rocks, arsenic in, 4, 17–18

Samples, arsenic
  analysis of, 258–59
  collection of, 255–56
  dissolution of, 256–57
  preparation of, 257–58
Scrubbers, for removing arsenic, 63
Seafood. See also Fish; Shellfish
  arsenic toxicity to, 132
  natural concentration of arsenic in, 225
  normal intake of arsenic in, 111
Seaweed, arsenic in, 95, 96, 97, 217
Sedimentary rocks, arsenic in, 17–18
Sediments, arsenic concentration in, 20, 23
Selenium poisoning, 179
  protective effect of arsenic against, 141–42, 143, 192, 221
Semiconductor technology, use of arsenic in, 42
Sewage sludge, arsenic waste from, 66
Shellfish, arsenic toxicity to, 132, 161–63
Skin
  absorption of arsenic through, 114, 116, 175
  effect of arsenic on, 14, 41, 153, 175
    abnormal pigmentation, 181, 182, 183, 184, 185, 189
    cancer, 182, 184, 185, 186, 195–97, 206–8, 223
    keratoses, 178–79, 182, 184, 185, 188, 191
Smelting
  arsenic-caused cancer from, 175, 187, 198–99, 200
  arsenic emission from, 32, 33, 56–57
  arsenic produced by, 26, 217
  arsenic residues in soil from, 45–46, 48–49

Index

cost of removing arsenic during, 27
disposal of arsenic from, 63
Snails, cacodylic acid accumulation in, 93, 94, 95
Sodium arsanilate, 151, 152, 153
Sodium arsenate
   as pesticide, 34–35, 217
   carcinogenicity of, 205–6
   chromosomal reactions to, 193–94
   effect on skin, 175
   for home-use products, 36
   teratogenic effects of, 192–93
Sodium arsenite, 36, 217
   carcinogenicity of, 205
   chromosomal reaction to, 195
   disposal of, 60, 65–66
   effect on birds, 167
   effect on plants, 119
   effect on skin, 175
   teratogenic effects of, 193
   translocation of, 82–83
Sodium cacodylate, 40
Soil
   arsenic concentration, 4, 18–19, 40
   arsenic residues in, 43–46, 103, 218
   effect on plants, 49–52
Solubility
   of arsenates, 9, 44–45
   of arsenic sulfides, 10
   of arsenic trioxide, 5–6
   of arsenites, 9
Spectrometry. *See* Mass spectrometry
Speiss, arsenic in, 72–73
Sulfides, arsenic in, 16, 18–19
Swine
   arsanilic acid in feed additives for, 151, 153
   effect of arsenic on, 155, 156, 157–58
Symptoms of arsenic toxicity
   in domestic animals, 146–47, 153–54
   in man, 173
      cardiac, 178, 188
      catarrhal, 177
      digestive, 177, 183
      in children, 180–81, 186–87
      in skin, 14, 41, 153, 175, 178–79, 182–83, 184–87
      neurologic, 177, 178, 183
      vascular, 181, 188
   in plants, 119, 120–25

Telangiectasia, from arsenic exposure, 184
Temperature, effect on arsenic toxicity in plants, 123, 124
Teratogenic effects of arsenic, 191–93, 222
   suggested research on, 228
Tetraarsenic tetrasulfide, 4
Tetrapotassium diarsenate, 9
Therapeutic use of arsenic. *See* Medicinal use of arsenic
Thiols
   effect on arsonic acids, 13
   interaction with enzymes, 13, 15
Threshold limit for arsenic, 25–26
Tobacco, arsenic content of, 48
Tolerance to arsenic
   by microorganisms, 119
   by plants, 49, 53
   by wildlife, 164, 165
Toxicity of arsenic. *See also* Arsenic poisoning; Symptoms of arsenic toxicity
   to aquatic organisms, 159–60, 220
   to domestic animals, 144–54, 220
   to laboratory animals, 128–44
   to man, 220, 222
      from contact, 174–76
      from exposure, 184–87
   to microorganisms, 117–18, 221
   to plants, 44, 120–25
   to wildlife, 164–69, 172, 220
Translocation of arsenic in plants, 81, 218–19
   by acid–arsenic method, 82
   from foliage to tubers, 83–85
Trimethylarsine, 11, 13, 45, 77, 217
Triorganyl arsenite, 9
Trivalent arsenic compounds, 10
   reaction with thiols, 13
   toxicity of, 8, 133–36
Tryparsamide, 41

Uptake, arsenic
   by algae, 92
   by plankton, 97
   by plants, 19, 49, 81
Urban areas, arsenic concentration in air, 56–57
Urinary arsenic, 25
   excretion, 105–7, 108, 110–11, 113, 132, 180

from occupational exposure, 175,
183–84, 188, 198

Valence, of arsenic, 113, 114
Vapor pressure, of cubic arsenic trioxide, 6
Vegetables, arsenic content of, 48–49, 52
Venereal disease, arsphenamine to treat, 2
Volatilization
  of arsenic, during smelting, 27
  to analyze arsenic samples, 258–59
Volcanic rock, arsenic-rich water from, 23

Warts, from arsenic exposure, 183, 187, 188
Wastes, arsenic. *See* Residues of arsenic
Wastewater, arsenic content of, 66
Water
  arsenic-caused cancer from, 202, 208
  arsenic concentration, 4, 46
    in fresh water, 21–22
    in groundwater, 20, 23
    in seawater, 20
    in sediments of, 20, 23
  arsenic poisoning from, 180, 183
  arsenic residues in, 47–48, 103
  emission of arsenic into, 76, 77
Weathering, arsenic, 69
Wet-vacuum pumps, for removing arsenic, 63
Wildlife
  effect of arsenic on, 164, 166, 167–68
  tissue arsenic concentration in, 169–71
Wood preservatives, arsenic used in, 38–39, 157

Zinc, interaction of arsenicals with, 126
Zinc arsenate, as pesticide, 34